MANUAL OF

Oculoplastic
Surgery

Fourth Edition

MANUAL OF

Oculoplastic Surgery
Fourth Edition

Mark R. Levine, MD, FACS

Emeritus Clinical Professor of Ophthalmology
Case Western Reserve University School of Medicine

Former Head of the Oculoplastic Section
Department of Ophthalmology
University Hospitals of Cleveland

Former Chief of Ophthalmology
The Mt. Sinai Medical Center

Staff Physician
Cleveland Clinic Foundation
Cleveland, Ohio

Past President of the American Society of Ophthalmic Plastic and Reconstructive Surgery
Wendell Hughes Lecturer
Emeritus Member of the Orbital Society

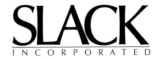

www.slackbooks.com

ISBN: 978-1-55642-897-5

Copyright © 2010 by SLACK Incorporated

Previous editions of *Manual of Oculoplastic Surgery* were published by Butterworth-Heinemann, an imprint of Elsevier Science.

The procedures and practices described in this book should be implemented in a manner consistent with the professional standards set for the circumstances that apply in each specific situation. Every effort has been made to confirm the accuracy of the information presented and to correctly relate generally accepted practices. The authors, editor, and publisher cannot accept responsibility for errors or exclusions or for the outcome of the material presented herein. There is no expressed or implied warranty of this book or information imparted by it. Care has been taken to ensure that drug selection and dosages are in accordance with currently accepted/recommended practice. Due to continuing research, changes in government policy and regulations, and various effects of drug reactions and interactions, it is recommended that the reader carefully review all materials and literature provided for each drug, especially those that are new or not frequently used. Any review or mention of specific companies or products is not intended as an endorsement by the author or publisher.

SLACK Incorporated uses a review process to evaluate submitted material. Prior to publication, educators or clinicians provide important feedback on the content that we publish. We welcome feedback on this work.

Published by: SLACK Incorporated
6900 Grove Road
Thorofare, NJ 08086 USA
Telephone: 856-848-1000
Fax: 856-853-5991
www.slackbooks.com

Contact SLACK Incorporated for more information about other books in this field or about the availability of our books from distributors outside the United States.

Library of Congress Cataloging-in-Publication Data

Manual of oculoplastic surgery / [edited by] Mark R. Levine. -- 4th ed.
   p. ; cm.
Includes bibliographical references and index.
ISBN 978-1-55642-897-5 (alk. paper)
1. Ophthalmic plastic surgery. I. Levine, Mark R.
[DNLM: 1. Ophthalmologic Surgical Procedures. 2. Eyelids--surgery. 3. Reconstructive Surgical Procedures--methods. WW 168 M294 2010]
RE87.M37 2010
617.7'1--dc22
               2009045845

Last digit is print number: 10 9 8 7 6 5 4 3 2 1

Dedication

To my wonderful family who are loving and supportive:
Teri, Marne, Lindsey, Phil, Jackson, and Zander.

In memory of my parents, Dorothy and Donald Levine,
who shared their wisdom, love, and encouragement.

Contents

Acknowledgments

I would like to thank SLACK Incorporated for undertaking and continuing the fourth edition. Their cooperation and flexibity has made redoing this book most enjoyable.

Contributing Authors

Meredith Brooke Allen, MD (Chapter 50)
Fellow
Ophthalmic Plastic and Reconstructive Surgery
New York Eye and Ear Infirmary
St. Luke's Roosevelt Hospital Center
New York, New York

Richard L. Anderson, MD (Chapter 20)
Center for Facial Appearance
Salt Lake City, Utah

Christine C. Annunziata, MD
(Chapter 48)
Oculofacial Plastic and Reconstructive Surgery
Los Angeles, California

Milton Boniuk, MD (Chapter 41)
Baylor College of Medicine
Houston, Texas

James R. Boynton, MD (Chapter 26)
Clinical Professor of Ophthalmology
University of Rochester School of Medicine and
    Dentistry
Attending Physician
Department of Ophthalmology
The Strong Memorial Hospital
Rochester, New York

Daniel E. Buerger, MD (Chapters 33, 34)
Clinical Instructor of Ophthalmology
University of Pittsburgh School of Medicine
Pittsburgh Oculoplastic Associates
Pittsburgh, Pennsylvania

David G. Buerger, MD (Chapters 33, 34)
Clinical Instructor of Ophthalmology
University of Pittsburgh School of Medicine
Pittsburgh Oculoplastic Associates
Pittsburgh, Pennsylvania

George F. Buerger, Jr, MD (Chapters 33, 34)
Pittsburgh Oculoplastic Associates
Pittsburgh, Pennsylvania

John A. Burns, MD, FACS (Chapter 17)
Clinical Professor, Department of Ophthalmology
Ohio State University
The Eye Center of Columbus
Columbus, Ohio

Kenneth V. Cahill, MD, FACS
(Chapter 17)
Clinical Professor, Department of Ophthalmology
Ohio State University
The Eye Center of Columbus
Columbus, Ohio

Mauricio R. Chavez, MD (Chapter 23)
Oculofacial Plastic & Reconstructive Surgery
Rocky Mountain Eye Center
Pueblo, Colorado

William P. Chen, MD, FACS (Chapter 12)
Clinical Professor of Ophthalmology
UCLA School of Medicine
Los Angeles, California
Eye Plastic Surgery Service
Harbor-UCLA Medical Center
Torrance, California

Roger A. Dailey, MD, FACS (Chapter 23)
Chief, Division of Oculofacial Plastic Surgery
Lester Jones Endowed Chair
Oregon Health & Sciences University
Portland, Oregon

Rodger P. Davies, MBBS, FRANZCO, FRACS,
FANZSOPS (Chapter 29)
Oculoplastic Surgeon
Eyelid, Tear Duct and Orbital Surgery
Hawthorn, Victoria, Australia

David A. Della Rocca, MD (Chapter 50)
Associate Adjunct Attending
Clinic Instructor
New York Eye and Ear Infirmary
New York, NY

Robert C. Della Rocca, MD (Chapter 50)
Professor of Clinical Ophthalmology
New York Medical College
Chairman, Department of Ophthalmology
St. Luke's-Roosevelt Medical Center
New York, New York

Richard K. Dortzbach, MD (Chapter 1)
Professor Emeritus
Department of Ophthalmology and Visual Sciences
University of Wisconsin Medical School
Department of Ophthalmology and Visual Sciences
University of Wisconsin Hospital and Clinics
Madison, Wisconsin

Essam A. El-Toukhy, MD, FRCOph (Chapters 30, 31)
Professor of Ophthalmology
Deputy Director
Head of Oculoplasty Division
National Eye Centre
Cairo, Egypt

Gil A. Epstein, MD (Chapter 40)
Assistant Clinical Professor
Nova Southeastern University
Ft. Lauderdale, Florida

Steven Fagien, MD, FACS (Chapter 27)
Aesthetic Eyelid Plastic Surgery
Private Practice
Boca Raton, Florida

Jill A. Foster, MD, FACS (Chapters 14, 17)
Associate Clinical Professor, Department of Ophthalmology
Ohio State University
The Eye Center of Columbus
Columbus, OH

Tamara R. Fountain, MD (Chapter 5)
Professor
Section Director, Oculoplastics
Rush University Medical Center
Chicago, Illinois
Ophthalmology Partners, Limited
Deerfield, Illinois

Constance L. Fry, MD (Chapter 37)
Associate Professor of Ophthalmology
The University of Texas Health Science Center at San Antonio
San Antonio, Texas

Perry F. Garber, MD (Chapter 50)
Associate Clinical Professor of Ophthalmology and Visual Science
Albert Einstein School of Medicine
New York, New York

Geoffrey J. Gladstone, MD, FACS (Chapter 8)
Clinical Professor of Ophthalmology
Michigan State University School of Medicine
East Lansing, Michigan
Assistant Clinical Professor of Ophthalmology and Otolaryngology
Kesge Eye Institute
Wayne State University School of Medicine
Detroit, Michigan
Co-Director, Oculoplastic Surgery
Department of Ophthalmology
William Beaumont Hospital
Royal Oak, Michigan
Consultants in Ophthalmic and Facial Plastic Surgery
Southfield, Michigan

Robert A. Goldberg, MD (Chapter 45)
Jules Stein Eye Institute
Los Angeles, California

Michael J. Hawes, MD (Chapter 25)
Clinical Professor of Ophthalmology
University of Colorado Health Sciences Center
Denver, Colorado

Jonathan Hoenig, MD (Chapter 9)
Assistant Clinical Professor of Ophthalmology
UCLA Medical Center
Jules Stein Eye Institute
Los Angeles, California

David E. E. Holck, MD (Chapter 14)
Wilford Hall Medical Center
San Antonio, Texas

John B. Holds, MD, FACS (Chapter 10)
Clinical Professor
Departments of Ophthalmology and Otolaryngology-Head and Neck Surgery
Saint Louis University
St. Louis, Missouri

Steven M. Houser, MD, FACS (Chapter 49)
Assistant Professor of Otolaryngology
Case Western Reserve University
Cleveland, Ohio

Catherine Hwang, MD (Chapter 9)
Jerome Comet Klein Fellow
Division of Orbital & Ophthalmic Plastic Surgery
Jules Stein Eye Institute/UCLA
Los Angeles, California

Thomas J. Joly, MD, PhD (Chapter 2)
Assistant Professor of Ophthalmology
Eastern Virginia Medical School
Ophthalmic Plastic Surgery
Virginia Eye Consultants
Norfolk, Virginia

*David R. Jordan, MD, FRCSC, FACS
(Chapter 20)*
Full Professor of Ophthalmology
University of Ottawa Eye Institute
University of Ottawa
Ottawa, Ontario, Canada

James Karesh, MD, FACS (Chapter 21)
Associate Professor
The Johns Hopkins Medical Institutions
The Wilmer Ophthalmologic Institute
Emeritus Chairman
The Krieger Eye Institute
The Sinai Hospital of Baltimore
Baltimore, Maryland

Don O. Kikkawa, MD (Chapter 48)
Professor
Chief, Division of Oculofacial Plastic and
    Reconstructive Surgery
UCSD Department of Ophthalmology
La Jolla, California

Jonathan W. Kim, MD (Chapter 47)
Director
Oculoplastic and Orbital Surgery
Codirector
Ocular Oncology Service
Stanford, California

Yoon-Duck Kim, MD (Chapter 7)
Department of Ophthalmology
Samsung Medical Center
Seoul, Korea

*Kimberly A. Klippenstein, MD
(Chapter 22)*
Assistant Professor of Ophthalmology
Vanderbilt University Medical Center
Nashville, Tennessee

*Bobby S. Korn, MD, PhD, FACS
(Chapter 48)*
Assistant Professor of Ophthalmology
Division of Ophthalmic Plastic and Reconstructive
    Surgery
UCSD Shiley Eye Center
La Jolla, California

Jacques G. H. Lasudry, MD (Chapter 1)
Clinical Assistant Professor
Université Libre de Bruxelles
Chief, Ophthalmic Plastic and Reconstructive
    Surgery
Department of Ophthalmology
Hôpital Universitaire Erasme
Brussels, Belgium

H. B. Harold Lee, MD (Chapter 6)
Oculofacial Plastic and Orbital Surgery
Indianapolis, Indiana
Louisville, Kentucky

Bradley N. Lemke, MD (Chapter 1)
Clinical Professor, Volunteer Faculty
Department of Ophthalmology and Visual Sciences
University of Wisconsin-Madison
Madison, Wisconsin

Alan M. Lessner, MD (Chapter 13)
Assistant Professor
Director of Oculoplastic Surgery
Department of Ophthalmology
University of Florida College of Medicine
Center for Plastic and Reconstructive Surgery
Faculty Surgeon
Departmen of Ophthalmology
Shands Teaching Hospital
Attending Surgeon
North Florida Regional Medical
Gainesville, Florida

Howard Levine, MD (Chapter 49)
Director
Cleveland Nasal Sinus & Sleep Center
Associate Staff
Head and Neck Institute
Cleveland Clinic
Cleveland, Ohio

Richard D. Lisman, MD (Chapter 39)
Professor of Ophthalmology
New York University School of Medicine
Director of Ophthalmic Plastic Surgery Services
New York University Medical Center
Institute of Plastic and Reconstructive Surgery
Manhattan Eye and Ear Hospital
New York, New York

William P. Mack, MD (Chapter 42)
Clinical Assistant Professor
Department of Ophthalmology
University of South Florida College of Medicine
Tampa, Florida

Joseph A. Mauriello, Jr, MD (Chapter 38)
Clinical Professor
Department of Ophthalmology and Visual Sciences
University of Medicine and Dentistry
New Jersey Medical School
Newark, New Jersey

Jill S. Melicher, MD (Chapter 47)
Cincinnati Eye Institue
Cincinnati, Ohio

Dale R. Meyer, MD (Chapter 46)
Ophthalmic Plastic Surgery
Lions Eye Institute
Albany Medical Center
Albany, New York

Kevin S. Michels, MD (Chapter 17)
Assistant Clinical Professor
Ohio State University
The Eye Center of Columbus
Columbus, Ohio

Thomas C. Naugle, Jr, MD
(Chapters 26, 37)
Clinical Professor of Ophthalmology
Tulane University
New Orleans, Louisiana

Jeffrey A. Nerad, MD (Chapter 47)
Cincinnati Eye Institue
Cincinnati, Ohio

Frank A. Nesi, MD, FACS
(Chapters 3, 4)
Associate Clinical Professor of Ophthalmology and
    Otolaryngology
Kresge Eye Institute
Wayne State University School of Medicine
Detroit, Michigan
Director, Oculoplastic Surgery
Beaumont Eye Institute
Dept of Ophthalmology
William Beaumont Hospital
Royal Oak, Michigan

William R. Nunery, MD (Chapter 6)
Clinical Assistant Professor
University of Louisville
Louisville, Kentucky
Clinical Assistant Professor
Indiana University
Bloomington, Indiana

Jay Justin Older, MD (Chapter 42)
Affiliate Professor of Ophthalmology
University of South Florida College of Medicine
Tampa, Florida

Julian D. Perry, MD (Chapters 14, 28)
Cleveland Clinic Cole Eye Institute
Cleveland, Ohio

Randal Pham, MD, FACS (Chapter 19)
Founder
Aesthetic & Refractive Surgery Medical Center
San Jose, California

Thu Pham, MD (Chapter 28)
Cleveland Clinic Foundation
Cleveland, Ohio

Allen M. Putterman, MD
(Chapters 11, 18)
Professor of Ophthalmology
Co-director, Oculofacial Plastic Surgery
University of Illinois College of Medicine
Chicago, Illinois

J. Earl Rathbun, MD (Chapter 15)
Emeritus Clinical Professor of Ophthalmology
University of San California, San Francisco
San Francisco, California

John G. Rose, Jr, MD (Chapter 1)
Clinical Instructor
Oculoplastics Service
Department of Ophthalmology and Visual Sciences
University of Wisconsin Medical School
Madison, Wisconsin

John W. Shore, MD, FACS (Chapter 43)
Adjunct Clinical Associate Professor of Ophthalmology
M.D. Anderson Cancer Hospital and University of Texas Health Science Center
Houston, Texas

Norman Shorr, MD (Chapter 9)
Clinical Professor of Ophthalmology
Jules Stein Eye Institute
Los Angeles, California

César A. Sierra, MD, FACS
(Chapters 3, 4)
Assistant Clinical Professor
Yale University School of Medicine
Department of Ophthalmology
New Haven, Connecticut

Charles B. Slonim, MD (Chapter 44)
Department of Ophthalmology
University of South Florida College of Medicine
Tampa, Florida

Robert G. Small, MD (Chapter 16)
Dean A. McGee Eye Institute
Department of Ophthalmology
Oklahoma City, Oklahoma

Thomas C. Spoor, MD (Chapter 46)
Professor Emeritus, Wayne State University School of Medicine
Director, Michigan Neuro-Ophthalmology and Oculoplastic Surgery
St. John Hospitals
Detroit, Michigan
Sarasota Retina Institute
Sarasota, Florida

Robert L. Tomsak, MD, PhD (Chapter 51)
Associate Professor, Department of Ophthalmology
Case Western Reserve University School of Medicine
Director, Division of Clinical Neuro-Ophthalmology, Department of Neurology
University Hospitals of Cleveland
Cleveland, Ohio

David T. Tse, MD, FACS (Chapter 24)
Professor of Ophthalmology
Dr. Nasser Ibrahim Al-Rashid Distin-guished Chair in Ophthalmic Plastic, Orbital Surgery and Oncology
Bascom Palmer Eye Institute
University of Miami Miller School of Medicine
Miami, Florida

Ralph E. Wesley, MD (Chapter 22)
Wesley & Klippenstein
Nashville, Tennessee

Eugene O. Wiggs, MD
(Chapters 32, 35, 36)
Clinical Professor of Ophthalmology Emeritus
University of Colorado Health Sciences Center
Denver, Colorado

Allan E. Wulc, MD, FACS (Chapter 14)
Associate Clinical Professor
University of Pennsylvania
Associate Clinical Professor
Drexel University
Philadelphia, Pennsylvania

Christopher I. Zoumalan (Chapter 39)
Division of Ophthalmic and Plastic Reconstructive Surgery
Department of Ophthalmology
New York University School of Medicine
New York, New York

Preface

This book is designed to provide ophthalmologists familiar with the surgical anatomy and principles of oculoplastic and orbital surgery with a concise guide for performing many of the basic surgical procedures. Each procedure is described in a step-wise fashion, as if the author of the chapter were assisting the reader-surgeon doing the procedure. It is assumed that the reader is well versed in the diagnosis, medical treatment, and surgical indications associated with the various procedures presented here.

This book is not intended to be a compendium of oculoplastic procedures; rather, it emphasizes the best and most up-to-date procedures for each clinical situation and anatomic region. This step-by-step approach to a procedure together with the selected illustrations should enable the surgeon to complete the surgical procedure successfully and with good results. Additional chapters of importance have been added and a number of chapters revised and supplemented.

I thank all of the authors for their excellent contributions and cooperation in this book's endeavor. A special thanks to the members of the American Society of Ophthalmic Plastic and Reconstructive Surgery for their pursuit of basic research, innovative ideas, and for acting as a forum for disseminating their knowledge to other societies, subspecialties, academic institutions, and patient information groups.

Two past authors will be missed by all of us, as they were productive members of our society as well as good friends to all. In memoriam Bernice Z. Brown and Albert Hornblass.

SECTION I

INTRODUCTION

CHAPTER 1

APPLIED SURGICAL ANATOMY
OF THE OCULAR ADNEXA

*Jacques G. H. Lasudry, MD; Bradley N. Lemke, MD; John G. Rose, Jr, MD;
and Richard K. Dortzbach, MD*

The order of presentation of this chapter follows the progression of a typical oculoplastic surgical procedure, from the more superficial to the deeper planes. Before an incision is made along appropriate skin lines, anesthesia is achieved through local infiltration and with regional nerve blocks. The superficial facial musculature and tissues supporting the eyelid are then examined according to their importance in eyelid stability, lacrimal pump function, and cosmetic appearance. Often, the position of the eyelid has to be adjusted by modifying the position of the retractors. In procedures addressing lacrimal outflow disturbances, endonasal anatomy is a keystone. Moving deeper, an orbitotomy is realized as soon as the septum is opened. The orbital fat pads invariably protrude into the field and must be respected as much as possible, even if they restrict access to the deeper planes. Last, the orbital bony structure comes into consideration in fracture repair, orbital decompression, or surgical exposure of the deep tissues of the orbit. The likelihood of anatomic variations of the deep neurovascular structures must always be kept in mind to avoid unnecessary iatrogenic sequelae. Only the common disposition is presented here.

Sensory Innervation of the Upper Face

From medial to temporal, the forehead and upper eyelid are supplied with the infratrochlear (ITN), supratrochlear (STN), supraorbital (SON), and lacrimal (LN) nerves, which are all branches of the ophthalmic division of the trigeminal nerve (V1) (Figure 1-1). The ITN exits the orbit beneath the trochlea and innervates the medial conjunctiva, the skin of the root of the nose, and the medial canthus as well as the canaliculi and the lacrimal sac. The STN exits the orbit with its homonymic artery and vein above the trochlea and innervates the skin and conjunctiva of the medial upper eyelid, the glabella, and the root of the nose. The SON, with its attendant artery and vein, exits through the supraorbital notch and distributes to the forehead and the central portion of the upper eyelid with the conjunctiva. The LN supplies the conjunctiva and skin of the lateral upper eyelid. The cutaneous tip of the nose is innervated by the external nasal nerve (ENN), which is the cutaneous termination of the anterior ethmoidal branch of the nasociliary nerve.

The lower eyelid, temple, malar eminence, side of the nose, and upper lip are supplied with the cutaneous distribution branches of the maxillary-division of the trigeminal nerve (V2). The infraorbital nerve (ION) exits with its homonymic artery and vein through the infraorbital foramen and innervates most of the inferior lid and conjunctiva, the lateral side of the nose up to the root of the nose, and the zygomaticolabial area. It is complemented in the temple by the zygomaticofacial nerve (ZFN) and zygomaticotemporal nerve (ZTN) erupting from their respective foramina. Considerable overlap exists between adjacent territories and also between V1 and V2 in both the medial canthal and lateral canthal areas. The remainder of the face is supplied with branches of the mandibular division (V3), except for the angle of the mandible, which is innervated by the cervical branches C2/C3.

CLINICOANATOMIC CORRELATIONS

The cutaneous branches of the trigeminal nerve cross the orbital rim and run deep to the plane of the orbicularis oculi muscle (OOM). The supratrochlear and infratrochlear branches traverse the muscle plane at approximately the eyebrow. The distribution territories of each cutaneous

Levine MR.
Manual of Oculoplastic Surgery, Fourth Edition (pp 3-14).
© 2010 SLACK Incorporated

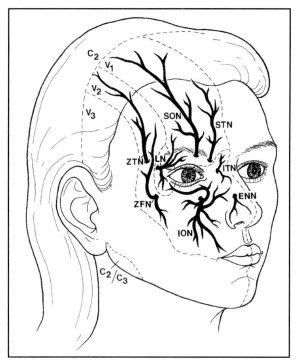

Figure 1-1.

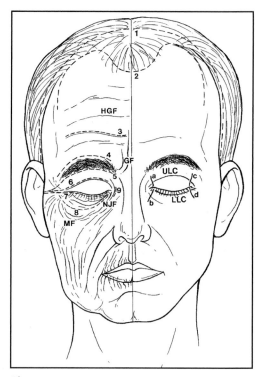

Figure 1-2.

branch are somehow overlapping, especially in the medial canthal area. Therefore, effective local nerve block is best realized deep to the orbicularis plane, with as many injections as there are tributaries to the surgical field.

The supraorbital notch is closed into a canal in 25% of people. During a bicoronal frontal flap procedure, care must be paid to this structure, which is palpable at the medial one third of the superior orbital rim, to avoid damage to the nerve. The infraorbital foramen is close to the orbital margin at birth and approximately 6 mm below the orbital margin in an adult. For practical purposes, the supraorbital notch, the infraorbital foramen, and the mental foramen almost fall in a vertical line passing the midpupil.

Cutaneous Landmarks of the Upper Face

The inferior border of the lower eyelid is demarcated by the nasojugal fold (NJF) medially and the malar fold (MF) laterally (Figure 1-2). The glabellar fold (GF) arises vertically at the medial aspect of the eyebrow, reflective of the corrugator superciliaris muscle activity drawing the eyebrow medially and inferiorly. The horizontal GFs (HGFs) reflect vertical depression of the medial eyebrow by the procerus and frontalis muscles (FMs). The upper lid crease (ULC) and lower lid crease (LLC) are caused by the eyelid retractors.

Usual elective skin incision lines are (1) transcoronal; (2) pretrichial; (3) midforehead; (4) suprabrow for eyebrow plasty; (5) infrabrow with a possible S-shaped prolongation in the lateral commissure and cantholysis; (6) in the upper eyelid crease; (7) infraciliary approximately 2 mm below the lashes; (8) in the lower eyelid crease or NJF, with or

without lateral prolongation, for anterior or lateral orbitotomy; and (9) vertical on the side of the root of the nose, in front of the insertion of the anterior limb of the medial canthal ligament for dacryocystorhinostomy.

In the eyelid, the skin and the subcutaneous fibroadipose tissue are very thin. Comparatively, the malar and glabellar areas are covered with a denser subcutaneous fibroadipose tissue and thicker skin. The transition between these areas is abrupt. Subcutaneous fat is absent in the pretarsal area and sparse in the preseptal region. The pretarsal skin is tightly adherent to the orbicularis muscle. Beyond the lid crease, the preseptal skin is loosely bound to the muscle plane.

CLINICOANATOMIC CORRELATIONS

The wrinkling pattern of the aging face follows naturally occurring creases generally perpendicular to the orientation of the underlying muscular fibers. These lines are most helpful in placing elective incision lines, as the underlying muscular activity helps wound closure. Incisions made perpendicular to the eyelid margin (see Figure 1-2, a-d) interrupt lymphatic drainage of the lid and increase postoperative lymphedema (especially c). The abrupt difference in skin thickness explains the often sharp demarcation of lymphedema in the eyelid from the malar area. The cilia of the upper half of the eyebrow are directed inferotemporally, whereas the cilia of the lower portion of the eyebrow are directed superotemporally. Medially, the cilia have a vertical orientation. Suprabrow incisions must be beveled in the same plane as the superior cilia follicles (ie, approximately 30° above the coronal plane) to minimize postoperative permanent loss. The converse is true for infrabrow incisions.

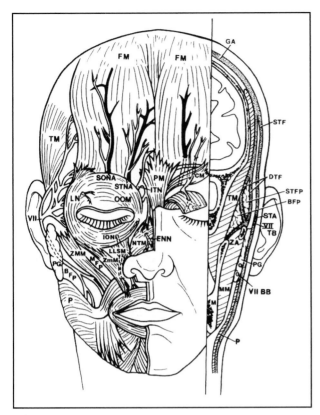

Figure 1-3.

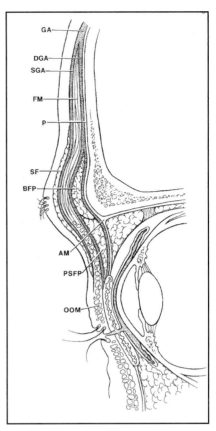

Figure 1-4.

Superficial Musculature of the Upper Face

The facial expression muscles are interconnected by the superficial musculoaponeurotic system (SMAS) (Figure 1-3). It is a fibrous fascial network that contains the facial muscles, divides the subcutaneous fat into 2 layers, and has fibrous septa extending to the skin. The fibers of the corrugator muscle (CM) and procerus muscle (PM) originate from the medial orbital rim and frontal bone to blend with those of the frontalis muscle (FM) into those of the OOM. The OOM is firmly attached to the orbital rim at the supraorbital ridge, the lateral palpebral raphe, the malar crease, and the naso-orbital region. The muscles of the midface are in the same plane as the orbicularis and comprise the nasalis transversus (NTM), levator labii superioris (LLSM), zygomaticus minor (ZmM), and zygomaticus major (ZMM) muscles. The malar fat pad (MFP) and buccal fat pad (BFP) are defined by these muscles and are the deep part of the SMAS. The temporalis muscle (TM) is a deep masticatory muscle and does not belong to the SMAS. In section, the galea aponeurotica (GA) covers the TM and splits along the muscle insertion into superficial (STF) and deep (DTF) temporal fascia. The deep fascia inserts onto the zygomatic arch (ZA) and coronoid apophysis of the mandible (M) and wraps around the superficial temporal fat pad (STFP) and the BFP. The STF covers the parotid gland (PG), masseteric muscle (MM), and the platysma (P) and on its deep surface conveys branches of the superficial temporal artery (STA) and the temporal branches of the facial nerve (V2TB).

CLINICOANATOMIC CORRELATIONS

A safe avascular plane is found between the galea aponeurotica and the periosteum and is used when raising a forehead flap or performing endoscopic forehead dissection. By remaining deep to the galea-SMAS and superficial to the deep temporalis fascia, damage to the temporal branches of the facial nerve can be prevented.

Foundations of the Eyebrow

The glabellar skin is thick and contains a high number of sweat and sebaceous glands. Under the skin, the eyebrow area is provided with some subcutaneous fat (SF) (Figure 1-4). In the scalp, the SMAS is represented by the galea aponeurotica (GA), which splits and ensheathes the FM. The superficial layer of the galea aponeurotica (SGA) represents the anterior muscle sheath of the FM and OOM muscles. The deep galea aponeurotica (DGA) is apposed to the periosteum (P). At the level of the eyebrow, the deep galea also splits and incompletely encloses the brow fat pad (BFP). The brow fat pad is in continuity with the preseptal fat pad (PSFP) in the upper eyelid and is also referred to as the ROOF (retro-orbicularis oculi fat). The ROOF is in the same anatomic plane as the MFP, which is also known as the suborbicularis oculi fat (SOOF).

CLINICOANATOMIC CORRELATIONS

Browpexy and reduction of brow fullness can be approached in the posterior plane of the ROOF. In this case, caution is necessary because the branches of the supraorbital vessels and nerves are located in this plane medially. The ROOF can be congenitally prominent or thicken in association with thyroid orbitopathy.

Motor Innervation of the Upper Face

The branching pattern of the facial nerve (VII) is particularly variable. Most commonly, it divides during its intraparotidian course into temporal (TB), zygomatic (ZB), buccal (BB), marginal mandibular (MMB), and cervical branches (CB) (Figure 1-5). The temporal branch is composed of 3 to 5 rami that cross the zygomatic arch in a zone located approximately 2 cm behind the anterior end of the zygomatic arch. While traveling in the same plane as the superficial temporal artery, it reaches the frontalis, procerus, corrugator, and orbicularis muscles by their temporal and posterior side. The orbicularis receives a second facial innervation supply through ZB, reaching the muscle by its inferior side.

CLINICOANATOMIC CORRELATIONS

The facial nerve is particularly vulnerable in its portion that crosses the zygomatic arch and above it, where it is subcutaneous. Biopsy of the superficial temporal artery must be performed outside this danger zone. Damage to the temporal branch results in paralysis of the frontalis, procerus, and CM with sparing of the orbicularis, which receives dual innervation. Ptosis of the eyebrow and asymmetric forehead animation are the clinical manifestation.

Arterial Supply of the Eyelids

The eyelids are richly vascularized by both the internal carotid and external carotid systems. From the internal carotid system, the ophthalmic artery supplies both lids through its lacrimal, supraorbital, supratrochlear, and dorsal nasal branches. Variations in the distribution of the ophthalmic artery are common. The dorsal nasal division exits the orbit below the trochlea and anastomoses with the angular artery. The supraorbital artery exits through the supraorbital notch with the nerve and a vein and sometimes gives off the supratrochlear branch before its exit. The lacrimal artery may receive a variable contribution from the middle meningeal artery through a recurrent branch entering the orbit by the meningeal foramen near the anterior end of the superior orbital fissure.

In the upper eyelid, the marginal and deep peripheral arcades are formed by several anastomoses between the lacrimal and dorsal nasal arteries before their exit from the orbit through the septum. The marginal arcade runs with an attendant vein 2 to 3 mm above the eyelid margin on the anterior surface of the tarsus, beneath the orbicularis muscle. The deep peripheral arcade lies just above the superior tarsal border between Müller's muscle and the levator aponeurosis. It supplies the superior fornix and bulbar conjunctiva and anastomoses with the anterior ciliary arteries near the limbus. The lower eyelid is provided with a less-developed double inferior marginal

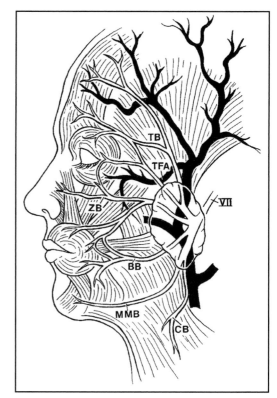

Figure 1-5.

arcade system, anastomosing branches of the dorsal nasal artery to variable contributions from the lacrimal, infraorbital, zygomaticotemporal, and zygomaticofacial arteries.

From the external carotid system, the 3 main arteries are the angular artery, superficial temporal artery, and infraorbital artery. The angular artery is the termination of the facial artery, which courses superficially on the side of the nose and in the nasolabial fold and originates from the external carotid under the angle of the mandible. The angular artery lies beneath the orbicularis muscle 6 to 8 mm medial to the medial canthus and 5 mm anterior to the lacrimal sac. It anastomoses with the dorsal nasal branch of the ophthalmic artery and supplies the orbicularis muscle and lacrimal sac, with a variable contribution to the lower eyelid. The superficial temporal artery courses from the preauricular area within the superficial temporal fascia in continuity superiorly with the galea aponeurotica. It supplies the lateral portion of both eyelids through 3 main branches: the frontal, which crosses the temple and anastomoses with lacrimal and supraorbital branches; the zygomatico-orbital, which runs along the upper border of the zygomatic arch and anastomoses with zygomatic and lacrimal branches; and the transverse facial, which runs forward below the zygomatic arch and anastomoses inferiorly with lacrimal and infraorbital branches. The infraorbital artery is a branch of the internal maxillary artery. It enters the orbit through the inferior orbital fissure and exits with infraorbital nerve and vein via the infraorbital canal. A small branch of the infraorbital artery can usually be found in the sutura notha at the insertion of the anterior limb of the medial canthal ligament.

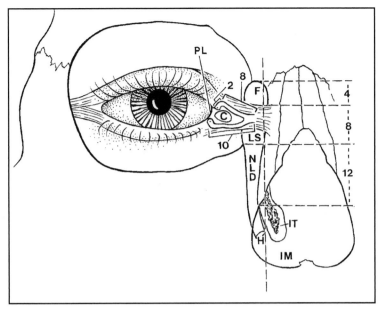

Figure 1-6.

CLINICOANATOMIC CORRELATIONS

During external dacryocystorhinostomy, significant bleeding can originate from the artery of the sutura notha. During a marginal fracture procedure, great care must be taken to incise the eyelid beyond the marginal arcade to avoid compromising the vascular supply of the lid margin. Dissection in Müller's muscle plane and severing of the levator horns can result in hemorrhage from the deep arcade.

Venous Supply of the Eyelids

The veins of the eyelids also determine anastomoses between the deep and superficial orbital systems. The frontal vein draining the glabellar area and the supraorbital vein running along the superior orbital margin deep to the orbicularis join into the angular vein on the bridge of the nose, where it is often visible under the thin skin 6 to 8 mm medial to the canthus. The angular vein receives nasal, superior palpebral and inferior palpebral, infraorbital, and zygomaticofacial veins and drains into the facial vein. The facial vein runs slightly lateral to the facial artery en route to the external jugular vein. Temporally, the supraorbital vein drains into a preauricular plexus through the superficial temporal vein. Via the deep facial vein, the facial vein communicates with the pterygoid venous plexus, which in turn communicates through the inferior orbital fissure with the inferior orbital vein and the cavernous sinus. The lymphatic drainage of the eyelids, conjunctiva, and anterior orbit follows 2 routes. The medial region lymph drains into the submandibular nodes. A larger lateral system drains into the superficial parotid nodes in the preauricular area. Both routes next drain into the deep cervical nodes.

CLINICOANATOMIC CORRELATIONS

Superficial facial infection can spread to the cavernous sinus through 2 routes. The first is via the anastomosis of the angular and supraorbital veins with the superior orbital vein. The second is via the deep facial vein anastomosis to the pterygoid plexus.

Lacrimal Excretory System

The lacrimal punctum is contained in the lacrimal papilla, which is a fibrous ring located at the level of the transition zone between the tarsus and the medial canthal ligament and is encased in pretarsal orbicularis fibers that insert onto the posterior lacrimal crest. The superior punctum faces the tear lake between the plica semilunaris (PL) and the caruncle (C), approximately 5 mm from the medial canthal angle, whereas the inferior punctum faces the tear lake lateral to the PL, approximately 7 mm from the medial canthal angle (Figure 1-6). The vertical portion of the canaliculi is 2 mm, ending in the ampulla. The horizontal portion is 8 mm for the superior and 10 mm for the inferior canaliculus and has a caliber of 0.5 mm. It is usually buried in orbicularis fibers, but may run immediately under the surface of the lid margin. After traversing the lacrimal fascia surrounding the lacrimal sac (LS), the 2 canaliculi join at an acute angle into a 1.2-mm common canaliculus in more than 90% of subjects. The junction determines an anterior angle of approximately 118°, whereas the common canaliculus enters the lateral aspect of the sac with an acute posterior angle of 58°, 2- to 3-mm deep and slightly superior to the medial canthi ligament. The lacrimal sac refers to the upper portion of the nasolacrimal duct (NLD) that lies in the lacrimal bone fossa. Its vertical dimension is 12 mm, 4 mm of which is the fundus (F) above the medial canthal ligament. It is 4 to 8 mm in its anteroposterior dimension and several millimeters wide. Intraosseous duct length averages 12.5 mm and ends with a 2- to 5-mm extension (Hasner's valve, H) into the inferior meatus (IM) under the inferior turbinate (IT).

Lateral inclination of the nasolacrimal duct in the frontal plane varies from 0° to 15° and practically follows a line drawn between the tear sac and the ala nasi. From superior to inferior, the duct has a 15° posterior inclination in the sagittal plane and practically follows a line drawn between the medial canthus and the first molar tooth.

CLINICOANATOMIC CORRELATIONS

After instrumentation, the fibrous ring will often exhibit continued enlargement, whereas the rest of the system is elastic. Ectropion of the punctum is diagnosed as soon as it is spontaneously visible. The lacrimal fossa is slightly narrower in women. Acute inflammatory swelling of the tear sac usually extends from its portion inferior to the medial canthal ligament. The orbital septum insertion along the posterior lacrimal crest prevents dacryocystitis from extending posteriorly to cause orbital cellulitis. Enlargement of the fundus is suggestive of a tumoral process.

The membranous lacrimal sac and upper nasolacrimal duct can be easily separated from bone, contrary to the lower portion of the duct. During probing, false passages can be distinguished by a progressive increase in resistance. A probe usually courses approximately 35 mm in adults and 25 mm in children before hitting the floor and is found approximately 30 mm posterior to the nasal vestibule.

Ten millimeters behind the insertion of the anterior limb of the medial canthal ligament, a distance of only approximately 8 mm separates the orbit from the anterior cranial fossa.

Endonasal Landmarks

The ethmoidal sinus (ES) is composed of 3 to 15 air cells that expand anteriorly up to the posterior lacrimal crest in 93% of subjects and enter the frontal process of the maxilla in 40% of subjects (Figure 1-7). The middle (MT), superior (ST), and inconstant supreme turbinates originate from the ethmoidal plate. The anterior tip of the MT corresponds to the projection of the lacrimal fossa (dotted line). The frontal nasal duct (FN) drains under the anterior portion and the ethmoidal ostia (EO) under the posterior portion of the middle turbinate. The maxillary sinus drains through its ostium (OMS) under the MT, just posterior to the bulla ethmoidalis (BE) and hiatus semilunaris (HS). The nasolacrimal duct opens under the inferior turbinate through a slit or a ±5-mm long mucosal flap valve (Hasner's valve, ONLD). The innervation of the endonasal cavity is mainly via the anterior ethmoidal nerve (a branch of nasociliary nerve, V1) and branches of the maxillary nerve (V2). The anterior and upper part of the nose is supplied with the terminal branches of the nasociliary nerve—that is, the ENN, later-

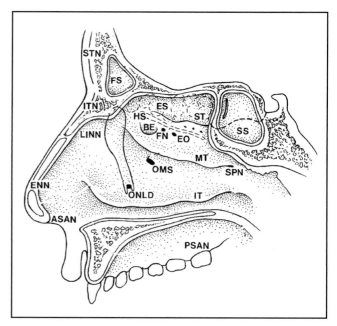

Figure 1-7.

al internal (LINN), and medial internal nasal nerves, and the ITN and STN nerves. From the maxillary nerve, the anterior superior alveolar (ASAN) and posterior superior alveolar (PSAN) nerves innervate the upper lip, maxilla, and front upper teeth and the posterior palate and the posterior upper teeth, respectively. The sphenopalatine nerve (SPN) distributes to the posterior nasal cavity.

Anatomy of the Eyelids

SUPERFICIAL LANDMARKS

The usual oculoplastic variables in White subjects are the following: The palpebral fissure in adults is 9 to 11 mm vertically and 28 to 30 mm horizontally. The highest point of the upper eyelid margin rests just nasal to the pupil, at the limbus in youths and 1.5 to 2 mm below it in adults, determining a margin reflex distance of 4 to 5 mm. The lowest point of the lower eyelid margin lies at the 6 o'clock limbus. Both medial canthi are separated by approximately 30 mm—that is, roughly the length of a third horizontal palpebral fissure. The lateral canthus lies approximately 2 mm above the level of the medial canthus in men and approximately 4 mm above the level of the medial canthus in women. The upper lid crease (ULC) is formed 7 to 8 mm above the eyelid margin in men and 10 to 12 mm above the eyelid margin in women. A less defined lower lid crease (LLC) is found 4 to 5 mm below the lower lid margin at midpupil and diverges from the margin temporally. The lateral canthus projects approximately 5 mm nasal to the lateral orbital rim. The medial canthus is approximately 5 mm wide and comprises the plica semilunaris and caruncle. The eyebrow arches approximately 1 cm above the level of the superior orbital rim, vertical to the 9 o'clock limbus.

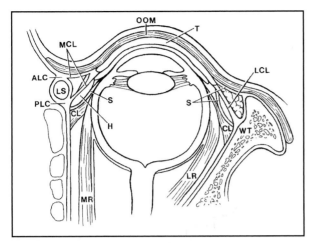

Figure 1-8.

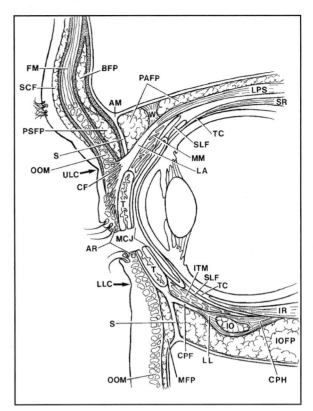

Figure 1-9.

CANTHAL LANDMARKS

Both the superior and inferior limbs of the medial canthal ligament (MCL) insert primarily onto the anterior lacrimal crest (ALC), around the lacrimal sac (LS), and onto the posterior lacrimal crest (PLC) (Figure 1-8). Horner's muscle (H) is composed of deep pretarsal orbicularis fibers inserting onto the PLC and lacrimal fascia around the sac. The superficial fibers insert with the MCL onto the ALC.

The lateral canthal ligament (LCL) inserts onto Whitnall's tubercle (WT) and is connected to the lateral rectus check ligament (CL). Superficial pretarsal orbicularis fibers fuse into a raphe, whereas deeper pretarsal fibers insert with the LCL onto WT. A small fat pocket is located between the septum (S) and the LCL.

CLINICOANATOMIC CORRELATIONS

The tarsoligament unit is subject to weakening and stretching with age. This is the pathophysiologic basis of the horizontal laxity component in lid instability conditions, such as ectropion and entropion.

Anatomy of the Eyelids and Retractors

ORBITAL

A variable fat pad is interposed between the preseptal orbicularis and the septum and is in continuity with the brow fat pad superiorly and the MFP inferiorly. The insertion of the septum follows the arcus marginalis (AM), corresponding to a thickening of the periosteum of the superior and inferior arches of the orbital rim. Medially, at the level of the insertion of the anterior limb of the medial canthal ligament, the septal insertion crosses the lacrimal sac and fascia to reach and follow the posterior lacrimal crest, where the septum covers the posterior aspect of Horner's muscle. Laterally, the portion of orbital septum posterior to the superficial orbicularis joins at the level of the lateral canthal ligament, whereas a sheath of sep-

tum posterior to the deep orbicularis muscle inserts onto Whitnall's tubercle behind the deep muscle heads.

The inferior portion of the septum inserts onto the inferior tarsus after fusing with the lower eyelid retractors approximately 4 to 5 mm below the inferior tarsal border. The superior portion of the septum inserts onto the levator aponeurosis 10 mm above the superior eyelid margin.

CLINICOANATOMIC CORRELATIONS

Considerable variation in septum strength prevails among individuals. It may attenuate with age, allowing the prolapse of orbital fat. This may be addressed by transseptal reduction of fat pads or by thermal sculpting of the septum. During surgical dissection to expose the septum, it can be identified by tugging on it to ascertain its firm attachment to the orbital rim.

LEVATOR APONEUROSIS

Deep to a reduced subcutaneous fat layer (SCF), the orbicularis oculi muscle (OOM) runs in continuity with other muscles of the SMAS (Figure 1-9). The denser fibers of its pretarsal portion are firmly bound to the tarsus (T) and to the levator aponeurosis insertion (CF). Its preseptal portion is underlined by the retro-orbicularis fascia or preseptal fat pad (PSFP), a fibrofatty layer in continuity with the brow fat pad (BFP) superiorly and the MFP inferiorly. The eyelid margin gray line corresponds to the arcade of Riolan (AR), a narrow bundle of orbicularis fibers running in the lid margin between the lash follicles and the tarsus. The ULC is located approximately 7 to 8 mm in men and approximately 10 to 12 mm in women above the lid margin at the level of the pupil. It results from the firm attachment of the levator aponeurosis (LA) onto the conjoined fascia (CF)/orbicularis interfascicular connective tissue and skin. Secondary insertion of the LA is onto the anterior lower third of the tarsal plate. In the levator palpebrae superioris (LPS), the transition zone between muscle fibers and aponeurosis fibers is located at approximately the level of Whitnall's superior transverse ligament (W), 14 to 20 mm from the anterior inferior tarsal border. The attachments of the LA to W are loose in the center and tighter laterally and medially. The levator complex is separated from the orbital roof and septum by the preaponeurotic fat pad (PAFP).

The superior tarsal muscle of Müller (MM) originates from the undersurface of the LPS approximately 15 mm from its insertion onto the superior tarsal border. It is tightly adherent to the conjunctiva but can easily be separated from the LA.

The less well-defined LLC is located approximately 4 to 5 mm below the lid margin. The inferior rectus muscle (IR) sheath forms an anterior expansion, the capsulopalpebral head (CPH), which wraps around the inferior oblique muscle (10) and condenses into Lockwood's ligament (LL) in front of it. From Lockwood's ligament, fibrous expansions extend anteriorly as capsulopalpebral fascia (CPF) fuse with the orbital septum (S) 4 mm below the inferior tarsal border and insert onto the tarsal plate, the orbicularis, and the skin. Sparse smooth muscle fibers are embedded in the fibrous fibers and compose the inferior tarsal muscle (ITM), which does not reach the tarsal border. The retractor complex is adherent to Tenon's capsule (TC) and is separated from the orbital floor and S by the inferior orbital fat pad (IOFP).

The depth of the fornix is 20 to 25 mm for the upper lid when the eye is closed and 13 mm when the eye is open, and 10 mm for the lower lid. The fornix is suspended over 360° by the suspensory ligament of the fornix (SLF) and the fascial extensions of the recti muscles. The marginal and peripheral arterial arcades anastomose with the anterior ciliary arteries, the circulus arteriosus iridis major, and the long posterior ciliary arteries.

CLINICOANATOMIC CORRELATIONS

For surgical purposes, the eyelid is divided into anterior and posterior lamellae. The anterior lamella is composed of the skin, orbicularis muscle, and lash follicles, whereas the posterior lamella is composed of the tarsus and conjunctiva. The tarsal plate is approximately 1 mm thick and has a maximum height of 10 to 12 mm in the upper lid and 3 to 5 mm in the lower lid. There are approximately 25 meibomian gland units in the upper tarsus and approximately 20 in the lower. These holocrine sebaceous glands are true epidermal appendages, and, as such, the openings of their ducts are keratinized. The mucocutaneous junction (MCJ) is thus just posterior to the meibomian orifices. Distichiasis is a condition, acquired or congenital, in which ectopic lashes arise from the meibomian glands resulting from metaplasia.

The palpebral conjunctiva is tightly adherent to the posterior surface of the tarsus, and pain is to be expected if anesthetics are injected in this plane. It is best to inject the palpebral conjunctiva beyond the tarsal border.

The vertical control of the eyelid position is controlled by the levator palpebrae superioris for the upper lid and by the lower lid retractors for the lower lid. With aging, the muscle belly and the aponeurosis can undergo lipoidic degeneration, leading to attenuation or disinsertion of their attachment to the tarsus and resulting in vertical laxity and instability for the lower eyelid and ptosis for the upper eyelid.

Müller's muscle activity accounts for approximately 2 mm of additional lift of the upper lid and the inferior tarsal muscle tone for approximately 1 mm of lower lid retraction.

PARTICULARS OF EYELIDS IN ASIANS

Compared with the eyelid skin in white subjects, the eyelid skin in Asians tends to be slightly thicker. In the upper lid, the postorbicularis fat pad, which connects with the brow fat pad (BFP), extends more inferiorly down to the superior tarsal border (Figure 1-10). In this same postorbicularis plane, a pretarsal fat pad is found anterior to the medial portion of the tarsus. The septum (S) may fuse with the levator aponeurosis (LA) well below the tarsal border, allowing the preaponeurotic fat pad (PAFP) to extend down to the superior tarsal border. The tarsal plate (T) is generally slightly smaller. The insertions of the LA onto the OOM at the level of the ULC are much less developed. As a result, the lid fold (LF) appears fuller, and the ULC is generally less defined, lower, or absent. An epicanthal fold generally completes the presentation.

Orbital Fat Pads

Technically, an anterior orbitotomy is created as soon as the septum is opened. In the anterior orbit, distinct fat compartments are identified. Behind the septum of the upper eyelid, the largest compartment is occupied by the preaponeurotic fat pad (PAFP) (Figure 1-11), which is yellow. Medial and inferior to the trochlea is the superior nasal fat pad (SNFP), which is firmer and lighter in color. Temporally, the orbital lobe of the lacrimal gland (LG) may prolapse in the wound and should not be mistaken for fat that can be removed. Behind the septum of the inferior lid, the inferior oblique muscle (IOM) divides the main fat pad into inferior nasal (INFP) and central compartments (CFP). An arcuate expansion of the inferior oblique extends to the orbital floor and, by so doing, separates a temporal fat pad (TFP).

CLINICOANATOMIC CORRELATIONS

In the superior nasal fat pad (SNFP) run the dorsal nasal artery and the ITN. Its removal during blepharoplasty usually requires deeper injection of anesthetics in the medial orbit. Dissection in this pad carries the risk of inducing a scar at the level of the trochlea (T) and subsequent Brown's syndrome or superior oblique palsy.

If the transconjunctival approach is chosen for inferior orbitotomy, the dissection plane transects the conjunctival fornix and lower lid retractors while remaining anterior to the inferior orbital fat and then progresses inferior to it.

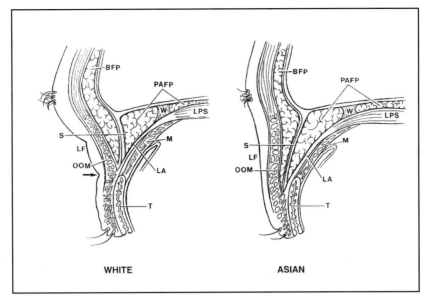

Figure 1-10.

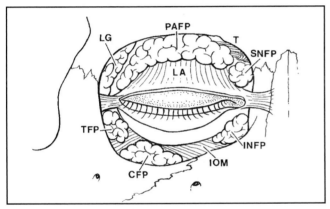

Figure 1-11.

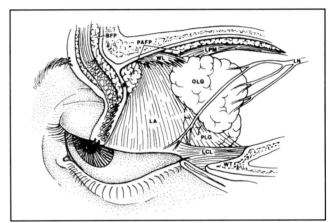

Figure 1-12.

Lacrimal Gland Relationships

The lateral horn of the levator aponeurosis (LA) indents the lacrimal gland into a larger orbital lobe (OLG) above and lesser palpebral lobe (PLG) below (Figure 1-12). The excretory ducts from the orbital lobe pass through the palpebral lobe or on its surface and drain with the palpebral lobe excretory ducts through Mutter's muscle into the superior fornix. Whitnall's superior transverse ligament (WL) is appended to the roof of the orbit and inserts onto the lacrimal gland fascia. The lacrimal gland receives its neurovascular supply through its posterior surface. Arterial supply and sympathetic fibers come with the lacrimal artery, which traverses the glandular parenchyma en route to the lateral canthal area. A variable contribution is provided by the recurrent meningeal artery. The lacrimal vein drains into the superior orbital vein. The LN (V1) travels apposed to the superotemporal periorbita, receives a branch from the zygomatic nerve (V2) carrying parasympathetic and sympathetic fibers, innervates the gland, and terminates into the lateral canthal area.

Fascial Orbital Structures

TENON'S CAPSULE AND LOCKWOOD'S LIGAMENT

Tenon's capsule (TC) fuses anteriorly with the bulbar conjunctiva slightly posterior to the limbus (see Figure 1-9). It is thickest anteriorly and between the anterior head of the recti muscles and thinnest at the emergence of the optic nerve. It is in continuity with the muscle fascia and extends between them as check ligaments. Inferiorly, the inferior rectus muscle (1R) sheath fuses with that of the inferior oblique muscle (10) and forms Lockwood's ligament (LL), which is a fibrous condensation extending from the medial orbital wall to Whitnall's tubercle and is strongest in front of the inferior oblique. It is connected inferiorly to the periorbita by means of fibrous septae. The extraocular muscle insertions onto the globe describe a spiral that parallels that of the orbital rim: The medial rectus is the closest to the limbus with a mean distance of 5.5 mm, whereas the superior rectus is the most posterior with a mean distance of 7.7 mm. Each of those distances varies over 3 mm.

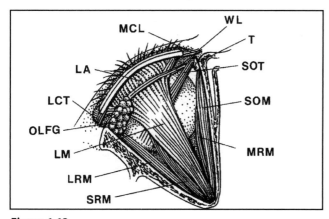

Figure 1-13.

CLINICOANATOMIC CORRELATIONS

Lockwood's ligament usually supports the globe in case of orbital floor fracture.

WHITNALL'S SUPERIOR TRANSVERSE LIGAMENT

Superiorly, Whitnall's superior transverse ligament (WL) fuses medially with the trochlear fascia, laterally with the lacrimal gland fascia (OLFG), and inferiorly with the intermuscular fibrous connections between the levator and the superior rectus muscles (Figure 1-13). The medial horn of the levator aponeurosis (LA) covers the superior oblique reflected tendon (SOT). The lateral horn splits the lacrimal gland into palpebral and orbital lobes and inserts onto Whitnall's tubercle (T). The lateral rectus check ligament inserts onto Whitnall's tubercle (T) and is slightly denser than the medial rectus.

Arterial Supply of the Orbit

Variations in the branching pattern of the ophthalmic artery are frequent. The arteries run independent of the orbital septa. The central retinal artery is the first branch and originates inferiorly to enter the inferior side of the optic nerve at a distance varying from 5 to 15 mm behind the globe. The medial and lateral long and short posterior ciliary arteries arise where the ophthalmic artery crosses the optic nerve and give approximately 15 to 20 branches to the globe around the optic nerve. The lacrimal artery travels with the LN along the upper margin of the lateral rectus, anastomoses with the recurrent meningeal artery passing through the superior orbital fissure, gives off zygomaticotemporal and zygomaticofacial branches that traverse the lateral orbital wall with the corresponding nerves, and terminates by supplying the palpebral arcades. Muscular branches are variable in number.

The branch for the lateral rectus also distributes to the superior rectus. Prolonging the muscular branches, usually 7 anterior ciliary arteries reach the globe through the insertion of the 4 recti muscles, 2 per muscle, except one for the lateral rectus. The superior orbital artery courses first medially to the levator palpebralis superioris, then between it and the orbital roof with the corresponding

nerve. In its medial position, it gives off an inconstant posterior ethmoidal artery. The ophthalmic artery then runs apposed to the medial orbital wall and gives off the anterior ethmoidal artery. After traversing the corresponding foramen with nerve and vein, its contribution follows the distribution of the nerve: lateral internal nasal, medial internal nasal, and external nasal arteries. The ophthalmic artery terminates by the dorsal nasal artery supplying the palpebral arcades, exiting the orbit beneath the trochlea, distributing to the root of the nose, and anastomosing with the facial artery. The lower portion of the orbit also receives branches from the infraorbital artery during its course in the infraorbital sulcus.

Venous Supply of the Orbit

The orbital veins travel within the septa. The superior ophthalmic vein is formed by the confluence of the supratrochlear and angular veins with anastomotic branches from the supraorbital vein. It courses backward beneath the superior rectus muscle, receives the vortex veins and other orbital and muscular venous branches, and drains through the superior orbital fissure into the cavernous sinus. An inconstant inferior ophthalmic vein may drain venous branches of the inferior portion of the orbit, the infraorbital vein, and anastomoses from the deep facial vein through the inferior orbital fissure. It may exit through the inferior orbital fissure and drain into the pterygoid plexus, or through the superior orbital fissure into the cavernous sinus, or into the superior orbital vein. To date, no true lymphatic vessel has been identified in the orbit.

Relationships of the Extraocular Muscles and Oculomotor Innervation

The 4 recti muscles originate from the fibrous annulus of Zinn. The levator palpebrae superioris and superior oblique originate slightly superonasally to it, from the lesser wing of the sphenoid. The medial rectus remains closely apposed to the lamina papyracea for two thirds of its length. In its anterior portion, the inferior rectus is separated from the floor by orbital fat and fibrous septa radiating from its muscle sheath. The inferior oblique originates from the orbital floor just lateral to the lacrimal fossa. It courses beneath the inferior rectus and inserts virtually without tendon onto the posterior pole of the globe 2.2 mm below the macula. These 3 extraocular muscles are innervated by the inferior division of the oculomotor nerve, which enters the orbit through the annulus of Zinn. The branch for the inferior oblique travels along the temporal side of the inferior rectus and gives an anastomotic twig to the ciliary ganglion carrying the efferent parasympathetic fibers from the Edinger Westphal nucleus. The superior rectus and levator palpebrae superioris receive their motor innervation from the superior oculomotor division. These 2 muscles have a fused medial sheath in their anterior portion. The nerve ramus to the levator passes medially around the superior rectus in 90% of subjects and through it in 10%. The superior oblique becomes tendinous before it reaches the trochlea, where it is reflected at a 54° angle.

It inserts beneath the superior rectus in the superotemporal quadrant. The trochlea is appended to the periorbita in a shallow fossa of the anteromedial aspect of the frontal bone. The trochlear nerve (IV) enters the orbit through the superior orbital fissure medially to the frontal trigeminal division (V). It courses outside the muscular cone, closely apposed to the orbital roof, and reaches its muscle in its posterior third.

The lateral rectus is separated from the lateral orbital wall by orbital fat. Its nerve, the abducens nerve (Vt), enters the annulus of Zinn and joins the muscle at the posterior third of its inner side. The lacrimal trigeminal division (V) and the superior ophthalmic vein also pass in the superior orbital fissure, whereas an inconstant inferior ophthalmic vein can be seen in the inferior orbital fissure.

Sensory Innervation of the Orbit

The trigeminal innervation of the deep orbital structures parallels the cutaneous distribution of the nerve (see Figures 1-1 and 1-7). The extraocular muscles are also provided with trigeminal proprioceptive innervation. The ophthalmic trigeminal nerve (V1) divides into its 3 branches in the lateral wall of the cavernous sinus. The LN enters the superior orbital fissure laterally. After receiving a branch from the ZTN (branch of V2), it supplies the lacrimal gland, conjunctiva, and lateral upper lid. The frontal nerve enters the superior orbital fissure, courses apposed to the orbital roof, and divides into the SON and STN. The nasociliary nerve enters the annulus of Zinn and crosses inward over the optic nerve with the ophthalmic artery to course forward between the superior oblique and the medial rectus. It has 4 branches: (1) the sensory root to the ciliary ganglion, reaching the globe via the short ciliary nerves; (2) the 2 (occasionally 3) long ciliary nerves; (3) the inconstant posterior and constant anterior ethmoidal nerves. The anterior ethmoidal nerve enters the intracranial cavity through the anterior ethmoidal foramen and the cribriform plate and penetrates the nasal cavity through the anterior nasal canal on the side of the crista galli. In the nose, it breaks off into a medial and a lateral internal nasal branch innervating the nasal cavity and terminates by the ENN, which exits between the nasal bone and the cartilage of the nose to innervate the tip of the nose; (4) the ITN, which runs below the superior oblique and anastomoses with the STN before exiting the orbit.

The inferior portion of the orbit is innervated by branches of the maxillary nerve (V2). In the pterygomaxillary fossa, it gives off branches to the sphenopalatine ganglion and the posterior superior alveolar nerves (PSAN). It then enters the inferior orbital fissure and divides into the zygomatic nerve and the ION. The zygomatic branch gives efferent parasympathetic fibers to the LN and terminates into the ZTN and ZFN. The ION courses in the infraorbital groove and canal, where it gives off the anterior superior alveolar branches (ASAN).

The sympathetic nerves enter the orbit via the ophthalmic artery and V1 and V2. The subsequent branches of the ophthalmic artery and of these sensory nerves supply sympathetic innervation to the ciliary ganglion, the globe, the orbital structures, and the forehead.

Retrobulbar Optic Nerve Relationships

The intraorbital portion of the optic nerve is 24 mm long, whereas the globe is 18 mm away from the optic foramen. This 6 mm of slack results in a gentle convex course inferotemporally. At its origin from the globe, the optic nerve is normally slightly bulbous. The axonal bundle is 3 mm in diameter and surrounded by pia mater, arachnoid, dura, and Tenon's capsule. In the subarachnoid space, the cerebrospinal fluid circulates freely within the intracranial cavity. Outside the dura, the optic nerve is closely surrounded by usually 5 or 6 short ciliary nerves entering from the ciliary ganglion located on the temporal side of the optic nerve approximately 15 mm behind the globe and accompanied by the short posterior ciliary arteries. Laterally and medially, 2 long ciliary nerves coming directly from the nasociliary nerve and bypassing the ciliary ganglion penetrate the posterior pole with 2 long posterior ciliary arteries and course anteriorly in a horizontal plane in the sclera and choroid. From the 4 quadrants, usually 4 but sometimes 5 or more vortex veins drain into the superior ophthalmic vein.

Landmarks of the Bony Orbit

The orbital rim is composed of the frontal (F), zygomatic (Z), and maxillary bones (M). In comparison, the orbital walls are much thinner. The posterior portion of the orbital plate of the M that is medial to the infraorbital groove is significantly thinner than the portion that is lateral to it (Figure 1-14). Also, the lamina papyracea of the ethmoidal bone (E) is the thinnest orbital wall, but it is somehow reinforced by the honeycomb structure of the ethmoidal cells. The anterior portion of the lacrimal bone and the posterior aspect of the frontal process of the maxillary bone define the lacrimal fossa, which is thinner than the posterior (PLC) and anterior (ALC) lacrimal crests.

At the apex, the optic canal (OC) traverses the lesser wing of the sphenoid bone and measures 6.5 mm in diameter and 8 to 10 mm in length. It is separated from the superior orbital fissure (SOF) by the optic strut. The inferior orbital fissure (IOF) extends more anteriorly than the SOF and ends approximately 20 mm behind the anterior orbital rim. Through it, the orbit communicates with the pterygomaxillary fossa.

The periorbita is the periosteum of the orbital walls and is in continuity with the dura of the optic nerve and canal at the apex, and with the intracranial dura through the superior orbital fissure. It is firmly attached to the suture lines, foramina, fissures, arcus marginalis, and lacrimal crests. Elsewhere, it is loosely attached to the bone. It is extensively vascularized. Its innervation depends on regional branches of the trigeminal ophthalmic and maxillary divisions. The posterior (PEF) and anterior (AEF) ethmoidal foramina are located 35 and 20 mm, respectively, behind the ALC.

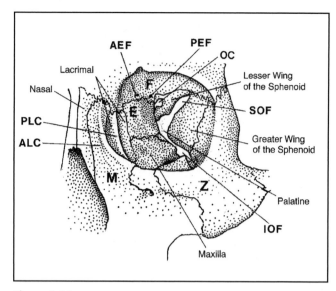

Figure 1-14.

Lateral Bony Wall of the Orbit

The facial buttress comprises laterally the thick zygomatic bone and the zygomatic process of the frontal bone. Posteriorly, the orbital plate of the greater wing of the sphenoid and the posterior portion of the zygomatic bone are much thinner, making the zygomaticosphenoid suture a convenient breaking point. Not more than 12 to 13 mm in men and 7 to 8 mm in women separate this point from the middle cranial fossa.

APPLIED ANESTHESIA

Thomas J. Joly, MD, PhD

Attended local anesthesia is the preferred method in most cases of oculoplastic surgery in adults. Procedures are relatively brief and can be performed with minimal hazard to the patient's general health. Topical anesthesia of the eye can be used for excision of minor conjunctival lesions or, in combination with local infiltrative anesthesia, to prevent irritation to the eye during preparation or surgery.

Anesthetic Agents

TOPICAL ANESTHETICS

The most widely used agents in topical anesthesia are proparacaine and tetracaine. Proparacaine is less irritating than tetracaine, but it has poor corneal penetration and a shorter duration of action. It is available in 0.5% to 2.0% solutions. Its anesthetic effect lasts 5 to 15 minutes after application.

Tetracaine, although more irritating than proparacaine, gives more prolonged anesthesia because of its better corneal penetration. It is available as 0.5% to 2.0% solutions.

LOCAL (INFILTRATION) ANESTHETICS

The most commonly used infiltration anesthetics are lidocaine (Xylocaine), procaine (Novocain), mepivacaine (Carbocaine), and bupivacaine (Marcaine). Hypersensitivity to procaine, tetracaine, and other ester-type anesthetics are fairly common. In contrast, lidocaine, mepivacaine, and bupivacaine are all amide-type anesthetics, to which hypersensitivity reactions are rare. Lidocaine has rapid penetration and an anesthetic effect that lasts 30 to 60 minutes. The maximum injectable dose in adults is

300 mg; however, if epinephrine is added to the solution, the maximum dose may be increased to 500 mg. The toxicity and side effects of lidocaine are more severe than those of other agents. Lidocaine is primarily used as 1% to 2% solutions.

A procaine injection takes effect in about 3 minutes, and anesthesia lasts up to an hour. The maximum injected dose in adults is 1000 mg. Procaine is primarily used as 1% to 2% solutions.

The addition of epinephrine (1:100,000; 1:200,000) to either lidocaine or procaine lengthens the duration of anesthesia and helps control bleeding.

Mepivacaine resembles lidocaine, but its action is more rapid in onset and somewhat more prolonged than that of lidocaine. It is available in 1% to 3% solutions.

Bupivacaine is a long-acting anesthetic agent, lasting 5 to 25 hours. It has low toxicity and is used in 0.25% to 0.75% solutions. A mixture of bupivacaine 0.5% and lidocaine 1% with epinephrine 1:100,000 produces rapid anesthetic effect, good hemostasis, and long postoperative analgesia.

In making the decision for local anesthesia, the metabolic state of the local tissue must be considered. Local anesthetics exist in an ionized, protonated form and a nonionized, unprotonated form depending on pH. It is in the unprotonated form that the anesthetic can penetrate the nerve cell membrane and exert its effect. Therefore, in inflamed tissue with a decreased pH, local anesthetic may be less effective; more anesthetic might be needed or the surgeon might better resort to a regional nerve block.

Local Infiltration

Local infiltration can be used for small lid lesions, such as papillomata, verrucae, chalazia, and xanthelasmata. The solution is injected subcutaneously before excision of

Levine MR.
Manual of Oculoplastic Surgery, Fourth Edition (pp 15-18).
© 2010 SLACK Incorporated

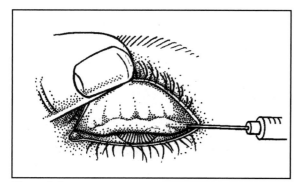

Figure 2-1.

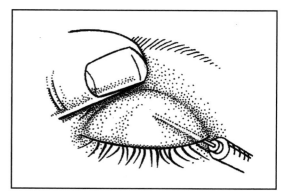

Figure 2-2.

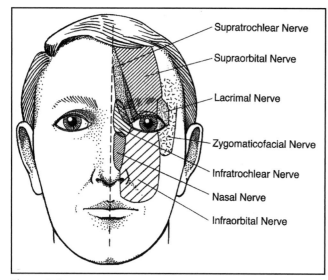

Figure 2-3.

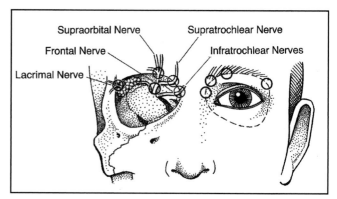

Figure 2-4.

lesions or subconjunctivally before excision of conjunctival lesions.

For removal of lid margin lesions and lesions requiring a full-thickness block resection of the lid (upper or lower), the following technique may be used:

Step 1

A few drops of topical anesthetic are applied to the eye, and the eyelid is everted.

Step 2

A fine-gauge (25, 27, or 30) needle is inserted through the conjunctiva at the upper (or lower, in a lower lid procedure) tarsal border. Approximately 0.5 mL of anesthetic solution is injected (Figure 2-1).

Step 3

With the needle in the same position as in Step 2, the lid is turned to its natural position, and the needle is advanced anteriorly and nasally to the subcutaneous space between the orbicularis and the orbital septum, where another 1 mL of solution is injected (Figure 2-2).

Regional Anesthesia

Nerve block anesthesia is useful (1) in cases in which large areas of lid and adnexal tissue are involved; (2) in cases of infected tissues; (3) in high-risk patients; or (4) to prevent distortion of tissue that can be caused by local infiltration. To achieve proper regional anesthesia, the surgeon must keep in mind that the sensory innervation of the face is supplied by the ophthalmic division and maxillary division of the trigeminal nerve. Blockage of its divisions (frontal, lacrimal, nasociliary, infraorbital, and zygomaticofacial) creates proper regional anesthesia for most oculoplastic surgical procedures.

LACRIMAL NERVE BLOCK

The lacrimal nerve is the temporal branch of the ophthalmic division of the fifth cranial nerve. It supplies the lateral third of the upper lid and the lacrimal gland (Figures 2-3 and 2-4). Block of this nerve is used in case of lesions of the temporal third of the upper lid and for lesions (cysts) of the lacrimal gland.

Step 1

With the upper lid closed, the needle is inserted along the superolateral orbital rim and advanced posteriorly. Adequate nerve block usually requires injection behind the lacrimal gland; however, care should be taken as the lacrimal artery may be hit, with consequential bleeding.

FRONTAL NERVE BLOCK

The frontal nerve is the middle branch of the ophthalmic division. It supplies the central and nasal portion of the upper lid, through its supraorbital and supratrochlear nerves (see Figures 2-3 and 2-4).

The supraorbital nerve emerges at the supraorbital notch, at the medial third of the superior orbital rim. It supplies the center of the upper lid, conjunctiva, eyebrow, forehead, and scalp.

Step 1

The supraorbital notch is palpated up to periosteum.

Step 2

The needle is inserted temporal to this area, going back 5 to 10 mm, and 1 mL of solution is injected (see Figures 2-3 and 2-4).

The supratrochlear branch of the frontal nerve exits above the trochlea, supplying the nasal part of the upper lid and eyebrow.

Step 1

The needle is inserted a distance of 5 to 10 mm under the orbital rim at the junction of the roof and medial orbital wall.

Step 2

An injection of 1 mL of anesthetic solution is given (see Figures 2-3 and 2-4).

A full frontal nerve block including both the supraorbital and supratrochlear branches may also be achieved by inserting the needle 20 mm under the center of the upper orbital rim, along the orbital roof. This, in combination with a lacrimal nerve block, anesthetizes the entire upper lid. This procedure is useful in surgery of the upper lid. In ptosis surgery, care must be taken as a motor block of the levator palpebrae may also be induced.

NASOCILIARY/INFRATROCHLEAR NERVE BLOCK

The nasociliary nerve is the medial branch of the ophthalmic division. It supplies the inner canthus, lacrimal sac, skin, and mucosa of the nose through its anterior and posterior ethmoidal and infratrochlear branches (see Figure 2-3).

Step 1

The needle is inserted under the trochlea or just above the medial canthal tendon, approximately 10 mm deep (posterior), and 1 mL of solution is injected for an infratrochlear block (see Figures 2-3 and 2-4).

Step 2

The needle is advanced 20 mm farther to block the posterior ethmoidal nerve for a more extensive nasociliary nerve block. This step is useful when a dacryocystorhinostomy is performed under local anesthesia. Care must be taken as the anterior and posterior ethmoidal vessels may bleed profusely.

INFRAORBITAL NERVE BLOCK

The infraorbital nerve is a branch of the maxillary division. It supplies the lower lid and conjunctiva and contributes innervation to the medial canthus and lacrimal sac area (Figures 2-3 and 2-5).

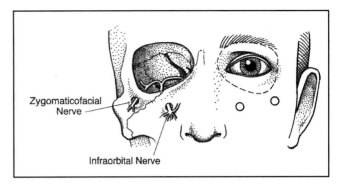

Figure 2-5.

Step 1

The infraorbital foramen is palpated at the medial third of a line drawn between the ala nasi and lateral canthus.

Step 2

An injection of 1 mL of anesthetic is administered into or around the infraorbital foramen.

Alternative 1

The needle is inserted above the orbital rim, hugging the orbital floor and 10 mm deep; 1 mL of solution is injected (see Figure 2-5).

Alternative 2

An intraoral approach can also be used; the needle is inserted in the maxillary gingiva between the canine and first premolar and passed superiorly along the face of the maxilla to the infraorbital foramen.

ZYGOMATICOFACIAL NERVE BLOCK

The zygomaticofacial nerve (a branch of the maxillary division) emerges from a foramen about 10 mm below the lateral canthus. It supplies the lateral canthal area and the outer part of the lower lid and shares innervation, in part, with the lacrimal nerve at the upper lid (see Figure 2-3).

Step 1

The zygomaticofacial foramen is palpated.

Step 2

An injection of 1 mL of solution is administered over the zygomaticofacial foramen (see Figure 2-5).

Complications and Management

The ophthalmologist must be aware of the potential complications that may arise with the use of topical or local anesthetics. If the anesthetic solution is inadvertently injected into a vein or into the highly vascular conjunctiva, blood levels may rise rapidly and cause stimulation or depression of the central nervous and cardiovascular systems by either the epinephrine or anesthetic agent in the anesthetic solution.

Stimulation of the central nervous system can produce anxiety, tremors, and agitation that may lead to convulsions, coma, and respiratory depression. The effect of the anesthetic solution on the cardiovascular system may cause bradycardia, irregular pulse rate, hypotension, and syncope.

To minimize toxic effects, a preoperative history of allergies to medications should be obtained. The solutions should be used in the minimal effective dosage (percentage and volume). Solution should be injected as the needle is advanced through the tissue, thereby lowering the possibility of injecting the agent into a blood vessel.

The addition of epinephrine to the anesthetic solution is an effective means of controlling oozing and of lengthening anesthesia time. This mixture should be administered carefully, as it may cause local tissue ischemia and an abrupt rise in blood pressure. The maximum dose should not exceed 0.5 mg (5 mL of 1:10,000 solution).

If surgery is performed as an office procedure, resuscitation equipment must be available. In cases of convulsions, 5 to 10 mg of intravenous diazepam (Valium) or a low dose of barbiturates should be administered. If asphyxia results from convulsions or respiratory depression, artificial respiration should be given. Hypotension and bradycardia are treated by placing the patient in a head-down position, increasing an intravenous infusion rate, and injecting alpha- or beta-stimulants (eg, ephedrine 10 mg) intravenously.

Systemic Anesthesia

Analgesia (loss of pain sensation), anxiolysis (loss of anxiety), sedation/hypnosis (loss of awareness), and amnesia (loss of memory) are 4 objectives of systemic anesthesia. Each goal may be fully or partially met with various systemic agents.

General anesthesia with inhalational agents and mechanical ventilation fully accomplishes all 4 anesthesia objectives. General anesthesia is indicated for some oculoplastic surgeries, including major orbital surgery, lacrimal surgery in which nasal bleeding is expected, and pediatric oculoplastic surgery; these cases are performed in consultation with an anesthesia specialist.

Monitored anesthesia care is indicated for many oculoplastic surgeries not requiring general anesthesia. Use of propofol, a benzodiazepine, and/or an opioid in combination with local or regional anesthesia can provide graded maintenance of each of the 4 systemic anesthesia objectives.

PROPOFOL

Propofol (Diprivan) is the most commonly used intravenous hypnotic agent in the current practice of monitored anesthesia care. It produces rapid anesthesia induction, with peak action within 1 minute and rapid recovery of 5 to 10 minutes after a single bolus. Induction dosing is 2 to 2.5 mg/kg, and sedation can be maintained with infusion rates of 100 to 200 µg/kg/min. Apnea, myocardial depression, and decreased vascular resistance are typical during induction, and excitatory phenomenon such as twitching or involuntary movements are not uncommon. Propofol has no analgesic properties and is typically used in conjunction with regional or local anesthetic injection.

Because of its rapid clearance, it has limited utility for sustained anxiolysis.

BENZODIAZEPINES

Benzodiazepines are anxiolytic and amnesic at low doses and more profoundly sedative at higher doses. Agents include midazolam (Versed), diazepam (Valium), and lorazepam (Ativan). Benzodiazepines have minimal cardiovascular depressant properties and less respiratory depression than propofol. However, patients should be monitored for these effects, especially when benzodiazepines are administered intravenously. Flumazenil, a benzodiazepine antagonist, is used to reverse benzodiazepine effects. Benzodiazepines do not have analgesic properties.

Midazolam is typically the preferred intravenous agent in the setting of monitored anesthesia care for oculoplastic procedures due to its rapid onset of action (<5 min). Sedation dose is 0.025 to 0.1 mg/kg.

Although diazepam can be administered intravenously, it is more often used an oral agent. Given orally, sedation dose is 0.1 to 0.2 mg/kg with peak effect at 15 to 60 minutes and duration of action of 2 to 6 hours. Lorazepam is longer-acting and, therefore, has less indication for oculoplastic procedures. Typical oral dose is 1 to 2 mg with peak effect at 2 hours and duration of 6 to 24 hours.

OPIOIDS

Opioids are primarily analgesic agents, although they can also have significant sedative effects. Sedative effects can be synergistic with benzodiazepines. Additionally, adequate pain control can certainly aid in anxiolysis. Agents commonly administered intravenously or intramuscularly for monitored anesthesia care include fentanyl (Sublimaze), meperidine (Demerol), and morphine. Opioids are respiratory depressants, and cardiovascular effects include bradycardia and decreased vascular resistance. Naloxone, an opioid antagonist, is used for reversal.

Fentanyl is the most commonly used intravenous agent in the setting of monitored anesthesia care. It is approximately 100 times more potent than morphine and has the additional advantages of rapid onset of action (within seconds) and short duration of action (less than 1 hour). Typical analgesia dose is 0.7 to 2 µg/kg. Morphine is typically dosed intravenously at 3 to 10 mg while the preferred route for meperidine is intramuscular at a dose of 50 to 150 mg, although either agent can be administered by oral, intravenous, intramuscular, or subcutaneous routes.

Several opioids are available orally in combination with acetaminophen for postoperative pain control, including codeine (Tylenol #3), hydrocodone (Vicodin, Lortab), oxycodone (Percocet, Tylox), and propoxyphene (Darvocet). With these agents, the opioid dose is limited by the amount of acetaminophen with which it is combined. The most common side effects are gastrointestinal, including nausea and constipation.

SECTION II

TRAUMA

CHAPTER 3

BASIC WOUND REPAIR
SURGICAL TECHNIQUES, FLAPS, AND GRAFTS

César A. Sierra, MD, FACS; Frank A. Nesi, MD, FACS; and Mark R. Levine, MD, FACS

An understanding of wound healing and basic surgical technique is important for optimum surgical results. Wound healing may be divided into 2 categories. Primary intention occurs when the skin edges are apposed. Secondary intention occurs in an untreated wound with or without tissue loss. In primary wound healing, there is an inflammatory phase, a fibroblastic phase, and a maturation phase. In the inflammatory phase, immediately after wounding, there is a release of cellular enzymes including amines, lymphokines, and other chemotactic factors. Initial vasoconstriction leads to a vasodilatation, increased capillary permeability, and recruitment of macrophages and lymphocytes. This establishes the environment for the process of wound healing and lasts from 4 to 7 days. In the well-sutured wound, a fibrin-platelet clot bridges the cut surface followed by migration and proliferation of epithelial cells toward the base of the wound until an epithelial bridge is formed in 12 to 24 hours. Epithelial hyperplasia with capillary vascular formation and epithelial reorganization occurs during days 10 to 15.

The fibroblastic phase is characterized by production of collagen by fibroblasts around day 3 after injury. Collagen is synthesized over the next 10 days with an increase in tensile strength over 4 weeks. The maturation phase is characterized by an alignment and restructuring of collagen fibers. During this phase, collagen synthesis is balanced by collagenolysis. This may continue for months.

Suture Techniques

Maximizing an optimum incision with minimal scarring requires good suture techniques and principles. First, it is important to place a skin incision along lines of facial expression or skin tension lines (Figure 3-1). Incisions made parallel to these lines tend to heal with less scarring than those that are oriented tangentially. Second, it is generally preferable to make the incision perpendicular to the skin surface. Beveled wounds retard healing and are more difficult to approximate. Beveled incisions, however, are often used in the eyebrow to minimize trauma to the eyebrow lash follicles. Third, it is important to relieve tension along the wound edge with properly placed deep sutures to facilitate compact scar formation. If this is ignored, the epithelial bridge will extend downward in an extended wound, and a depressed wide scar will occur. Fourth, delicate tissue handling with minimal crush injury to wound edges will reduce the inflammatory phase. Fifth, it is important to have slight eversion of the wound edges. This compensates for contraction during wound healing and avoids or minimizes depressed scar formation (Figure 3-2). Interrupted sutures offer great safety in that if one suture breaks or unties, remaining sutures may prevent dehiscence. Because a running suture distributes the tension relatively evenly along the entire extent of the suture, interrupted suturing techniques may better maintain tension for a curved incision or complex laceration. Sixth, wound eversion can be exaggerated by a vertical mattress that provides good deep support and wound edge eversion (Figure 3-3). A horizontal mattress suture distributes the coaptive tension of the suture along a greater length of the wound. This may be of value when closing a wound with friable wound edges (Figure 3-4).

Suture Material

Suture material may be absorbable or nonabsorbable and may best fit certain situations depending on the age of the patient, type of incision, location, amount of wound tension needed, and suture handling characteristics.

Levine MR.
Manual of Oculoplastic Surgery, Fourth Edition (pp 21-26).
© 2010 SLACK Incorporated

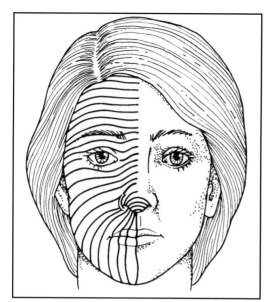

Figure 3-1.

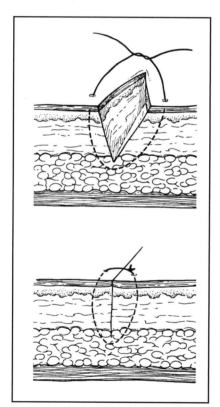

Figure 3-2.

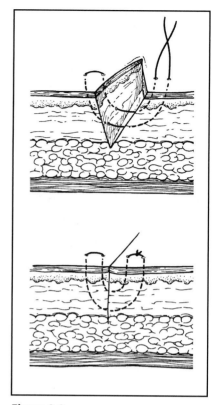

Figure 3-3.

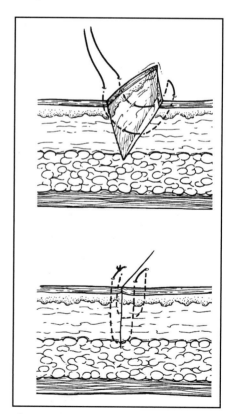

Figure 3-4.

Fast-absorbing gut suture comes from the intestinal mucosa of a sheep. The sutures lose 50% of the tensile strength in 3 to 5 days. It should only be used in wound closure that has little or no tension. Plain gut sutures lose half of the tensile strength in 7 to 10 days, whereas chromic catgut sutures, which have been treated with chromic oxide solution, lose 50% of tensile strength in 10 to 14 days. Synthetic sutures such as polyglycolic acid (Dexon) and polyglactin (Vicryl) are braided sutures and are less reactive than gut and lose 50% of their tensile strength over 2 to 4 weeks. Nonabsorbable sutures include silk, Dacron, nylon, and Prolene. Silk is a naturally occurring braided suture that is very surgeon friendly, and it maintains its tensile strength over 2 years. Mersilene (Dacron) is a synthetic braided suture that holds its tensile strength for 2 years. Nylon is a monofilamentous synthetic suture that maintains 70% of its tensile strength over 2 years. It does not lay down as well as silk but it is easier to remove because it is monofilamentous. Prolene is a synthetic monofilamentous suture with 100% tensile strength over 2 years. Finally, the most inert suture material is stainless steel wire with little tissue reactivity.

Periocular Flaps and Grafts

Tumor excision may result in a defect that is larger or more complicated than estimated in the preoperative evaluation. The oculoplastic surgeon must be able to adapt to different, unexpected intraoperative situations that can arise with these procedures. Small skin defects may be closed by direct apposition and closure of the wound edges. Free skin grafts and vascularized skin flaps are commonly used in larger defects. Flaps may be used to minimize the tension during closure of an adjacent or nonadjacent skin defect or to release tension of contracted scars. A myocutaneous flap is designed pre- and intraoperatively according to the size, shape, and location of the defect or scar. Occasionally, a simple skin flap does not provide adequate closure due to the size or location of the defect. A free skin graft may be harvested from a more distant site, minimizing the extent of tissue mobilization and deformity. The donor choice will depend on the size and depth of the defect as well as the integrity of the blood supply in the recipient bed. Recruitment of available tissue with retention of its vascular supply through an unaltered base makes a flap superior to a free graft in circumstances where skin needs to be mobilized over an area of compromised arterial supply, such as free grafts or exposed bone. The right blood supply is also helpful, decreasing the risk of infection and ischemic necrosis of the mobilized tissue. In other words, the survival of the tissue is dependent on the degree of perfusion, which in turn is proportional to the size and length of the flap. Hemostasis is important but should be achieved with judicious cautery to prevent vascular compromise. Meticulous and proper handling to avoid crushing of the furthermost edge of the flap is vital because this is the area most susceptible to ischemia. Blanching due to poor vascular supply is an indication, especially in large flaps, for a delayed procedure until revascularization occurs.

A flap reduces the morbidity by using available neighboring tissue. Contracture of a flap is significantly less than in a free skin graft. However, overcorrection is still recommended to provide for the expected amount of contracture of the donor tissue. It also allows a better match in color and texture of the skin. The major disadvantage over a graft is the higher incidence of subcutaneous hypertrophy that could mask the recurrence of a malignant tumor.

There are several general rules that need to be followed when creating a flap. First, it is vital that the surgeon fully understands and feels comfortable with the facial anatomy. This is especially important when reconstructing danger zones such as the area overlying the zygoma between the tragus of the external ear and the tail of the brow where the facial nerve becomes more superficial. Incisions should be made parallel to the relaxed skin tension lines to minimize the tension during the healing period of the wound. Flaps in the lower lid should displace the tissue in a horizontal vector to prevent retraction of the eyelid caused by cicatricial displacement. The amount of undermining and mobilization required to close a defect depends on the laxity of the surrounding tissues. Younger patients with tighter, unyielding skin and large defects are usually more challenging to reconstruct. A flap should have minimal tension, but its length should not surpass 3 times the span of the base unless exceptional perfusion is observed at the most distal edge. Judicious cautery and careful handling of the tip of the flap is essential for its survival. Torsion, as well as tension, at the base of the flap should be minimal to ensure adequate arterial support. Different types of periocular flaps will be discussed in this chapter. Sliding, advancement, rotation, and transposition flaps are used to close a variety of anterior lamella defects. Others, such as the Z-plasty and V-Y-plasty, are commonly used to reduce the tension in contracted scars.

SLIDING FLAP

The sliding flap is the simplest form of tissue recruitment for wound closure. This technique is effective in closing small elliptical defects. The tissue surrounding the defect is undermined with sharp dissection. The edges of the wound are then gently drawn together with toothed forceps to determine the amount of residual tension. Care should be taken to avoid damage to the skin with the forceps. If the wound edges are still under tension, further dissection should take place to take on more tissue (Figure 3-5).

ADVANCEMENT FLAP

A more advanced technique should be planned when a simple sliding flap does not provide sufficient mobilization. An advancement flap is generally used to close rectangular or square defects. The skin next to the defect is undermined, and relaxing incisions parallel to the edges of the wound are created to advance the tissue. As previously mentioned, the length of the flap should not exceed 3 times the size of its base unless there is evidence of perfect arterial flow. Burrows triangles need often to be released at the base of the flap to reduce tension and to prevent irregular cicatrization. Advancement flaps are commonly used as part of other eyelid reconstructive

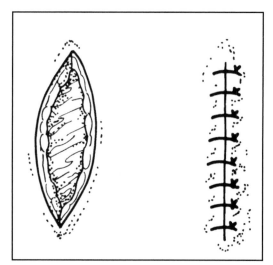

Figure 3-5. (Redrawn from FA Nesi, et al. [eds], *Smith's Ophthalmic Plastic and Reconstructive Surgery* [2nd ed]. St. Louis, MO: Mosby; 1998;90. Virginia Hoyt Cantarella, Medical Illustrator.)

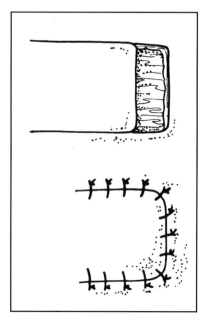

Figure 3-6. (Redrawn from FA Nesi, et al. [eds], *Smith's Ophthalmic Plastic and Reconstructive Surgery* [2nd ed]. St. Louis, MO: Mosby; 1998;90. Virginia Hoyt Cantarella, Medical Illustrator.)

procedures such as Hughes and Cutler-Beard procedures (Figure 3-6).

ROTATION FLAP

The rhomboid rotational flap is used moving tissue around a stationary base to close an adjacent defect. A flap is created as in an advancement flap and is rotated on its own axis to fill in the defect. The corners of the flap are used as landmarks to begin the closure. The puckered tissue created by the rotation of the skin can be excised as triangles before closure of the wound. Examples of

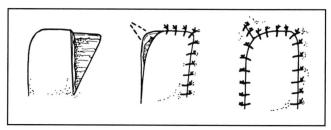

Figure 3-7. (Redrawn from FA Nesi, et al. [eds], *Smith's Ophthalmic Plastic and Reconstructive Surgery* [2nd ed]. St. Louis, MO: Mosby; 1998;90. Virginia Hoyt Cantarella, Medical Illustrator.)

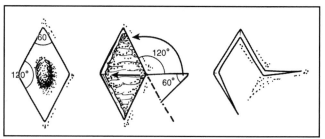

Figure 3-8. (Redrawn from FA Nesi, et al. [eds], *Smith's Ophthalmic Plastic and Reconstructive Surgery* [2nd ed]. St. Louis, MO: Mosby; 1998;90. Virginia Hoyt Cantarella, Medical Illustrator.)

advanced reconstructive techniques that incorporate the use of rotation flaps are the Tenzel semicircular flap and Mustarde flap (Figure 3-7).

RHOMBOID FLAP

The rhomboid rotational flap is a very useful variation of the standard rotation flap. This technique is used to close diamond-shaped defects especially in the cheek, temple, and lateral canthal areas. The flap should be created on the side of maximum skin availability and laxity by extending an incision at a 120° angle with one of the edges of the rhomboid defect. The dimensions of the sides of the flap should be equal to the sides of the defect. A second incision is made at the end of the first incision. This should be placed parallel to the defect and 60° from the first incision. Meticulous undermining of the flap provides sufficient mobilization to fill in the defect with minimal tension. The donor area should be closed first because it is the site where most of the tension is located following rotation of the flap. Subcutaneous sutures may be used to further reduce the tension exerted on the wound closure (Figure 3-8).

TRANSPOSITION FLAP

A transposition flap may be used to close a large anterior lamella defect when adjacent tissue is not available. This technique requires the transposition of the nonadjacent flap over normal tissue. Once the flap is created and the surrounding area undermined, it is pivoted into position. Care should be taken to avoid tension at the base of the transposed flap to preclude strangulation of the blood supply. Transposition flaps from the glabellar, temporal, or nasolabial fold areas generally possess excellent vascular supply. Transposition flaps are often used to

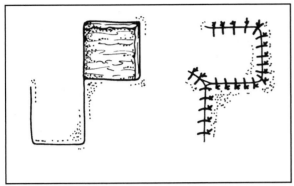

Figure 3-9. (Redrawn from FA Nesi, et al. [eds], *Smith's Ophthalmic Plastic and Reconstructive Surgery* [2nd ed]. St. Louis, MO: Mosby; 1998;90. Virginia Hoyt Cantarella, Medical Illustrator.)

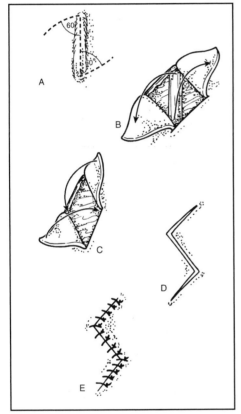

Figure 3-10. (Redrawn from FA Nesi, et al. [eds], *Smith's Ophthalmic Plastic and Reconstructive Surgery* [2nd ed]. St. Louis, MO: Mosby; 1998;90. Virginia Hoyt Cantarella, Medical Illustrator.)

reconstruct medial canthal defects in which the glabellar flap becomes the donor tissue. The patient should be aware that further debulking might be necessary due to the high incidence of hypertrophy of the flap (Figure 3-9).

Z-PLASTY

The Z-plasty is a variation of the transposition flap used to relieve tension in contracted scars. The central arm of the Z-plasty should correspond to the line of

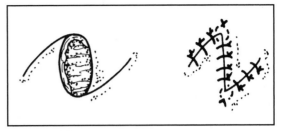

Figure 3-11. (Redrawn from FA Nesi, et al. [eds], *Smith's Ophthalmic Plastic and Reconstructive Surgery* [2nd ed]. St. Louis, MO: Mosby; 1998;90. Virginia Hoyt Cantarella, Medical Illustrator.)

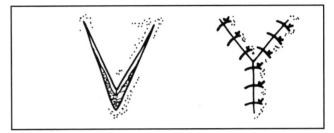

Figure 3-12. (Redrawn from FA Nesi, et al. [eds], *Smith's Ophthalmic Plastic and Reconstructive Surgery* [2nd ed]. St. Louis, MO: Mosby; 1998;90. Virginia Hoyt Cantarella, Medical Illustrator.)

maximum tension of the scar. The 2 side incisions of the Z should be placed at 60° from the central arm. This creates 2 mirror-image triangles with equal dimensions and angles, allowing a straight-forward closure. A longer Z incision with angles larger than 60° amplifies the lengthening of the cicatrix but is more challenging to close. Extensive undermining of the 2 triangular flaps and the available surrounding skin allows proper closure with minimal tension on the incision. Both flaps are transposed and sutured into their new recipient location. The central arm of the Z will rotate 90° from its original position, decreasing the tension of the scar. Closure should take place first at the apex of the flaps with subcutaneous sutures to further decrease the incisional tension (Figure 3-10). The O-Z-plasty combines the elliptic excision of a scar or mass with a Z-plasty–like closure. The mass should be included within the central incision. Curved offset incisions are created to close the defect with 2 advancement flaps (Figure 3-11).

V-Y-PLASTY

This technique is especially useful in the treatment of lateral and medial canthal deformities. The V-Y-plasty is another approach to the contracted scar. The axis of the contraction should be bisected by the V-shaped incision. The skin is undermined to release the flap and the available surrounding tissue. As the tissue is mobilized, the released V-shaped flap becomes a Y, releasing the tension on the axis of the scar (Figure 3-12). When the technique is reversed, a Y-V-plasty results, advancing the tissue toward the long axis of the Y.

SPLIT-THICKNESS SKIN GRAFTS

Split-thickness skin grafts are rarely used in oculoplastic surgery. They are usually harvested with a dermatome and consist of epidermis and a portion of dermis. In general, a split-thickness skin graft is inadequate for eyelid reconstruction due to its poor thickness, texture, and color match as well as for its marked tendency to contract. The main advantage is its ability to survive in areas with poor vascular supply, such as periosteum and bone following orbital exenteration.

FULL-THICKNESS SKIN GRAFTS

In the case of a full-thickness skin graft, the epidermis and dermis are well-preserved for transfer. These can be used to repair small defects measuring up to 5 cm. When possible, the tissue should be obtained from the contralateral eyelid for an optimal color, thickness, and texture match between the graft and the host site. Other donor choices, in order of preference, are the preauricular, retroauricular, and supraclavicular areas. The recipient bed should possess an intact vascular supply for the graft to survive. Hemostasis should be performed in a meticulous manner to ensure proper apposition of the donor and recipient sites.

A template made of nonadhesive dressing should be fashioned to match the size and shape of the defect. This is transferred to the area where the graft is to be harvested. The outline of the graft should be approximately 20% larger than the actual template to allow for the expected contracture. The skin graft is then excised, and the subcutaneous tissue is removed to allow revascularization of the full-thickness skin graft. After closure of the wound, small draining incisions can be made and a cotton bolster secured, placing gentle pressure over the graft.

Full-thickness skin graft survival depends on the vascularity of the recipient bed, careful removal of the subcutaneous tissue in the graft, and direct apposition of the tissues in the absence of an interface created by hemorrhage.

CHAPTER 4

EYELID LACERATION AND LID DEFECTS

César A. Sierra, MD, FACS and Frank A. Nesi, MD, FACS

Eyelid reconstruction is a common challenge that ophthalmic and plastic surgeons encounter. Facial trauma, tumors, and congenital colobomas are examples of instances when such procedures are required. Knowledge of the anatomy of the periorbital tissues is crucial for the precise repair of the involved structures to ensure proper lid function and to prevent excessive cicatrix formation. The surgeon should be able to choose the appropriate technique and should be familiar with the step-by-step plan in order to prevent loss of excessive tissue. Different approaches will be discussed with emphasis on eyelid trauma. However, all these can be applied to periocular tumor excision and reconstruction as well.

A complete history should be taken when possible to establish the circumstances of the injury. Information should be collected regarding the composition of the material involved in the injury (ie, organic matter, metal, sharp, blunt) as some of these can be devastating with sudden-onset vision-threatening consequences from penetrating eye injury. Imaging studies are often necessary to identify the mechanism of injury and to rule out the possibility of neurological or other major ocular damage, including rupture of the globe or intraocular foreign bodies.

Every examination should start with visual acuity and pupil exam followed by a thorough inspection of the globe and periocular tissues. A meticulous external and ocular examination must be performed in every patient regardless of the reason for reconstruction. Frequently, eyelid lacerations are deeper than they appear on initial inspection and give the false impression of being smaller and shallower. The thin eyelid skin and the rapid onset of edema have the tendency of concealing the true depth and extent of a wound. As a consequence, injury to the underlying ocular surface is frequently unnoticed by the referring source. With gentle handling of the eyelids, slit-lamp biomicroscopy and indirect ophthalmoscopy should be completed to exclude the possibility of ocular injury. Unmistakably, a penetrating eye injury takes priority and should be treated first. In such a case, the eyelid laceration should be gently rinsed, and antibiotic ointment applied. Repair of the eyelid should be delayed and planned as the ocular injury heals.

As a general rule, if the septum orbitalis is violated and/or the preaponeurotic fat can be visualized within the depths of the wound, the levator complex is suspected to be injured until proven otherwise. These need to be explored carefully prior to closure and after ophthalmic evaluation as previously mentioned.

When there is injury to the medial canthal area, particular attention is paid to the puncta and canalicular system. External signs of possible canalicular damage include rounding of the medial canthi in the case of avulsion. More commonly, the laceration is just medial to the punctum and presents as lateral displacement of the punctum. There is no tarsus at this position, and the eyelid tends to be weaker at this point. Probing and irrigation of the system should be performed to assess the continuity of the canaliculus if injury is suspected but not evident.

Orbital examination is essential in patients with periocular trauma. Potential entrapment of the muscles by a concomitant orbital fracture is ruled out with evaluation of the extraocular movements and diplopia in all fields of gaze. Abnormal position of the globe; hypoesthesia of the cheek; pain upon movement of the mouth; or deformity of the orbital rim, cheek, or malar eminence are also signs of concurrent orbitofacial injury and should prompt further assessment with computed tomography imaging with axial and coronal views of the orbit.

The excellent vascular supply that explains the abrupt inflammation commonly seen in these cases also accounts

Levine MR.
Manual of Oculoplastic Surgery, Fourth Edition (pp 27-32).
© 2010 SLACK Incorporated

for the very low risk of infection when repair is delayed. In fact, most canalicular lacerations and complex eyelid laceration with apparent tissue loss are better treated after the swelling dissipates and there is less need for tissue mobilization. The repair of the levator complex is also significantly enhanced when the inflammatory reaction has resolved completely, allowing the surgeon to better judge the eyelid position intraoperatively.

The elasticity of the skin and thinness of the eyelid dermis accounts for the illusion of apparent tissue loss commonly seen in traumatic lacerations. After careful exploration of the wound, most of these can be repaired with direct skin closure. It is crucial to initiate the repair by realigning the facial and periocular landmarks (ie, eyebrow line and apices of the wounds) when treating a stellate laceration. Generally, the tissue previously thought to be avulsed is present and viable following the apposition of such landmarks.

Full-thickness eyelid lacerations can be repaired by direct closure as long as the wound has smooth, even margins and there is no tension. Commonly, the wound edges are crushed and irregular. In such instances, a full-thickness pentagonal resection is preferred as long as there is enough laxity of the tissues. The wound can then be repaired using the classic 3-suture technique or the vertical mattress suture approach. Both of these provide a secure closure and sufficient eversion of the eyelid margin to prevent a deformity of the eyelid margin. Lacrimal stenting with silicone tubes and canalicular anastomosis using 7-0 absorbable sutures should take place prior to closure of the wound in cases where the canaliculus is lacerated.

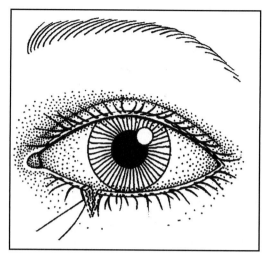

Figure 4-1.

Repair of
Full-Thickness Eyelid Defects

Step 1

Preoperative evaluation will dictate the method of reconstruction. In general, defects smaller than one quarter of the eyelid length can be closed directly depending on the degree of laxity. Using 2 toothed forceps, the edges of the wound are gently apposed to evaluate the amount of resistance. A 3-suture technique has classically been used when there is a full-thickness defect through the lid margin and the evaluation shows absence of tension. Alternatively, a vertical mattress ("far-far, near-near") suture can be used with equal precision.

If there is a crushed injury and the defect is markedly irregular, especially at the tarsal plate, the edges should be trimmed to create a full-thickness pentagonal excision while trying to preserve as much tissue as possible. This will provide for a smoother lining of the eyelid and prevent irritation of the cornea (Figure 4-1).

Step 2

In the 3-suture technique, 6-0 silk sutures are placed at equal distance and contain the same amount of tissue on both edges of the defect. Each suture is placed parallel to each other through the eyelash line, meibomian gland line, and the con-

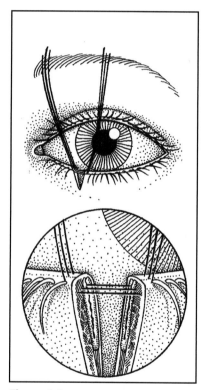

Figure 4-2.

junctival-epithelial junction. The first suture is placed through the line connecting the meibomian gland orifices. The other 2 are passed anterior and posterior. The sutures are not tied until the surgeon confirms the margin is perfectly aligned.

The silk provides adequate strength with moderate reactivity. Other nonabsorbable suture materials of the same caliber would sever or "cheese-wire" through the tissue (Figure 4-2).

An alternative to full-thickness eyelid margin laceration repair is to use a vertical mattress suture. This approach is not only relatively easy and fast but also takes advantage of the excellent wound eversion provided by the suture. A 6-0 silk is placed

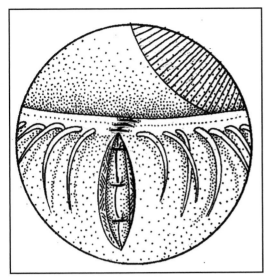

Figure 4-3.

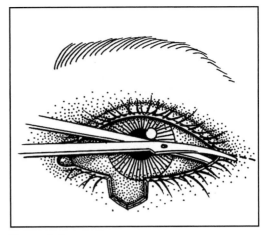

Figure 4-4.

through the gray line using the meibomian glands and the eyelashes as a guide to properly realign the margin. The suture is tied when there is sufficient eversion of the wound edges to prevent a depression of the eyelid margin in the postoperative period.

Step 3

The tarsal plate is then perfectly aligned so both edges are absolutely parallel to each other. Interrupted sutures of 6-0 polyglactin (Vicryl) are passed in a partial-thickness fashion to prevent corneal irritation. One suture is usually enough to secure the tarsus of the lower lid while 2 or more of these are needed in the upper tarsal plate. It is crucial to confirm that the suture is not exposed at the conjunctival side, especially in the upper eyelid where the suture can irritate the cornea. As with margin sutures, the placement of the tarsal sutures should be equidistant to avoid a kink at the tarsal wound. At this point, there should be accurate apposition of the tarsal plates and relief of the tension at the eyelid margin (Figure 4-3).

Step 4

In the case of the 3-suture technique, the surgeon goes back to the margin sutures, and the middle lid margin suture is then tied. At this point, the margin is re-evaluated for precise alignment, apposition, and contour. If not accurate, the sutures should be removed and replaced. Finally, the posterior and anterior sutures are tied permanently. The 3 silk sutures are incorporated into the anterior most skin suture knot to avoid corneal contact. The eyelid margin is confirmed to be everted to allow for wound contraction to create a smooth eyelid margin contour. The position of the posterior most sutures should always be evaluated because the close proximity to the cornea could irritate the ocular surface. This, in turn, could cause blepharospasm that can lead to dehiscence by creating excessive and repetitive tension on the wound.

Step 5

Finally, the skin is closed with 6-0 absorbable gut sutures. The underlying orbicularis muscle can be closed with buried 6-0 polyglactin sutures if needed to reduce wound tension on the skin.

Step 6

Ophthalmic antibiotic ointment and a 24-hour mild pressure patch are recommended for comfort and prevention of injury, especially while asleep.

Canthotomy and Cantholysis

Step 1

Sometimes, it is impossible to directly close an eyelid defect. These cases can be due to absence of lid laxity in younger patients, significant tissue loss, or swelling. The surgeon needs to know the several options depending on the size of the defect and the degree of lid laxity. A canthotomy and cantholysis may be required in cases where the defect is too large for direct transmarginal suturing and is smaller than 40% of the eyelid length (Figure 4-4). The lateral canthus is crushed with a hemostat and then incised to relax some of the tension.

Step 2

Additional relaxation of the lid is obtained by incising the corresponding inferior crus of the lateral canthal tendon. Depending on the amount of canthal fibers released from its attachment is the amount of mobilization up to a maximum of approximately 5 mm (Figure 4-5).

Step 3

Finally, the lateral aspect of the eyelid is swung medially, and the defect is closed in the manner described for the 3-suture technique for full-thickness eyelid defects.

Step 4

A new epithelial-cutaneous junction and lining to the new lateral eyelid is created by advancing

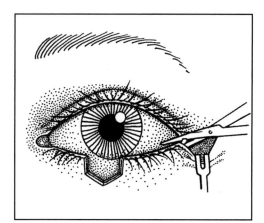

Figure 4-5.

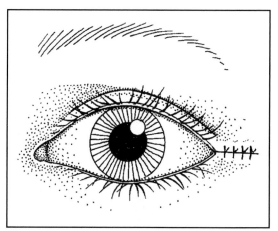

Figure 4-6.

the conjunctiva with 7-0 polyglactin sutures in a buried, interrupted manner. A single circular 6-0 plain gut suture is used to reconstruct the lateral angle by going through the subcutaneous tissue of the lower lid then through the lower lid grey line, back through the upper lid grey line into the subcutaneous tissue and tied. Care is taken to prevent the suture knot from rubbing against the globe (Figure 4-6).

More complicated reconstruction is necessary in cases of full-thickness defects larger than 40% of the eyelid. Other techniques for more advanced full-thickness eyelid reconstruction include Tenzel semicircular advancement flap, Hughes lower lid tarsoconjunctival reconstruction, and Cutler-Beard upper lid tarsoconjunctival reconstruction.

Tenzel Semicircular Advancement Flap

The mobilization of further tissue for closure of defects in both the upper and lower eyelids can be accomplished by semicircular advancement flaps. The incisions are placed at the lateral canthal angle and followed in a semicircular fashion toward the opposing eyelid (see Chapter 34 for more details).

Step 1
The defect should be trimmed to become a pentagon before mobilization of the tissues. Two forceps are used to hold the edges of the wound and to determine if more tissue needs to be mobilized.

Step 2
A semicircular incision line is marked from the lateral canthal angle and is extended in the opposing direction of the involved eyelid. Thus, for a lower lid defect, the curved line should arch superiorly; for an upper lid defect, it should arch inferiorly.

Step 3
A #15 blade is used along the markings to make the incision through skin and orbicularis muscle. Dissection takes place in the suborbicularis plane to mobilize the flap.

Step 4
A canthotomy and cantholysis of the corresponding crus of the lateral canthal tendon is performed with Westcott scissors. The lateral aspect of the eyelid should be freely rotated at this point to release all the tension in the wound and fill the defect adequately.

Step 5
Once the wound edges are apposed without tension, the defect can be closed as described for the transmarginal 3-suture technique as a first fixation point.

Step 6
The new lateral canthal angle is created by a second fixation point suturing the orbicularis of the semicircular flap to the periosteum laterally with a 5-0 polyglactin suture a couple of times. A 6-0 polyglactin suture is then passed through the normal lateral edge of the opposing eyelid as a full-thickness pass, and then passed as a full-thickness bite through the newly formed eyelid.

Step 7
A conjunctival flap should be carefully undermined and advanced to line the newly formed eyelid as its posterior aspect is orbicularis muscle. The conjunctival flap is advanced using 7-0 polyglactin sutures in a buried, interrupted manner to prevent them from irritating the globe. Other options for lining the flap include buccal mucous membrane, conjunctival, and amniotic membrane graft.

Hughes Tarsoconjunctival Flap

A tarsoconjunctival flap is the choice for lower lid reconstruction when there is a larger defect that cannot be closed directly or by advancement of sliding tissue. The flap is brought from the opposing upper lid to create the posterior lamella and a skin-orbicularis flap or full-thickness skin graft used as the anterior lamella (see Chapter 35 for more details).

Step 1

The defect is prepared for the procedure by removing devitalized tissue and fibrin with a #15 blade to make smooth edges. Care should always be taken to preserve as much viable tissue as possible.

Step 2

Both edges of the wound are held with forceps and brought closer together without tension to be able to evaluate and measure the real width of the wound with calipers. Then, the opposing upper lid is everted with a Desmarres retractor to reveal the conjunctival side and to mark the flap to be made using the same dimensions of the defect.

Step 3

The incision should be made with a #15 blade 4 mm above and parallel to the lid margin. The vertical incisions are made on both sides and high into the fornix. With the use of blunt Westcott scissors, the flap is carefully dissected in the potential space between Müller's muscle and the conjunctiva. Once the flap is positioned, the integrity of the conjunctival vessels and the lack of tension are confirmed as this is essential for its survival.

Step 4

The margins of the defect should be incised to separate the posterior lamella from the anterior lamella. This will provide a groove that will accept the flap. The tarsoconjunctival flap is sutured to the margins of the defect with a 6-0 double-armed silk suture in vertical mattress fashion and tied over a rubber bolster. The suture is passed through the posterior lamella of the margin of the defect, then through the flap, and finally through the anterior lamella of the margin of the defect.

Step 5

The inferior edge of the flap is sutured to the conjunctiva with 7-0 polyglactin sutures.

Step 6

A skin flap is advanced from the eyelid and cheek if there is adequate laxity of the tissues. Vertical incisions are made inferiorly, and the skin is undermined with scissors. A full-thickness skin graft is a better option when there is tension or insufficient tissue laxity to provide for a good skin flap without the risk of retraction. The skin flap can be advanced and secured with 6-0 plain gut suture.

Step 7

Hughes procedure—stage II. The tarsoconjunctival flap can be opened as early as 2 weeks depending on the individual. The cornea should always be protected as the flap is severed at the level of the lower eyelid margin. Any irregularities in the level of the margin can be resurfaced with thermal cautery at the end of the procedure.

Eyelid Lacerations Involving the Levator Aponeurosis

Anatomically, the eyelid layers 4 mm above the superior edge of the tarsus moving from the surface inward are (1) skin, (2) preorbital orbicularis muscle, (3) septum orbitalis, (4) preaponeurotic fat, (5) levator palpebrae, (6) Müller's muscle, and (7) conjunctiva. As a rule, a laceration in the upper eyelid deep enough to expose preaponeurotic fat will involve the levator complex until proven otherwise with exploration of the injured lid.

A patient with a laceration involving the levator palpebrae complex will present with significant ptosis and a severely affected levator function. Occasionally, patients with lacerations and no involvement of the levator will initially present with the same findings due to severe swelling. Although, once the inflammation resolves and the levator function remains normal, the same rule applies to the latter case.

If the possibility of a foreign body has been excluded with a thorough history and/or imaging, exploration and repair of these lacerations is better performed when the swelling decreases but generally within 48 to 72 hours. An attempt to repair the eyelid and levator laceration should be made to prevent severe ptosis. The preferred method of anesthesia in a cooperative patient is local infiltration of appropriate anesthesia with light sedation. This allows the patient to be alert and work together with the surgeon as the eyelid height is assessed and adjusted.

Step 1

The patient is appropriately sedated for the infiltration of the eyelid with local anesthetic containing epinephrine for hemostasis. Then, the eyelid is cleansed and explored to determine the depth and extent of the wound. Remember that, as the name implies, the preaponeurotic fat lies over the levator complex and serves as a key landmark.

Step 2

Once the septum orbitalis is open with scissors or cautery, the fat pad is identified, and the anatomy becomes clearer. With the fat gently retracted, the aponeurosis should be visible as a white shiny band and the muscle observed superior to it. There may be a hematoma in the area as the laceration through the levator could have penetrated the underlying peripheral vascular arcade. The patient is instructed to look from downgaze to upgaze to identify the levator. The surgeon may gently grasp the levator with forceps as the patient changes from one gaze to another.

Step 3

Once the levator laceration and both edges are identified, it should be approximated with a 5-0 or 6-0 nonabsorbable suture like silk or polypropylene. The same type of suture can be used if the aponeurosis has dehisced from the tarsus. Care should be taken to avoid additional advancement of the levator resulting in overcorrection and eyelid retraction. The patient should be asked to open both eyes, and the eyelid height and contour should be evaluated for symmetry.

Step 4

The septum should never be closed but permitted to close on its own. The herniated fat can be partially removed if necessary by clamping with a hemostat and carefully cauterizing the stump before letting the fat retract into the orbit. In these cases, we leave as much fat as possible to act as a "lubricating agent" to avoid excessive scarring between the injured levator and the overlying septum and skin. The skin is usually closed with interrupted 6-0 absorbable or nonabsorbable sutures with low inflammatory potential.

The postoperative care is similar to that for a full-thickness laceration. Ophthalmic antibiotic ointment is prescribed. An eye shield may be used, especially during sleep, to avoid accidental injury. The sutures are removed in 5 to 7 days, if needed. The healing and scarring process may occasionally improve the residual ptosis on its own. A period of at least 6 months is allowed to elapse before the diagnosis of persistent residual ptosis and any further surgical decision is made.

CHAPTER 5

MANAGEMENT OF
CANALICULAR TRAUMA

Tamara R. Fountain, MD

The location of the proximal lacrimal drainage system makes it particularly vulnerable to direct and indirect trauma of the medial eyelid. Prompt evaluation of the globe and adnexal structures is necessary to rule out intraocular, intraorbital, and even possibly intracranial injury. Once life- or vision-threatening diagnoses have been ruled out, thorough evaluation of the lacrimal drainage system should focus on the presence of lid lacerations/avulsions and possible canalicular compromise.

Once a canalicular laceration has been identified, most lacrimal surgeons would advocate that direct primary repair be offered to the patient. One exception might include patients with an established history of chronic dry eye. Repair can generally be undertaken up to 48 or 72 hours after injury, and this delay may provide the added benefit of reduced wound swelling and improved visualization.

Historically, repair of either canaliculus involved bicanalicular intubation with intranasal retrieval of stent tubing, often under general anesthesia. There are now a number of commercially available stent products that allow a wide range of flexibility in surgical approach. The choice of stent tubing and surgical approach will be dictated by location of the laceration, patient anatomic features, and surgeon preference. Despite the potential choices, there are general measures that will be taken in the repair of most canalicular lacerations.

General Intubation and Lid Closure Techniques

Step 1

Preoperative cold compresses and/or systemic steroids to decrease medial canthal edema.

Step 2

Irrigation of the wound and removal of any particulate foreign matter, if present.

Step 3

Meticulous inspection of the wound to identify the distal cut edge of the canaliculus. The operating microscope or use of surgical loupes and bright lighting will greatly aid in this step. Adjunct maneuvers like dye irrigation or air injection into a submerged wound or retrograde probing via the opposite canaliculus with a pigtail probe may be used as needed.

Step 4

Passage of stent material to effect an end-to-end anastomosis of the lacerated canaliculus.

Step 5

The cut ends of the canalicular tissue can be directly sutured with 2 or 3 7-0 polyglactin sutures but will often appose naturally around the stent material with closure of the surrounding soft tissue (Figure 5-1).

Step 6

Close the lid laceration using buried 6-0 polyglactin suture through tarsal plate, 6-0 silk at the margin, and 6-0 suture of choice to close the skin.

Step 7

Topical antibiotics may be prescribed postoperatively.

Step 8

The stent is usually left in place at least 6 weeks and removed in the office.

Levine MR.
Manual of Oculoplastic Surgery, Fourth Edition (pp 33-38).
© 2010 SLACK Incorporated

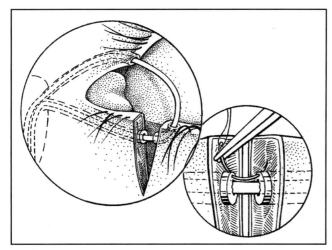

Figure 5-1.

Specific Canalicular Intubation Techniques

* Proximal (outer two thirds) laceration of one canaliculus using the Mini Monoka self-retaining monocanalicular stent (FCI Ophthalmics, Marshfield
Hills, MA).

Step 1
Dilate the involved punctum.

Step 2
Identify the distal cut edge of the canaliculus.

Step 3
Introduce the Mini Monoka stent via the punctum
and retrieve from the proximal cut edge of the canaliculus.

Step 4
Use a punctal plug inserter to seat the collar of the
tube in punctal ampulla.

Step 5
Trim the end of the Mini Monoka, if necessary, leaving at least 5 mm to seat in the distal canaliculus.

Step 6
Reintroduce the monocanalicular stent into the distal edge of the cut canaliculus (Figure 5-2).

Step 7
Close the canaliculus, lid margin, tarsus, and skin
as in steps 2 through 5 "General Intubation and Lid
Closure Techniques."

Step 8
Tube can be removed 2 to 6 months after injury by
grasping the collar at the punctum with a blunt forceps and pulling.

* Laceration of one canaliculus using monocanalicular transnasal Monoka or Mono-Crawford (FCI
Ophthalmics) silicone intubation.

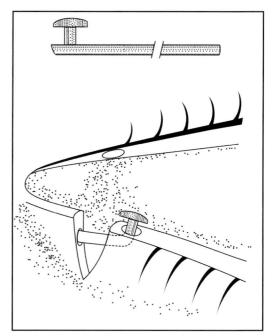

Figure 5-2.

Step 1
Induce general or monitored assisted care anesthesia.

Step 2
Anesthetize and decongest the inferior meatus and
anterior nasal vestibule with subcutaneous local
anesthesia combined with epinephrine.

Step 3
Further decongest the nasal passageways by packing the inferior meatus with cottonoids soaked in
vasoconstrictive agents like 4% xylocaine with
oxymetazoline (Afrin) or 4% cocaine.

Step 4
Dilate the involved punctum.

Step 5
Using Monoka or Mono-Crawford stent, thread malleable steel guide into the punctum, retrieve from
the proximal cut end, and reintroduce via distal cut
end of lacerated canaliculus.

Step 6
Advance the steel guide across the lacrimal sac and
down the nasolacrimal duct.

Step 7
One may retrieve the steel guide from beneath the
inferior turbinate under direct visualization with
the aid of an endoscope. The Mono-Crawford guide
has an olive tip that can also be grasped with a
Crawford hook (Figure 5-3A), while the rounded
end of a Monoka may be retrieved with the aid of a
grooved director (Figures 5-3B and 5-3C). The cuff
of the tubing is seated in the ampulla of the punctum with a punctal plug inserter.

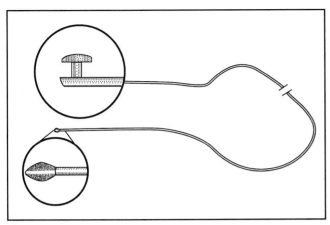

Figure 5-3A.

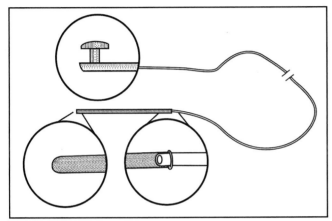

Figure 5-3B.

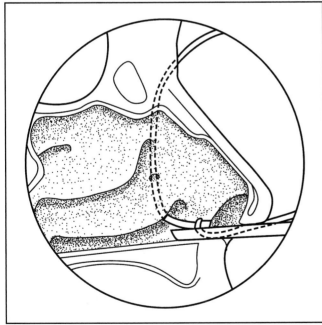

Figure 5-3C.

Step 8
Trim tubing within the nasal vestibule.

Step 9
Close canaliculus, lid margin, tarsus, and skin as in steps 2 through 5 of "General Intubation and Lid Closure Techniques."

Step 10
Tubing can be removed 2 to 6 months after placement by grasping the collar at the punctum with a blunt forceps and pulling.

* Laceration of one canaliculus using monocanalicular transnasal Ritleng self-threading Monoka (FCI Ophthalmics).

Step 1
Follow steps 1 to 4 of previous Monoka or Mono-Crawford technique above.

Step 2
Thread prolene guide suture into punctum and retrieve from the proximal cut end of the canaliculus.

Step 3
Introduce Ritleng probe into the distal cut end of the canaliculus. Advance across the sac and down the nasolacrimal duct to the floor of nasal fossa. Guide the plateau of Ritleng probe so that the inferior opening is directed forward toward the nostril.

Step 4
Thread the prolene suture emerging from the proximal cut end of canaliculus into the probe (Figure 5-4A). Withdraw the probe slightly to facilitate emergence of the prolene loop into the nasal cavity. Advance so a wide loop of prolene will lie flat on the nasal fossa.

Step 5
The prolene thread can be recovered under direct visualization with the aid of an endoscope or with a Ritleng hook (FCI Ophthalmics) (Figure 5-4B).

Step 6
Back the Ritleng probe out of the canaliculus.

Step 7
Separate the probe from the tubing by sliding the narrow section of prolene thread through the slit on the probe (Figure 5-4C).

Step 8
Pull the prolene suture to guide the silicone tubing down the nasolacrimal duct and out of the nose.

Step 9
Insert the collar into punctum with the punctal plug inserter.

Step 10
Trim tubing within the nasal vestibule.

Step 11
Close the canaliculus, lid margin, tarsus, and skin as in steps 2 through 5 "General Intubation and Lid Closure Techniques."

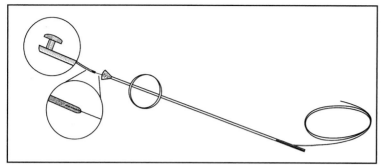

Figure 5-4A.

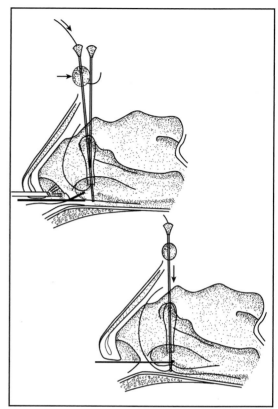

Figure 5-4B.

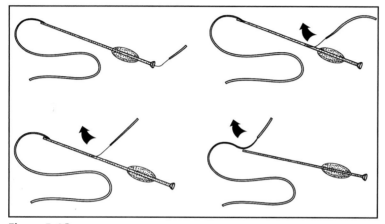

Figure 5-4C.

Step 12

Tubing can be removed 2 to 6 months after placement by grasping the collar at the punctum with a blunt forceps and pulling.

✳ Laceration of one canaliculus using bicanalicular non-nasal silicone intubation (Goldberg cerclage) (FCI Ophthalmics). (This is useful for distal canalicular lacerations where passage of the Mini Monoka is difficult. This requires the presence of a single, common canaliculus and familiarity with and use of a pigtail probe).

Step 1

Dilate both punctae.

Step 2

Identify the prolene suture end of the Goldberg cerclage that is swaged onto the overlying silicone tubing (Figure 5-5A). Pass this end into the involved punctum, and retrieve it from the proximal cut end of the canaliculus.

Step 3

Introduce a pigtail probe with an eyelet via the uninvolved punctum.

Step 4

Rotate the pigtail probe so the tip emerges from the distal cut edge of the lacerated canaliculus.

Step 5

Thread the prolene emerging from the proximal end (see step 2) into the pigtail probe eyelet (Figure 5-5B).

Step 6

Back the pigtail probe out of the uninvolved punctum, pulling the prolene and silicone sleeve with it.

Step 7

With the silicone sleeve completely spanning the canalicular system, trim the silicone if necessary (without cutting underlying prolene by nicking tubing then pulling), and tie the prolene suture to itself, forming a loop of tubing. Place the knot in the tubing and rotate the knot and cut the silicone end into canaliculus (Figure 5-5C).

Step 8

Close the canaliculus, lid margin, tarsus, and skin as in steps 2 through 5 of "General Intubation and Lid Closure Techniques."

Step 9

Tubing can be removed 2 to 6 months after placement by cutting the tube between punctae and pulling.

✳ Laceration of one or both canaliculi using bicanalicular transnasal silicone intubation.

Traditional bicanalicular silicone intubation may be performed using the smooth tipped, olive tipped, or Ritleng systems for mono- or bicanalicular trauma using the same steps as described above for transnasal monocanalicular intubation.

Step 1

With both ends of the tube projecting out of the nose, a square knot or 3 half throws are securely

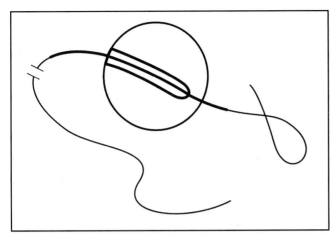

Figure 5-5A.

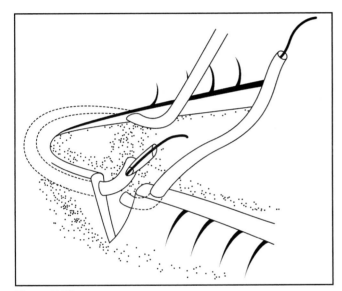

Figure 5-5B.

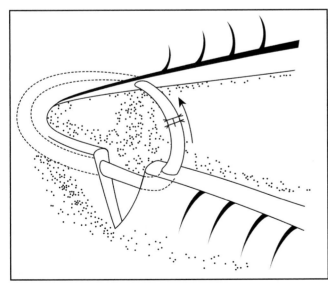

Figure 5-5C.

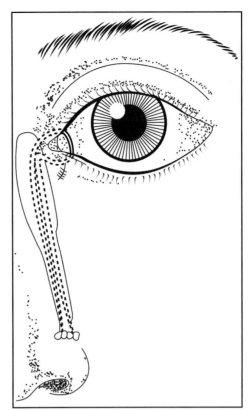

Figure 5-6.

placed in the silicone, taking care to leave enough slack in the loop such that no tension is placed on the punctae. The ideal placement of the knot is just below the inferior turbinate in the anterior nasal vestibule so no tubing is visible outside the nose.

Step 2

A 5-0 prolene suture is passed through the loop of silicone tubing and tied snugly to the lateral nasal vestibule to prevent the tubing from being inadvertently pulled out of the punctae (Figure 5-6).

Step 3

Tubing can be removed after the wound has re-epithelialized, generally no sooner than 2 months after injury. Many surgeons suggest leaving tubes in at least 6 months. When ready to remove, the prolene knot is cut inside the nostril, and then the tubing is cut between the punctae. The knot of tubing can then be pulled gently from the nose.

Step 4

If the loop of tubing is not readily seen at the nostril, forceful blowing of the nose while occluding the other nostril often will bring the tubing into view.

Step 5

If the tubing cannot be found in the nose or if the tubing prematurely extrudes from the punctae, the loop can be cut between the punctae and the remainder of the loop, and the knot can be removed with a deliberate pull from the punctum opposite the site of the original canalicular trauma.

Complications of canalicular repair are few but include premature extrusion of stent material with obstruction of canaliculus, cheese-wiring of silicone tubes at level of the punctum, pyogenic or foreign body granuloma formation, and epistaxis. The benefits of maintaining tear drainage generally far outweigh the risk of these potential complications.

With the available armamentarium of lacrimal drainage system stent materials, surgeons have a wealth of choices when approaching the sometimes challenging repair of canalicular lacerations. When successful, the reward is a happy patient with normal tear drainage and no excessive tearing.

ORBITAL FLOOR FRACTURES

William R. Nunery, MD and H. B. Harold Lee, MD

Orbital floor fractures often occur when blunt force is applied to the orbit. Two mechanisms play a role. The first is hydraulic compression of the globe and orbital contents, leading to an explosion of orbital soft tissue through the weakest part of the bony orbit—usually along the medial portion of the orbital floor and the inferior portion of the medial wall of the orbit. The second mechanism consists of buckling forces transmitted to the posterior orbital walls by compression of the stronger and more fracture-resistant orbital rims.

Orbital floor fractures may lead to restrictive diplopia from entrapment of orbital soft tissue along fracture lines. Fractures may also cause enophthalmos as a result of injury and atrophy of the orbital fatty tissue or of herniation of orbital soft tissue into the maxillary or ethmoid sinuses. General indications for repair of orbital floor fractures are restrictive diplopia, the presence of a large fracture with enophthalmos, and a large asymmetrical blowout fracture with more than 50% of the floor involved.

Patient Evaluation

HISTORY

The history should include the mechanism of injury to predict the most likely location of fracture and the likelihood of an orbital foreign body being present. If the patient has noticed a subjective loss of vision, the onset of vision loss should be noted. An immediate loss of vision more likely indicates direct injury to the globe or optic nerve. A later or more gradual onset indicates possible compression secondary to hematoma.

A history of numbness of the ipsilateral cheek, nose, or upper gum line suggests injury to the infraorbital nerve. Although the infraorbital nerve is not universally associated with an orbital floor fracture, it is a commonly associated finding, and its absence calls the diagnosis of orbital floor fracture into question. When diplopia exists, the history of horizontal diplopia suggests medial wall fracture, and the history of vertical diplopia suggests orbital floor fracture. However, either fracture location may cause restrictive, concomitant ocular deviations in horizontal or vertical versions.

The patient should be questioned regarding pain in the temporomandibular joint and whether the dental occlusion has changed. These findings suggest possible maxillary, mandibular, zygomatic, or Lefort-type fractures.

PHYSICAL EXAMINATION

The most important aspect of orbital examination includes vision and associated ocular injury. Second, proptosis or enophthalmos should be noted. Proptosis suggests an increase in intraorbital pressure from hemorrhage. Enophthalmos is rare in acute orbital trauma patients, but the incidence increases dramatically over the 3 to 6 months after the fracture. When enophthalmos is present, it suggests an enlarged orbit resulting from out-fracturing of the orbital floor or medial wall.

The pupillary examination should particularly note a Marcus Gunn afferent pupillary defect, which may indicate injury or compression of the optic nerve. A third nerve pupil may indicate intracranial injury or local intraorbital injury to the pupillary pathways. Traumatic iritis, sphincter tears, or a ruptured globe may be considered if the pupil is irregular and if anterior chamber reaction or a hyphema is present.

A decrease in motility may be paralytic or restrictive. Paralytic motility loss conforms to a pattern of involvement of cranial nerves III, IV, or VI and is not associated with an increase in the intraocular pressure in the field of duction of the involved muscle.

Levine MR.
Manual of Oculoplastic Surgery, Fourth Edition (pp 39-46).
© 2010 SLACK Incorporated

Restrictive diplopia is usually in both vertical directions or both horizontal directions. It usually has a double diplopia pattern in which diplopia is present in one extreme position of gaze and is reversed in the opposite position of gaze. An island of single binocular vision is usually present between the 2 areas of diplopia. Restrictive diplopia is also associated with increased intraocular pressure in the field of duction of the involved eye. This test can be done easily with a Goldmann tonometer. An increase in intraocular pressure of more than 4 mm in the involved field is highly suggestive of restrictive myopathy. The differential intraocular pressure test is more objective and easier to perform than the forced duction test.

Evaluation of binocular visual fields with the Goldmann perimeter permits objective measurement of diplopia and assessment of improvement on follow-up. Infraorbital nerves should be tested with pin, light touch, or both. The orbital rims, zygoma, and temporomandibular joints should be palpated for associated fractures.

RADIOLOGIC EVALUATION

Plain films may be obtained during the initial screening of facial and orbital injury patients. Opacification of the ipsilateral maxillary sinus suggests an orbital floor fracture. Associated fractures of the maxilla, zygoma, orbital rims, and mandible may be noted on plain films. Orbital floor fractures, however, can be missed on plain films, and the absence of a definite fracture does not rule out the existence of orbital floor or medial wall injury.

Computed tomographic (CT) scanning of the orbit is more accurate and definitive in localizing orbital fractures. The coronal view is especially helpful in determining the location of either a medial wall or floor fracture, the size of the fracture, and the degree of tissue herniation through the fracture.

The orbital CT scan may be ordered to (1) diagnose an orbital fracture in a patient with a suggestive physical examination but no definitive fracture on plain films, (2) define the size of a fracture previously noted on plain films, or (3) determine whether repair should be undertaken in a patient with an orbital fracture who does not initially have enophthalmos or diplopia. Whereas the third indication is not universally accepted, a fracture larger than 50% of the orbital floor with evidence of tissue herniation should be repaired even in the initial absence of enophthalmos because the likelihood of cosmetically significant enophthalmos is high in patients with a fracture that is larger than 50% of the orbital floor.

PREOPERATIVE MANAGEMENT

After an orbital floor fracture requiring surgical repair has been diagnosed, the patient is instructed to report any change in visual acuity or field immediately and to avoid performing Valsalva's maneuvers or blowing the nose until after the orbital repair has been completed. (Valsalva's maneuver may force air into the orbit, which could compress the optic nerve.) Cessation of anticoagulation therapy should be managed with the patient's internist or cardiologist. The patient's systemic medical condition and suitability for general anesthesia are assessed.

Between 3 and 5 days after injury, ocular motility and enophthalmos are reassessed. Repeat evaluation of binocular Goldmann diplopia fields can be helpful in assessing improvement in ocular motility. Motility photographs are also important in documenting the degree of restriction and in assessing postoperative improvement.

Patients need not necessarily remain in the hospital during the interval between initial injury and surgical repair. Orbital fracture repair may be done on an outpatient basis, if suitable arrangements are made for follow-up soon after surgery, if close monitoring of the orbit for 12 to 14 hours can be accomplished, and if the patient and the patient's family are reliable.

Anesthesia

General anesthesia with endotracheal intubation is the ideal for patient comfort and the prevention of aspiration. Lidocaine (concentration of 0.5% to 1.0%) mixed with epinephrine at a ratio of 1:100,000 units is injected through a 25-gauge needle. The solution is injected slowly to minimize the risk of inadvertent intra-arterial injection and retrograde embolization. Epinephrine in the solution improves hemostasis during the procedure and prolongs the effect of the anesthesia. Halothane is avoided as an inhalation agent because epinephrine combined with halothane may potentiate cardiac arrhythmia.

Surgical Procedure

PREPARATION OF THE PATIENT

The entire face is prepared, usually with povidone-iodine (Betadine) solution. If hexachlorophene (pHisoHex) is used, care should be taken to avoid direct application to the cornea because this may be toxic to the corneal epithelium. Chlorhexidine (Hibiclens) has occasionally caused corneal opacification as a result of severe corneal toxicity and should not be used near the eyes.

A head drape combined with a thyroid split sheet provides excellent coverage with retention of a full facial field. Plastic corneal protectors are placed over the globes to decrease the risk of injury to the eyes. Lighting is provided by a fiberoptic headlight to illuminate the posterior orbit.

SELECTION OF SURGICAL APPROACH

Surgical approaches to the orbit include (1) lateral canthal-inferior fornix, (2) subciliary, (3) orbital rim, and (4) Caldwell-Luc incisions (Figure 6-1). The lateral canthal-inferior approach is preferred for orbital fracture repair. It provides the greatest orbital exposure and the greatest flexibility in dealing with fractures, as well as the most favorable cosmetic result of all orbital approaches.

Subciliary incisions, orbital rim incisions, and the Caldwell-Luc maxillary sinus approaches are to be avoided as primary treatments for orbital fractures. The subciliary approach may lead to lower lid retraction, postoperative lymphedema, and an unnecessary eyelid scar. An oral, upper gingival approach may be a useful

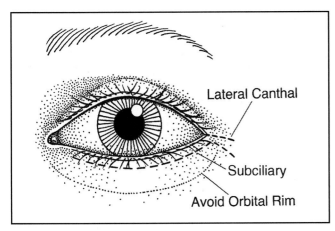

Figure 6-1.

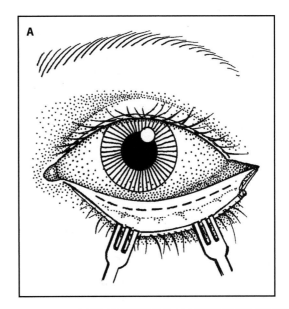

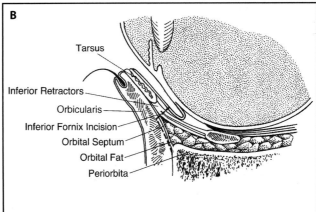

Figure 6-2.

adjunctive approach, particularly with zygoma fractures, but exposure to the orbit is limited and placement of an orbit implant is difficult through this approach. The orbital rim approach may lead to postoperative eyelid lymphedema and leaves an unnecessary facial scar.

If an associated medial wall fracture is present, both the orbital floor and medial wall can be addressed through a combined transconjunctival and medial orbitotomy approach. The medial wall is exposed through a 1-cm vertical incision created just anterior to the medial canthal tendon. This transcutaneous approach provides optimal exposure along a continuous subperiosteal plane to visualize both the inferonasal strut of the orbit as well as any associated nasal fractures. Sharp dissection is carried to the periosteum, which is subsequently elevated along with the medial canthal tendon and lacrimal sac. Dissection is carried posteriorly to approach the medial wall fracture. This dissection can be carried inferiorly to connect the orbital floor and medial wall fracture sites in a continuous plane.

LATERAL CANTHAL APPROACH

Step 1

Canthal incision: A #15 Bard-Parker blade incision is made at the lateral canthus precisely in the lateral canthal angle. The incision is carried laterally approximately 5 mm. Sharp dissection with straight iris scissors is then carried down to the lateral orbital rim periosteum. The inferior ramus of the lateral canthal tendon is identified, and the lateral canthal support between the lateral lower lid tarsus and the periosteal orbital rim is severed with straight iris scissors. The lower eyelid can then be everted freely and retracted anteriorly.

Step 2

Fornix incision: An incision is made between the lower border of tarsus and the inferior fornix (Figure 6-2). This incision is usually made with blunt-tipped Westcott scissors and is usually carried nasally to a position just lateral to the caruncle. After the conjunctiva and the inferior retractor layer are opened, the tarsal conjunctiva is retracted anteriorly with small rake retractors. A #15 Bard-

Parker knife blade is used to make a deeper incision through the inferior fornix. The first direction of the incision is slightly anterior to achieve a preseptal tissue dissection plane. The orbital septum, as well as the retroseptal fat tissue, is retracted with a malleable ribbon retractor. The small rake retractors on the tarsal conjunctiva are replaced with 2 Cinn retractors for deeper retraction, and further dissection is continued with the #15 Bard-Parker knife blade.

Step 3

Exposure of the orbital rim and floor: The dissection plane is carried anteriorly to the orbital septum to a position immediately anterior to the crest of the infraorbital rim (Figure 6-3). Care is taken to avoid making the dissection plane posterior to the orbital rim. The insertion of the inferior oblique is carefully avoided along the nasal aspect of the lower orbit. Whereas the proper dissection plane will permit an approach to the orbit immediately anterior to the orbital rim, care should be taken to avoid injury to the infraorbital foramen, which lies approximately 4 to 5 mm anterior to the crest of the

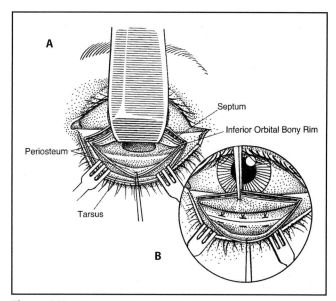

Figure 6-3.

infraorbital rim across the entire portion of the rim. The orbital floor periosteum is then elevated with a Tenzel periosteal elevator. The tip of the elevator is rounded and slightly sharper than a Freer or Coddle elevator.

Step 4

Location of fracture: The orbital floor periosteum is retracted gently with the malleable ribbon and periosteal elevator after being elevated from its original position (see Figure 6-3A). A medium rather than a small malleable retractor is used. A small or thin malleable ribbon retractor (less than 5/8-inches in width) may be easily placed dangerously far posteriorly in the orbit and may increase the risk of inadvertent injury to the optic nerve or superior orbital fissure structures. A wider ribbon retractor is not as likely to be placed dangerously far posteriorly in the orbit. Bleeding from vessels penetrating the orbit floor may be controlled with bone wax. The infraorbital canal along with the infraorbital neurovascular bundle is identified. This usually lies in a posterior-to-anterior direction along the orbital floor, usually lateral to the midline. Most orbital floor fractures begin immediately nasally to the infraorbital canal and often involve the neurovascular bundle of the infraorbital canal.

Step 5

Hemostasis: Care is taken to avoid retraction on the infraorbital neurovascular bundle. If bleeding from the neurovascular bundle is encountered, this may be controlled with absorbable gelatin sponge (Gelfoam) saturated with topical thrombin. If this is not adequate for hemostasis, gentle and superficial electrocauterization may be used, but great care should be taken to avoid thermal injury to the infraorbital nerve. In the anterior nasal aspect of the orbit, care is taken to avoid injury to the origin of the inferior oblique muscle.

Step 6

Reduction of herniated tissue: After the fracture is located, usually in the medial half of the orbital floor and lower ethmoidal wall, the herniated orbital tissue is gently elevated through the fracture site. This is done only with blunt dissection and in a slow and gentle manner. Care should be taken to avoid sharply cutting any orbital tissue because the soft tissue may contain extraocular muscle or nerve tissue. If the fracture is repaired within 2 weeks of the original injury, the mucosal tissue from the sinus separates easily from the orbital tissue. If the fracture has healed a longer time, differentiation between sinus mucosa and entrapped orbital tissue may be more difficult.

The entrapped tissue should be gently pulled free of the fracture line until the entire rim of the fracture can be identified. If the tissue elevates with resistance, a medium Kerrison rongeur may be introduced to enlarge the fracture slightly and free the orbital tissue from its bony entrapment. After the orbital tissue has been elevated, bony fragments herniating into the maxillary sinus can be gently removed with a hemostat or Kerrison rongeur. Large bony fragments are used for floor reconstruction, but small fragments are removed and discarded. Old blood clotted in the maxillary sinus is removed with suction. During the disengagement of orbital tissue from the fracture line, considerable care should be taken not to confuse the infraorbital neurovascular bundle with entrapped orbital tissue.

Also, care should be exercised to avoid compression of the orbital apex structures by the malleable ribbon retractor or by introducing the periosteal elevator more posteriorly than 35 mm from the orbital rim. Fractures extending along the ethmoidal wall may be reached through the inferior fornix incision provided the fracture is in the lower half of the ethmoidal wall. If the fracture is higher than this position, ethmoidal fractures may be reached through a second medial orbitotomy incision anterior to the medial canthal tendon (Figure 6-4). The combination of medial orbitotomy incision and inferior fornix incision provides excellent flexibility in reaching any fracture of the medial orbital wall and orbital floor.

Step 7

Orbital implant: After release of the orbital tissue from orbital fracture sites, an orbital implant is placed to prevent reherniation of orbital tissue or adhesions forming between the raw surface of the sinus mucosa and orbital tissue. I prefer to use sheets of nylon (Supramid) foil, which come in a variety of thicknesses. The foil can be cut at the time of surgery to fit the shape and size of the orbital fracture. In cases in which structural support of the orbital floor is not diminished by the fracture, a 0.2-mm Supramid foil sheet may be used. If the implant must provide orbital support as well as separation of tissue, a 0.4-mm Supramid foil is a better choice. Other possible implant choices include

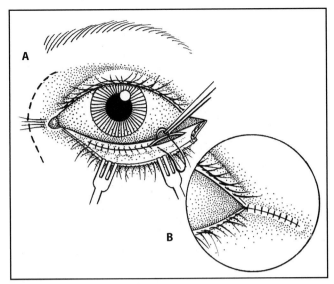

Figure 6-4.

Medpore plates, silicone elastomer (Silastic), or preformed polytetrafluoroethylene (Teflon) orbital plates. Silastic, however, has the disadvantage of providing less tensile strength than Supramid. Teflon plates are thicker, and less flexibility is possible in altering the plate to the fracture dimensions.

In cases of combined ethmoidal and orbital floor fractures, a 0.4-mm Supramid foil sheet may be wrapped entirely from the ethmoidal wall superiorly to the lateral aspect of the orbital floor to provide excellent orbital support. This is placed by cutting a large 0.4-mm Supramid foil plate and attaching a 4-0 suture through the medial edge. The suture is then passed from the orbital floor incision internally up to the medial orbitotomy incision with a hemostat. After recovery of the suture, the plate can then be pulled through the orbital floor up to the medial orbital wall and placed in the desired position. The traction suture is then removed from the plate.

Step 8

Anchoring the implant: After the orbital implant has been satisfactorily positioned and the adequacy of hemostasis and freedom of all previously entrapped tissue reassessed, the orbital implant may be fastened anteriorly by making a small trap door or flap at the anterior aspect of the implant and tucking this flap into the previous fracture line. If the implant rests securely in position, however, fixation to the bone may not be necessary. The likelihood of orbital implant extrusion is very low, even when the implant is not fixated.

Step 9

Closure of the conjunctiva: The inferior fornix incision is closed with a 6-0 plain catgut or mild chromic suture through the inferior fornix mucosa and conjunctiva just inferior to the tarsal plate (Figure 6-4A).

Step 10

Closure of the lateral canthus: The lateral canthi tendon is replaced with a 5-0 polyglactin (Vicryl) suture through the cut edge of the lateral tarsus into the inner aspect of the lateral orbital rim periosteum approximately 1 or 2 mm above the original insertion site. This directs the lower eyelid posteriorly behind the lateral orbital rim and overcorrects the lateral canthal position slightly to allow for slight downward contracture during the healing process. The internal suture can be reinforced with an external 5-0 Prolene or Vicryl suture through the myocutaneous portion of the lower eyelid, through the external portion of the lateral rim periosteum, and through the upper skin edge. The remainder of the lateral canthal skin incision is closed with one 6-0 gut suture (Figure 6-4B).

ZYGOMATIC FRACTURES

The zygoma is a thick, sturdy bone providing major supportive and protective functions for the mid-face and orbit. Because of its prominent location at the cheek, it is commonly involved in facial fractures. The primary sites of articulation with other facial bones are (1) superiorly with the frontal bone at the frontozygomatic suture, (2) laterally with the temporal bone at the zygomaticotemporal suture along the zygomatic arch, (3) inferomedially with the maxillary bone at the zygomaticomaxillary suture, and (4) internally through the zygomaticosphenoidal junction at the lateral wall of the orbit. In addition to segments of the lateral and inferior orbital rims, the zygoma provides the anterior portion of the lateral orbital wall and the lateral part of the orbital floor. When the zygoma is fractured, the fracture line rarely extends through the body of the zygoma itself. Rather, the zygoma separates along the primary articulation sites described previously, producing the so-called tripod or trimalar fracture.

The clinical findings of a tripod fracture may be minimal or extensive, depending on the severity and direction of the causative force. The zygoma is typically displaced inferiorly and posteriorly with downward rotation of the lateral segment of the inferior orbital rim. This produces flattening of the malar eminence, which may not be immediately apparent because of acute edema or hemorrhage. Palpable step-offs along the inferior and lateral orbital rims are common. Because the orbital septum emanates from the orbital rim, lower eyelid retraction may occur when the inferior rim is displaced. With inferior displacement of the lateral rim, malposition of the lateral canthal angle is present. Lateral impact to the zygoma may cause depression of the zygomatic arch. The arch may then impinge on the coronoid process of the mandible and cause malocclusion or pain in the temporal fossa when jaw closure is attempted.

Tripod fractures absorb the impact in trauma and thereby protect the globe. For this reason, the frequency and severity of ophthalmic injuries are somewhat less with tripod fractures than with orbital blowout fractures. Ocular injuries, however, still may occur with zygoma fractures, and ophthalmic examination is required as part of the initial management of zygoma fractures. In

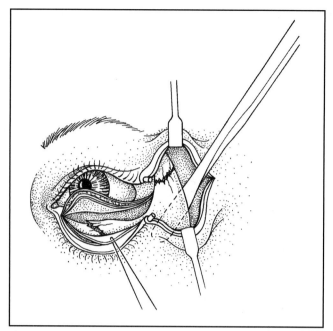

Figure 6-5.

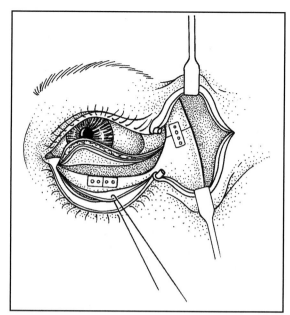

Figure 6-6.

addition, because the zygoma forms the major portion of the orbital floor and lateral wall, restrictive motility disturbances and enophthalmos may result from zygoma fractures. With extensive displacement of the fracture, the globe may be displaced inferiorly, even into the maxillary sinus. Bony lateral wall fragments may be displaced into the orbit, causing direct compression of the optic nerve or other apex structures.

Patients also frequently report numbness of the cheek, nasolabial fold, upper lip, and upper teeth on the injured side. This results from trauma to the infraorbital and alveolar nerves traveling in the orbital floor and anterior maxillary wall. The hypesthesia is usually transitory, although it may take several months to resolve. CT provides the most detailed information regarding zygoma and other orbital fractures. Axial scans are useful for imaging the lateral orbital wall, medial orbital wall, and the orbital apex. Also, the axial scan shows the degree of posterior displacement of the malar eminence. Coronal views show the orbital floor and roof and allow estimation of the degree of inferior displacement and rotation of the zygoma.

The surgical reduction of zygoma fractures is easiest 3 to 7 days after the injury. This allows soft tissue edema and hematoma to partially resolve. Closed reduction techniques are rarely adequate. Optimum results are obtained with open reduction and internal fixation using titanium plates along the external orbital rims.

SURGICAL REPAIR OF ZYGOMA FRACTURES

The optimal repair of zygoma fractures is accomplished through the fornix-lateral canthal approach described previously for orbital floor fractures. In addition, the superior ramus of the lateral canthal tendon is severed, and the upper lid is retracted superiorly to expose the zygomafrontal fracture line. The lateral orbital periosteum is also opened along the rim and elevated to connect the lateral and superior dissection area to the floor and infraorbital rim area. The zygomatic periosteum is then elevated laterally until the arch fractures are exposed. This allows the entire zygoma fracture fragment to be observed and reduced in continuity with direct exposure. Reduction is accomplished by placing a periosteal elevator or urethral sound behind the frontal process of the zygoma and beneath the body of the zygoma (Figure 6-5). With constant and forceful elevation and some intorsion of the elevator, complex zygomatic fractures are reduced. Placing a small periosteal elevator at the fronto-zygomatic suture assists in the reduction of the upper portion of the zygomatic fracture.

If the fracture becomes unstable, a screw may be placed in the body of the zygoma. With a hemostat pulling up on the screw, microplate fixation may begin. Fixation of the zygomatic fracture is secured at the zygomaticalfrontal and inferior orbital rim fracture sites with mini- or microplate fixation (Figure 6-6). In addition, the inferior aspects of the zygomatic fracture on the maxillary buttress may be exposed and stabilized through a superior intraoral gingival buccal incision line.

PLATE FIXATION

A wide variety of micro- and miniplate fixation plates are available for orbital fracture repair. Materials are usually titanium (Leibinger or Synthes) or Vitallium (Luhr) based. Vitallium has a slightly higher tensile strength and resists screw breakage more than titanium. Titanium, however, induces less artifact on subsequent CT scanning or magnetic resonance images.

I prefer low-profile (1.0-mm hole diameter) titanium microplates for lateral and inferior orbital rim fractures. Slightly more rigid plates (1.3- to 1.5-mm hole diameter) are useful for zygomatic arch and inferior zygomaticomaxillary buttress fracture plating. New plating systems (Synthes Midface Matrix) combine the benefits of lower profile dimensions (0.4 mm in thickness) and ease of operation (a single screw size for all plate thicknesses).

Complications

Most significant complications after orbital fracture repair include direct injury to the optic nerve, compressive hemorrhage in the orbit, eyelid malposition, and persistent diplopia.

Direct injury to the optic nerve occurs with posterior dissection along the floor or medial wall. Avoidance requires constant awareness of the position of the nerve, discontinuing dissection 35 mm from the anterior orbital rim, and avoiding placement of small retractors, which might compress the optic nerve.

Compressive hemorrhage may cause blindness secondary to central retinal artery occlusion or direct pressure on the optic nerve. Compression is best avoided by discontinuing anticoagulants if allowable based on cardiac risk factors. Hemostasis is achieved in surgery with Gelfoam and thrombin. After surgery, the patient should be monitored for pain, a decrease in vision, and proptosis. When orbital hematoma is suspected, the lateral canthal tendon is released for decompression. If necessary, the lateral orbital wall may also be removed until orbital pressure returns to normal.

Eyelid malposition occurs more frequently after subciliary incision than inferior fornix incision. To avoid malposition, care is taken to replace all eyelid layers in their original position and avoid downward pulling on the eyelid. A Frost tarsorrhaphy suture with upward traction, taped to the forehead, may prevent lower lid contracture. Treatment consists of artificial tears, massage, and time. The lower lids may require later elevation through inferior retractor muscle recession or extensive full-thickness skin grafting.

Residual diplopia may occur as a consequence of residual extraocular muscle entrapment or secondary to extraocular muscle fibrosis. Residual diplopia can be avoided by relatively early intervention (3 to 5 days) and careful release of all entrapped tissue with placement of a nonadhering Supramid implant. We avoid bone, hydroxyapatite, titanium, and all other implants that may fibrose to extraocular muscle. When residual diplopia occurs, the orbit may be re-explored for residual entrapment, or extraocular muscle may be readjusted to minimize diplopia in the primary position.

Postoperative Care

RECOVERY ROOM

After general anesthesia, the patient should be watched in the recovery room for 2 or 3 hours. Antiemetics may be useful in preventing orbital hemorrhage caused by vomiting. Pain medication should not include aspirin or other pain relievers that would interfere with platelet function. The patient should be observed for any evidence of hemorrhage behind the eye or loss of vision.

PATIENT AND FAMILY INSTRUCTIONS

Outpatient surgery should only be done if the patient is reliable and has easy access to the surgeon and to the hospital. Postoperatively, the patient should be attended by someone who is instructed to be alert for orbital pain, evidence of hemorrhage, or increasing proptosis. The patient should be instructed to avoid Valsalva's maneuver or blowing the nose. Instructions against lifting and bending and the use of aspirin are also given. The patient should know where to contact the surgeon immediately if any orbital pain, hemorrhage, or a decrease in vision occurs. If the surgeon doubts the patient's reliability or suspects orbital hemorrhage or complications, the patient should be admitted to the hospital.

FOLLOW-UP EXAMINATION

The patient should be called on the telephone the morning after surgery and should be re-examined within the first week after surgery. At that time, ocular motility exercises are prescribed. The patient is asked to move the eye into the extreme ductions that were restricted preoperatively. This should be done 30 to 40 times and repeated 3 or 4 times a day. If there is no evidence of orbital or ocular complication, the sutures are removed 5 to 7 days after surgery.

DACRYOCYSTORHINOSTOMY

Mark R. Levine, MD, FACS and Yoon-Duck Kim, MD

Dacryocystorhinostomy (DCR) is a drainage procedure that bypasses the site of obstruction in the nasolacrimal duct system. This procedure is performed in adults or children who have chronic epiphora or dacryocystitis secondary to partial or complete nasolacrimal duct obstruction or failed previous probings and silicone intubations.

A DCR should not be performed on a patient with acute dacryocystitis, which should be treated first with local and systemic antibiotics and warm compresses. An incision and drainage of the lacrimal sac may be necessary to resolve the acute process. A reassessment of the patient's symptoms and clinical findings based on lacrimal diagnostic tests will point to the site of obstruction and technical variations in the standard DCR. These tests include a Schirmer test with anesthesia, a dye disappearance test, and irrigation and probing of the upper and lower lacrimal system. Before surgery, it is mandatory to rule out nasal pathologic conditions such as a deviated septum, polyps, or tumor that could compromise the end result.

Preoperative Management

Step 1

To avoid bleeding, the patient is advised not to take anticoagulants such as aspirin, Plavix, or Coumadin or anti-inflammatory drugs for 10 days to 2 weeks.

Step 2

Hypertension should be well controlled in hypertensive patients.

Step 3

A determination of partial thromboplastin time should be ordered in patients suspected of having any bleeding problems.

Step 4

Patients with discharge from the sac are advised to massage the sac and use topical antibiotics for several days before surgery.

Anesthesia and Skin Marking

General anesthesia or attended local anesthesia may be used. We prefer attended local anesthesia because it has the advantage of excellent hemostasis and patients are not sick afterward. The middle meatal area in front of the middle turbinate adjacent to the lacrimal fossa is packed with cotton soaked in 4% cocaine or xylocaine 4% and 0.25% phenylephrine hydrochloride (Neo-Synephrine). The bayonet forceps should be directed to the medial canthus to place the pack properly. Placement of the packing in the posterior nasal cavity has no effect.

Methylene blue dye is used to mark the proposed surgical site. A line is drawn 10 to 12 mm medial from the medial canthal angle, beginning at the level of the medial canthal tendon (MCT), extending downward and laterally in a straight line into the nasal jugal fold for a distance of 15 mm (Figure 7-1). It is important to confine the incision to the thicker nasal skin and not to curve the incision to involve the thinner eyelid skin because postoperative contracture will result in a bowstring scar. An alternative surgical site is a blepharoplasty-type incision parallel to the lid and canaliculus extending into the medial canthal area. Lidocaine 1% with 1:100,000 dilution of epinephrine, 0.75% bupivacaine (Marcaine), is injected in the operative site below the MCT along the lacrimal crest and in the region of the infratrochlear nerve above the MCT. An additional injection is given above the MCT along the medial orbital wall to approximately 13- to 15-mm deep. This anesthetizes the anterior ethmoidal nerve, which gives sensation to the nasal

Levine MR.
Manual of Oculoplastic Surgery, Fourth Edition (pp 47-54).
© 2010 SLACK Incorporated

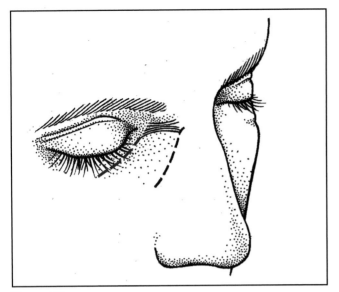

Figure 7-1.

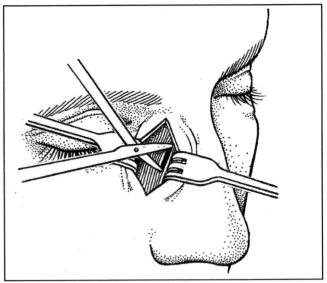

Figure 7-2.

mucosa. A temporarily dilated pupil or medial rectus muscle paralysis is not unusual.

After these injections, the eyes and face are prepared and draped. The nose and face are left open so there is access to the nose for nasal inspection or to retrieve the silicone stent during surgery. Loupes and fiberoptic headlights are essential.

Surgical Procedure

SKIN INCISION

Step 1

Diluted methylene blue is injected into the punctum and canaliculus. This stains the inside of the lacrimal sac blue for identification purposes.

Step 2

A skin incision over the preplaced mark is made with a #15 Bard-Parker blade. The incision is carried to the subcutaneous fascia.

Step 3

With the skin edges tented up by forceps, the remaining strands of superficial fascia are cut with Stevens scissors.

Step 4

Curved Stevens scissors penetrate the orbicularis muscle fibers just nasal to the anterior lacrimal crest, and the blades are spread vertically over the crest (Figure 7-2). Blunt dissection of the muscle fibers with a scissors rather than incising them with a scalpel minimizes bleeding and severing of the angular vein. When the angular vessels are identified, they are retracted away with a rake retractor.

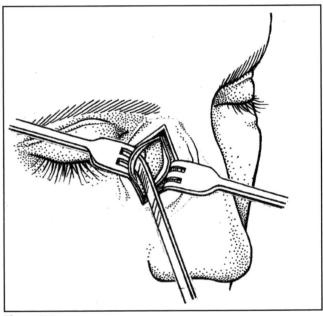

Figure 7-3.

Step 5

If the angular vessels are severed, significant hemorrhage may occur. This is best managed by ligating or cauterizing each end of the cut vessel.

PERIOSTEUM

Step 6

With a lacrimal retractor in place, an incision is made with a #15 Bard-Parker blade through the periosteum 3 to 4 mm anterior to the anterior lacrimal crest from the MCT to the inferior orbital rim (Figure 7-3). The entire anterior arm of the MCT and periosteum is reflected with a Freer periosteal elevator, past the anterior lacrimal crest into the lacrimal sac fossa, elevating the sac and periosteum

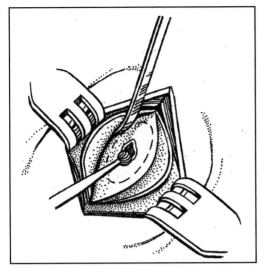

Figure 7-4.

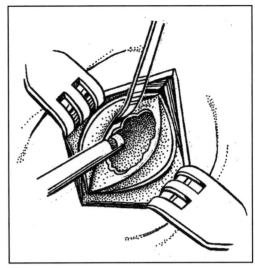

Figure 7-5.

from the fossa. It is important to reflect as much of the MCT as possible to expose the maximum vertical lacrimal sac dimensions. There is no fear of telecanthus because the posterior attachments and frontal attachments of the MCT are not disturbed. The periosteum anterior to its line of incision is also elevated a few millimeters so that it will not be excised during bone removal.

OSTEOTOMY

Step 7

Bone removal should include the anterior lacrimal crest down to the nasolacrimal duct and the bone medial to the sac and just superior to it. Care must be taken not to reach the cribriform plate. Bone removal can be accomplished with a Hall dental drill (Figure 7-4) with an assortment of dental burrs. The area of bone removal will vary according to the patient's anatomy. The osteotomy opening is approximately 15 mm x 15 mm, with the boundaries extending anteriorly to approximately 5 mm anterior to the anterior lacrimal crest, posteriorly to the posterior lacrimal crest, superiorly under the reflected portion of the MCT, and inferiorly to the inferior orbital rim.

Step 8

The tip of the dental burr is placed against the anterior lacrimal crest below the MCT, and the bone is circumferentially burred away toward the nasal mucosa with large circular movements so that the operator does not work into a small hole. The high-speed burr requires constant irrigation with saline to reduce heating. With the lacrimal sac retracted laterally with a Freer elevator, the operator should burr toward the posterior lacrimal crest. Once nasal mucosa is visible, drilling should stop to avoid tearing the mucosa, which will be used as a flap and can bleed. A Freer elevator is then used to separate nasal mucosa from the bony opening. A small Kerrison bone punch is used to remove addi-

tional bone (Figure 7-5), enlarging the osteotomy to the desired dimensions.

Step 9

An alternate, easier way to initiate a bony opening is to take a Freer elevator or curved mosquito forceps and push through the lacrimal bone, which is often rarified to nasal mucosa. This is posterior to the anterior lacrimal crest of the maxilla, which is solid and impenetrable by this means. The Kerrison punch is then used as described. This procedure, our preferred way, is simple and time- and cost-effective.

Step 10

If mucosal bleeding is encountered, 1% lidocaine with epinephrine (1:100,000) is injected into the mucosa to provide hemostasis. In addition, thrombin with absorbable gelatin sponge (Gelfoam) is placed against the mucosal surface for hemostasis. The last piece of bone to be removed is the medial wall of the bony nasolacrimal canal. Removal of the osseous ridge exposes the nasal cavity with the membranous nasolacrimal duct and the lacrimal sac, which is important for the ultimate success of the procedure. It is extremely important in Jones tube placement, so the Jones tube can be positioned anterior-inferior.

INCISION INTO THE SAC

Step 11

After the bony opening is completed, a 0 Bowman probe is inserted through the superior punctum into the sac so that the tip tents the medial wall of the lacrimal sac. A #11 Bard-Parker blade is then used to cut over the probe the entire length of the sac, going under and slightly above the anatomic position of the MCT.

The tip of the probe should come through, and methylene blue should be visible, staining the sac mucosa. This ensures a full-thickness cut

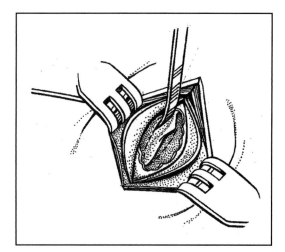

Figure 7-6.

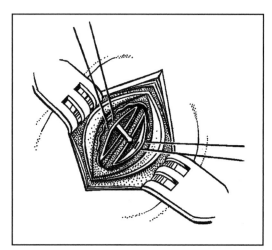

Figure 7-7.

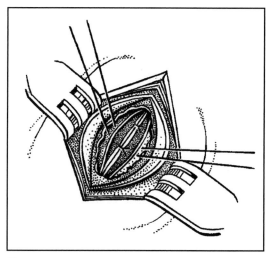

Figure 7-8.

through the periosteal and mucosal layers of the medial wall of the lacrimal sac (Figure 7-6). The incision is placed on the anterior side to leave the posterior flap slightly larger. The blade of a Westcott scissors is inserted through the lacrimal sac opening, and the incision is enlarged in a superior and inferior direction from the top of the fundus of the sac to the nasolacrimal duct. The inside of the sac should be examined for dacryoliths or tumors. A #0 Bowman probe is inserted through the canaliculus and common canaliculus or internal punctum (Figure 7-7). If there is a membrane or stricture of the common canaliculus, a common canaliculostomy is done by tenting the common canaliculus with a probe and cutting the tissue over the probe. Silicone tubes must be inserted to prevent strictures or complete closure. There should be a 4- to 5-mm margin from the common canaliculus to a bony margin to ensure success.

INCISION OF THE MUCOSA

Step 12

The nasal mucosa is then incised with a #11 Bard-Parker blade the length of the osteotomy. The incision is made along a line directly opposite the lacrimal sac incision. Westcott scissors can extend the mucosal incision superiorly and inferiorly to make anterior and posterior flaps with similar dimensions to those of the lacrimal sac flaps. The preplaced nasal packing can be seen through the mucosal incision, verifying the proper position of the incision. The nasal packing is then removed from the nostril with a bayonet forceps. Sometimes, the middle turbinate blocks or is close to the osteotomy opening. The postoperative edema after the cocaine and 0.25% phenylephrine hydrochloride wear off may result in blockage of the osteotomy opening. If this is the case, an anterior middle turbinectomy is accomplished by crushing the anterior turbinate with a hemostat for hemostatic control, then excising it with pituitary forceps or a Kerrison punch.

ANASTOMOSIS OF THE POSTERIOR FLAPS

Step 13

The posterior flaps of the sac and nasal mucosa are closed with 6-0 polyglactin (Vicryl) sutures if possible. Extreme care should be taken to avoid tearing the flaps (Figure 7-8).

PLACEMENT OF THE SILICONE STENT

Step 14

One end of the Crawford probe is inserted in the upper canaliculus through the newly created ostium and into the middle meatus. The tip of the

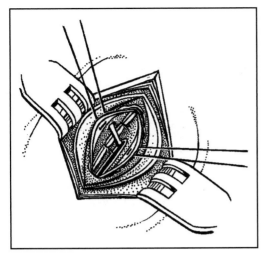

Figure 7-9.

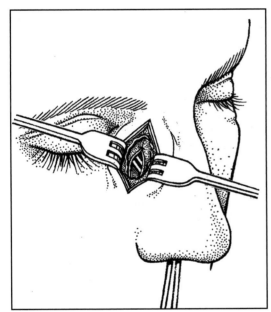

Figure 7-10.

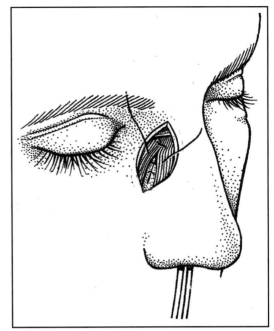

Figure 7-11.

ANASTOMOSIS OF THE ANTERIOR FLAPS

Step 15

After the silicone stents are placed, the anterior lacrimal sac flaps are sutured to the anterior nasal mucosa flap with a 5-0 Vicryl mattress suture (Figure 7-10). The flaps should be taut enough not to collapse and block the common canaliculus or adhere to the posterior flap anastomosis. In reality, anterior and posterior flaps are not necessary for success. We prefer a simple anterior flap anastomosis.

SKIN CLOSURE

Step 16

The lacrimal retractor is removed, and a few 6-0 catgut sutures are used to reapproximate the orbicularis muscle (Figure 7-11). The skin incision is closed with 6-0 plain catgut suture in an interrupted or a continuous fashion.

Postoperative Management

Antibiotic steroid ophthalmic ointment is placed on the incision site once a day until the sutures are removed in 5 to 7 days. Antibiotic steroid solution is placed in the eye 4 times a day for 2 weeks and then is tapered off over the following 2 weeks. A 1-week course of systemic antibiotics is given in cases with mucopurulent discharge. The patient is discharged the day of surgery and told to use ice-cold compresses for the first 8 to 10 hours. Any nasal packing, other than thrombin and Gelfoam, placed at the time of surgery for hemostasis is removed over the next 2 to 3 days. The bacitracin impregnated in the gauze helps prevent it from adhering to the mucosal surfaces, thereby minimizing bleeding. A nasal decongestant is used twice

probe is extracted with a Crawford hook (Figure 7-9) and withdrawn from the external nose with the silicone tubing trailing. The procedure is repeated through the lower canaliculus so that both ends of the tubing are delivered out the nose. The tubing is tied tightly with 4 to 5 knots in the external naris and reinforced with a 6-0 silk suture. The tube is cut close to the knots and placed in the middle meatus area. A 6-0 silk suture is also used to tie together both Crawford tubes as they enter the osteotomy away from the common canaliculi to avoid loop displacement into the lacrimal lake. If there is significant mucosal ooze of blood that does not respond to cautery, a bacitracin-impregnated gauze (0.25 to 0.50 in) is placed in the lacrimal sac area, osteotomy site, and middle meatus to minimize the oozing. Lesser amounts of mucosal oozing can be controlled with thrombin and Gelfoam.

a day for 1 week if needed, and the patient is told not to blow the nose for 4 weeks, except very gently if needed, to avoid subcutaneous emphysema in the medial orbit. The silicone stent is removed in 2 to 6 months, depending on the degree of surgical difficulty, especially when associated with stenosis of the common caniculus. Postoperative bleeding is uncommon, but if it occurs, the wound may require repacking with bacitracin gauze or surgery. Postoperative infection is also uncommon. This may require warm compresses and systemic antibiotics.

Complications

The most common complication is a failure to drain. This may be caused by stenosis of the common canaliculus secondary to injudicious probing. If this occurs, placement of Crawford tubes, if not previously used, will re-establish drainage. In addition, closure of the rhinostomy site during the cicatricial phase of wound healing (6 to 8 weeks) necessitates placement of Crawford tubes, if they were not used during the operative procedure. Poor drainage with Crawford tubes in place may occur because of excess scar tissue and may necessitate endoscopic removal of intranasal scar tissue. Poor drainage with Crawford tubes in place may also be a result of the hydrophobic nature of the tubes or an inflammatory reaction to the silicone tubes. Removing the Crawford tubes and placing the patient on antibiotic steroid drops should correct this condition.

Other, less common causes of drainage problems are anterior displacement of the ethmoids with secondary ethmoiditis and secondary inflammation of the lacrimal sac and common canaliculitis. Computed tomographic scans of the sinus can be used to diagnose the problem, and decongestants and systemic antibiotics can alleviate it.

It is always helpful to send a specimen of the lacrimal sac for pathologic examination to rule out conditions such as sarcoidosis, lymphoma, leukemia, and intrinsic lacrimal sac neoplasms.

Dacryocystorhinostomy With Jones Pyrex Tubes

GOALS AND PRINCIPLES

DCR with Jones tubes is performed after a failed DCR and subsequent revision, severe stenosis of the common canaliculus, and canalicular obstruction. The aim of the procedure is to directly bypass the canaliculus and lacrimal system. The Jones tube sits at the site of the excised caruncle and is situated in the middle meatus anterior to the middle turbinate, not hitting the nasal septum. Before surgery, it is mandatory to rule out a deviated septum, which would compromise fit and function. The procedure is as described previously up through the incision of the mucosa (see Step 12).

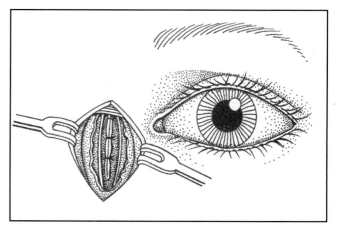

Figure 7-12.

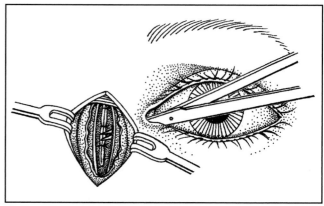

Figure 7-13.

ANASTOMOSIS OF POSTERIOR FLAPS

Step 1

The posterior flaps of the sac and nasal mucosa are closed with 6-0 Vicryl sutures if possible (Figure 7-12).

Extreme care should be taken to avoid tearing the flaps. After anastomosis of the posterior flap, the caruncle is injected with 1% lidocaine with a 1:100,000 dilution of epinephrine, and the caruncle is excised. A Stevens scissors is used to penetrate the site of the excised caruncle beneath the orbicularis muscle anterior to the posterior flap anastomosis, into the osteotomy site (Figure 7-13). A straight Kirschner (K)-wire is inserted beneath the scissors in the exact tract, and a 15- to 19-mm Jones Pyrex tube is placed onto the K-wire and placed in an anteroinferior dependent drainage position (Figure 7-14). The length of the Pyrex tube is adjusted by nasal inspection such that the tube does not butt against the nasal septum or the middle turbinate. A partial turbinectomy may be required if anteriorly situated. The K-wire is then removed (Figure 7-15).

Step 2

The anterior flaps are anastomosed, and the orbicularis muscle and skin are closed as described.

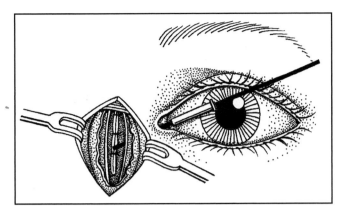

Figure 7-14.

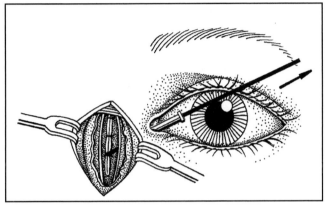

Figure 7-15.

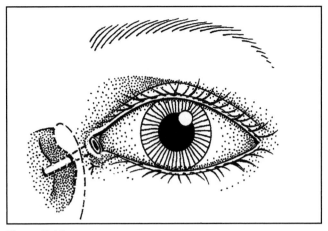

Figure 7-16.

Postoperative Management

In addition to the routine postoperative care, the tube may necessitate change if it is too long or too short. This is best accomplished in an office setting 6 to 8 weeks after the surgery by giving a medial canthal injection of 1% lidocaine with a 1:100,000 dilution of epinephrine. Cetacaine nasal spray is used in the nose for anesthesia.

A K-wire is placed down the Pyrex tube, and the Pyrex tube is removed and exchanged for the appropriate length. The Pyrex tube is kept clean and patent by having the patient use artificial tears twice a day, holding the nose and gently inhaling, which clears the tube.

Step 3

A 6-0 Vicryl suture is tied around the collar of the Pyrex tube with both arms going beneath the orbicularis and exiting the skin in the area of the medial canthus. This ensures tube position and prevents accidental displacement (Figure 7-16).

ENDOSCOPIC LACRIMAL SURGERY

Geoffrey J. Gladstone, MD, FAACS

Endoscopic Dacryocystorhinostomy

Endoscopic dacryocystorhinostomy (EDCR) is a surgical procedure that bypasses an obstruction of the nasolacrimal duct. It is usually performed to alleviate excessive tearing or discharge secondary to this partial or complete obstruction. It can be performed after a failed previous DCR or in a patient without previous surgery.

An EDCR can be performed in a patient with an acute dacryocystitis because a skin incision is not necessary. However, an attempt to resolve the acute dacryocystitis with oral antibiotics is typically made prior to surgical intervention. An endonasal examination using an endoscope is performed prior to surgery to look for septal deviation and intranasal tumors. A significantly deviated nasal septum may require a septoplasty prior to the EDCR. Insufficient intranasal room makes the EDCR procedure difficult. Prior to surgery, various tests are performed to evaluate the lacrimal system. These include lacrimal irrigation and probing of the canaliculi, basic secretor testing, and palpation of the lacrimal sac looking for discharge.

PREOPERATIVE MANAGEMENT

Step 1

To minimize bleeding during surgery, it is ideal to stop a variety of medications prior to surgery. These include aspirin, cox-1 nonsteroidals, Coumadin, Plavix, and any other medications that inhibit hemostasis.

Step 2

When prescribed by another physician, these medications should not be stopped without his or her consent. It is important to ascertain how long the patient may be off these medications and how soon after surgery it is necessary to re-start them.

ANESTHESIA

The patient is asked to clear his or her nasal passage approximately 30 minutes prior to surgery. Two sprays of a nasal decongestant, 0.05% oxymetazoline, are administered to the nasal cavity on the surgical side. After 5 minutes, administration of the nasal decongestant is repeated. The patient is then brought into the operating room and sedated. While most patients tolerate the procedure under monitored intravenous sedation, some patients require general anesthesia. Under sedation, 18 inches of 0.5-inch gauze soaked in 4% cocaine solution is packed in the area of the middle turbinate for 5 minutes. After removal of gauze, local anesthesia using a 50:50 mixture of 2% lidocaine with 1:100,000 epinephrine with 0.75% bupivacaine with 1:200,000 epinephrine is injected into the submucosa of the anterior middle turbinate, uncinate process, and lateral nasal wall. The injection is given under direct visualization with the endoscope, and blanching of the mucosa is noted. With the endoscope, another strip of cocaine-soaked gauze is placed between the lateral nasal wall and the middle turbinate for at least 5 more minutes. This will further shrink the mucosa and provide more working area during surgery. Hemostasis is the most important factor in maintaining an excellent view during endoscopic lacrimal surgery.

MUCOSA REMOVAL

Step 1

The nasal packing is removed, and the endoscope is placed within the nose. Occasionally, the middle turbinate is infractured with the blunt end of a periosteal elevator to enable an unobstructed view of the uncinate process and avoid blocking of the ostium. This maneuver is performed gently to avoid potential cerebrospinal fluid (CSF) leaks, as the

Levine MR.
Manual of Oculoplastic Surgery, Fourth Edition (pp 55-58).
© 2010 SLACK Incorporated

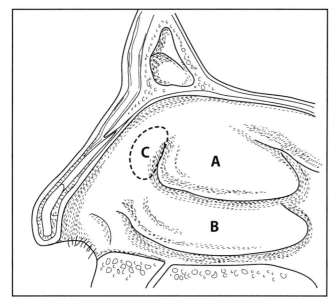

Figure 8-1. Intranasal anatomy showing (A) middle turbinate, (B) inferior turbinate, and (C) area of bone and nasal mucosa that will be removed.

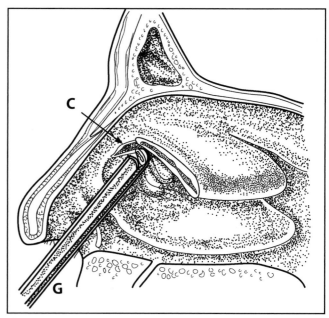

Figure 8-2. Kerrison rongeurs (G) removing bone (C).

middle turbinate attaches directly to the cribriform plate superiorly (Figure 8-1).

Step 2

The sharp end of the periosteal elevator is used to incise the mucosa at the anterior border of the uncinate process. This demarcates the posterior border of the osteotomy.

Step 3

In preparation for the osteotomy, the mucosa overlying the lacrimal fossa is cauterized with a guarded monopolar cautery. The boundaries for cautery extend 10 mm anterior to the uncinate process and 10 mm inferior to the root of the middle turbinate. Care is taken to avoid cautery of the middle turbinate.

Step 4

Once cauterized, the mucosa is removed with the sharp edge of a periosteal elevator in a downward motion, exposing the underlying bone. A Blakesley forceps is used to clear any mucosal fragment still in the way. Clearing the mucosa reduces bleeding during bone removal.

OSTEOTOMY

Step 5

Bone removal begins at the posterior edge of the exposed bone using a medium-sized 90° Kerrison rongeur. This site corresponds to the site of the previous incision over the uncinate process. Several bites with the rongeur anteriorly and superiorly expose the underlying lacrimal sac (Figure 8-2).

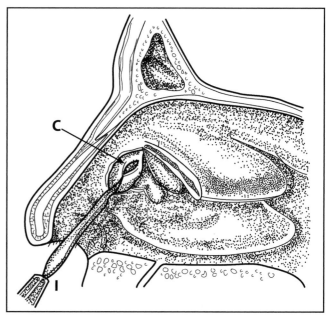

Figure 8-3. Sickle blade (I) incising the lacrimal sac (C).

LACRIMAL SAC INCISION

Step 6

After punctal dilation, a 1-Bowman probe passes through the upper canalicular system and tents the posterior wall of the lacrimal sac. The tented sac is then incised vertically with a sickle blade (Figure 8-3).

Step 7

Enlargement of the sac opening is performed with the same blade or by gently tearing the mucosa with Blakesley forceps.

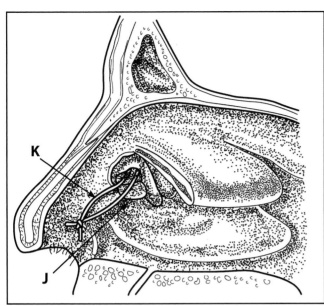

Figure 8-4. Silastic tubing (K) protruding through bony ostium and overlying a flap of nasal mucosa (J).

PLACEMENT OF THE SILICONE STENT

Step 8

Silastic tubing is passed through both canaliculi, the ostium, and the nose. Under mild tension, tubes are tied in a square knot. A 3-mm section of a Robinson catheter may be tied over this knot to facilitate repositioning in the event of tube prolapse. No dressing or medication is required postoperatively (Figure 8-4).

POSTOPERATIVE MANAGEMENT

Postoperative care for EDCR is rather simple. The main precaution is to avoid eye rubbing, which can displace the tube. The patient is asked to not blow his or her nose for the first week because this can cause bleeding. After the first week, he or she is asked to use saline nasal spray multiple times per day on the operative side and to then blow his or her nose. This helps remove intranasal debris and makes the nose feel less congested. This can be stopped after 1 or 2 weeks. Ideally, the tube should be left in place for at least 3 months. At this time, the tube is cut at the canthus, and the patient forcefully expels the tubing by blowing his or her nose. Occasionally, the tube will need to be manually retrieved. Retesting of the lacrimal system is now performed with irrigation.

COMPLICATIONS

If the silastic tubing prolapses, the patient can try to blow the nose forcefully while occluding the opposite nostril. After a few unsuccessful attempts, the tubing can be temporarily taped to the nose or cheek to avoid ocular irritation. In a cooperative patient, the tube can be repositioned easily. Minor prolapse is sometimes amenable to external feeding of the tube back into the nose. When this is attempted with more significant prolapse, the tub-

ing will often curl into the lacrimal sac and later recoil. In this instance, the tube should be pulled back into the nasal cavity using bayonet forceps. An endoscope aids in tube localization, but, often, the Robinson catheter is visible with only a speculum. Prior to entering the nose, a nasal decongestant can be used to shrink the mucosa and help with minor bleeding. In addition, an inhaled mucosal anesthetic can be used for comfort. Ideally, the tube should be left in place for at least 3 months.

Endoscopic Conjunctivodacryocystorhinostomy With Modified Jones Tube

GOALS AND PRINCIPLES

A complete bypass of the lacrimal system may be indicated in several instances. These include failed dacryocystorhinostomy, canalicular blockage, and lacrimal pump failure secondary to facial nerve paralysis. This procedure bypasses the entire lacrimal system, taking the tears from the caruncular area directly to the nose.

SURGICAL PROCEDURE

The surgical procedure for endoscopic conjunctivodacryocystorhinostomy entails the steps of endoscopic DCR, starting with patient preparation to removal of bone overlying the lacrimal sac (see Step 5). Opening of the posterior sac wall is not necessary.

Step 1

Once the osteotomy is created, a tract for the Jones tube is formed with a 12-gauge angiocath. A bend is placed in the angiocath prior to placement to assist anterior placement of the tube. In a 45-degree inferomedial direction, the angiocath is advanced through the middle of the caruncle. Excision of the caruncle is not recommended, as this promotes internal migration of the Jones tube. Endoscopic visualization is used as the needle passes through the lacrimal fossa and into the nasal cavity. Adjustments in position are made at this time. The needle is retracted, leaving the plastic catheter in place.

Step 2

A 9-inch 20-gauge guide wire is passed through the catheter and held securely, and the plastic catheter is then removed.

Step 3

A 4-mm x 19-mm Gladstone-Putterman modified Jones tube is then passed over the wire. This tube was designed with an internal flange 4 mm distal to the external flange. The added flange functions like an arrowhead to secure the tube against internal and external migration or ejection with forceful nose blowing, sneezing, or coughing. The modified tube inserts in a similar fashion as the original design, except that a palpable click is felt when the internal flange traverses the medial canthal tissues.

Both thumbnails are used on the external flange to effectively lock the tube into position. Ideally, the distal end of the tube is situated midway between the lateral wall and septum. In the event tube length is not appropriate, a longer or shorter tube may be inserted with the guide wire in place. Tube exchange is done carefully to avoid shattering the glass tube. If forceps do not deliver the tube easily, a 2-0 silk suture may be wrapped around the proximal end to aid in gentle extraction. Once the proper tube is inserted, the guide wire is removed.

Step 4

To encourage the tube to heal without internal migration, a 6-0 double-armed silk suture is double-wrapped around the external flange. Both needles are passed through the medial canthus and tied over skin with a sterile rubber band bolster. The bolster and suture are removed 1 week postoperatively. No dressing or medications are needed postoperatively.

SPECIAL SURGICAL CONSIDERATIONS

Occasionally, the distal end of the Jones tube may be too close to the middle turbinate. This situation risks tube occlusion and external migration. Intraoperative partial middle turbinectomy avoids these complications. Local anesthetic is injected into the substance of the turbinate. The posterior extent of the turbinate to be removed is crushed with a small curved hemostat. Bounding the offending portion of the turbinate, the hemostat is applied to the superior border, attempting to join the compressed areas. Following the crushed lines, curved endoscopic turbinate scissors incise the portion of turbinate. Persistent connections often require gentle twisting with a Blakesley forceps for amputation of the piece.

POSTOPERATIVE MANAGEMENT

The patient is asked to not blow his or her nose for the first week because this can cause bleeding. After this time, he or she is asked to place a finger over the proximal end of the modified Jones tube whenever he or she blows the nose, sneezes, or coughs. This avoids externally displacing the tube. The rubber band bolster is removed 1 week after surgery.

COMPLICATIONS

Poor postoperative drainage results from misplacement or displacement of the tube. Tears cannot enter a tube that is displaced anteriorly. The course of action is to reposition the Jones tube more posteriorly. The tube must be removed, usually by wrapping a 2-0 silk suture around the external flange to minimize tube breakage. Contraction of medial canthal tissues around the tube can necessitate the use of Westcott scissors to release the tube. The 12-gauge angiocatheter re-enters the caruncular tissues posteriorly in relation to previous placement. Jones tube insertion follows as previously described.

Similarly, posterior placement of a tube is repositioned more anteriorly. Exaggerated posterior position of the Jones tube causes ocular irritation and risks conjunctival blockage of the proximal tube opening.

Internal migration of the tube also causes obstruction of the proximal end, and possibly the distal end, of the Jones tube. When caruncular tissues are needlessly excised, inward displacement is more likely. Removing these tubes can be challenging. Sometimes, a soft instrument is used intranasally to coax the tube outward. Westcott scissors are used to release contracted medial canthal tissues overlying the external flange. Once the tube is exposed, 2-0 silk suture can aid in extraction. Dissection should be purposeful to cause minimal disruption of the medial canthal tissues. In the event of extensive tissue manipulation, subsequent replacement of the tube should await adequate healing. This will reduce the probability of repeated internal migration.

External displacement of the tube precludes tear entry and may cause eyelid or ocular irritation. Occasionally, manual pressure can re-lock the Jones tube in position. Intranasal examination may reveal a treatable cause of this migration. Possibilities include contact with the nasal septum, which requires placement of a shorter tube. As mentioned previously, partial turbinectomy is necessary if the middle turbinate pushes on the distal end of the tube.

Sometimes, even a perfectly placed Jones tube can be blocked by redundant conjunctiva. Simple chemosis may resolve with a depot steroid injection, but resection of excessive tissue can also be curative. Topical or depot steroid may be used to quiet irritation of the medial canthal tissues.

SECTION III

COSMETIC

BROW LIFT

Norman Shorr, MD; Catherine Hwang, MD; and Jonathan Hoenig, MD

Eyebrow ptosis occurs in older people as a result of a syndrome produced by the effects of gravity. Tissues of the forehead, eyelids, and upper face develop laxity with time, permitting the eyebrow to move inferiorly. As a person ages, the normal, delicate attachments of the eyebrow to the periosteum become attenuated. As the eyebrow moves inferiorly, the frontalis muscle is recruited to elevate the eyebrow, which may result in deep horizontal forehead furrows. The lateral eyebrow lacks deep structural attachments to the periosteum and is especially susceptible to laxity. Furthermore, the frontalis muscle fibers do not extend to the lateral brow, and, thus, despite maximum frontalis contraction, lateral eyebrow ptosis often persists. In severe cases, the lateral eyebrow may actually encroach on the eyelid space.

Patients with eyebrow ptosis may complain of dermatochalasis. However, when the eyebrows are raised to their normal position, there is often much less redundant upper eyelid skin than anticipated. Thus, the eyebrow position must be evaluated before an upper blepharoplasty is performed. Patients with eyebrow ptosis also show horizontal and vertical redundancy in the multicontoured areas of the medial and lateral canthi. These redundancies are a challenge for the aesthetic surgeon and are poorly rectified by an upper blepharoplasty alone.

It is imperative that the surgeon and patient understand that excision of tissue above the eyebrow raises the brow. Excision of tissue beneath the brow (ie, the eyelid) lowers the eyebrow. Thus, if a patient with eyebrow ptosis has an upper blepharoplasty, the eyebrow position will be further lowered.

The normal position of the medial eyebrow is approximately 1 cm above the medial aspect of the superior orbital rim. In women, a high eyebrow arch is present, with the apex of the arch located over the lateral limbus. In men, the eyebrow takes a gentler curve and is straighter, more diffuse, and located more inferiorly. By manually raising the medial and lateral aspect of the eyebrow during an examination, the normal anatomy as well as improvement of the tissue redundancies of the medial and lateral canthi can be demonstrated to the patient. The surgeon must be careful to preserve the structural integrity of the eyebrows and the eyelids. After eyebrow and upper eyelid surgery, the patient should be able to simultaneously raise the eyebrows and close the eyelids. For this reason, eyebrow elevation should be performed before upper blepharoplasty.

There are 9 general types of eyebrow elevation procedures: (1) standard direct eyebrow elevation, (2) paralytic eyebrow lift (variation of direct eyebrow lift), (3) gull-wing direct eyebrow lift, (4) orbicularis plication, (5) mid-forehead eyebrow lift, (6) temporal eyebrow lift, (7) coronal forehead and eyebrow lift, (8) internal eyebrowpexy and trans-eyelid eyebrow lift, and (9) endoscopic eyebrow lift.

Direct Eyebrow Lift

The direct eyebrow lift affords the greatest elevation per millimeter of tissue excised. This approach is useful in those men in whom coronal or temporal lifts are not advised because of the tendency toward, and progression of, male pattern baldness or in patients who do not want to undergo endoscopic surgery. The standard direct brow lift is excellent for lateral segmental brow lift in men and women. It does not address medial brow ptosis, nor does it reduce horizontal or vertical glabellar folds.

Paralytic Eyebrow Lift (Variation of Direct Eyebrow Lift)

Eyebrow ptosis may also be seen in patients with seventh nerve palsies. Surgical intervention is indicated

Levine MR.
Manual of Oculoplastic Surgery, Fourth Edition (pp 61-74).
© 2010 SLACK Incorporated

when the brow ptosis is long standing and reinnervation of the nerve has not occurred. Because lagophthalmos is often present with many seventh nerve palsies, it is imperative that the brow not be overelevated. This would worsen the lagophthalmos. The essential part of paralytic eyebrow surgery is a direct eyebrow lift, with placement of permanent sutures between the eyebrow and the periosteum to overcome the effects of gravity.

Gull-Wing Direct Eyebrow Lift

Modification of the standard direct brow lift by extension of the incision into the glabellar region, in a gull-wing fashion, can also correct medial brow ptosis and the glabellar folds. The incision in the glabellar region is hidden in the horizontal fold created by the action of the procerus muscle. This procedure achieves excellent elevation of the entire brow and glabellar region. However, it is reserved for patients who wear spectacles or who are willing to tolerate a scar in the glabellar region.

Orbicularis Plication

Orbicularis plication is useful in patients who need brow stabilization while undergoing blepharoplasty. A small, horizontal, 1.5-cm incision is made above the lateral two-thirds brow junction in a horizontal fold. The orbital portion of the orbicularis muscle is plicated superiorly to the periosteum. This is an elegant technique that can be used on a patient who does not want to undergo a more involved procedure or who has minimal brow ptosis.

Mid-Forehead Eyebrow Lift

The mid-forehead lift is also effective in correcting eyebrow ptosis and glabellar folds. The incision can be hidden in a prominent forehead furrow. Because the procedure may lower the frontal hairline, it is reserved for men with prominent forehead furrows and a high, sparse frontal hairline. Patients with no forehead furrows may be poor candidates for this procedure because a prominent scar may be seen.

Temporal Eyebrow Lift

The temporal eyebrow lift is especially useful in patients with lateral eyebrow ptosis and lateral canthal ptosis. The incision is hidden within the hairline and is useful in young women where only the temporal eyebrow has become ptotic. There is no elevation of the medial brow, and a slight elevation of the temporal hairline may occur with this procedure.

Coronal Forehead and Eyebrow Lift

The coronal eyebrow and forehead lift is a very effective brow lift. It successfully raises the medial and lateral brow, reduces glabellar folds, and smooths the forehead. The incision is placed entirely within the hair-bearing scalp, camouflaging the scar. The procedure is most appropriately used in women or men older than 55 years of age who have no familial tendency toward male pattern baldness. In men, the coronal incision is modified to a gull-wing configuration (do not confuse this with the gull-wing direct eyebrow lift). The hairline may be slightly elevated by this procedure. In a woman with a low hairline, this often improves the aesthetic appearance of the face. In men or women who are concerned with elevation of the hairline, the anterior portion of the incision may be placed along the hair line, effectively lowering it. This is called the pretrichial coronal eyebrow and forehead lift. Hair loss and persistent numbness posterior to the incision are potential significant limitations of this procedure.

Internal Eyebrowpexy and Transeyelid Eyebrow Lift

Internal browpexy is useful in patients undergoing concurrent blepharoplasty. This procedure plicates the eyebrow at or above the level of the superior orbital rim through an upper blepharoplasty incision. Internal browpexy is often combined with blepharoplasty and debulking of the sub-brow fat pads. The main advantage of the browpexy is that it limits postblepharoplasty eyebrow descent. The main disadvantage is that tenderness and dimpling of the brow can occur in the region of the plication. The internal browpexy is usually used as a stabilizing suture (ie, "brassiere" suture), and actual brow lifting is difficult to produce without pleating. A modification involves suturing the superior cut edge of the orbicularis muscle to the superior, lateral arcus marginalis. Usually 2 to 3 absorbable sutures are placed, which achieves fullness to the lateral brow and prevents descent of the roof fat pad.

Endoscopic Eyebrow Lift

Endoscopic eyebrow and forehead lifting has become one of the primary means of raising the eyebrows and forehead. This method is accomplished through easily hidden incisions in the hair-bearing scalp. Endoscopic forehead lift can achieve many goals, including elevation of the eyebrows and glabella, smoothing forehead furrows, and decreasing glabellar folds. Like the coronal lift, this technique is most appropriate in women and men who do not have a predilection for male pattern baldness. The advantages of the endoscopic forehead lift over the coronal methods include smaller incisions, decreased risk of alopecia, and decreased postoperative recovery time and discomfort. Various incision patterns may be used, with the most traditional being 5 incisions within the hair-bearing scalp. Titrated dissection in the glabella and lateral brow, including differential release of the periosteum and arcus marginalis, combined with strategic fixation of the degloved scalp to the underlying frontal bone provide effective means of restoring brow symmetry. Myriad fixation techniques are used, including the use of titanium or resorbable screws, fibrin glue, and suture with or without bone tunnels. Surgeons are encouraged to try various techniques and find the ones that give the best result in their hands. The authors have used all of the

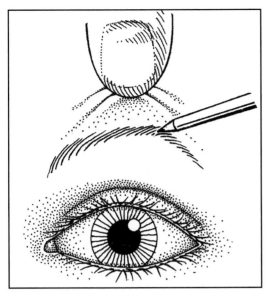

Figure 9-1.

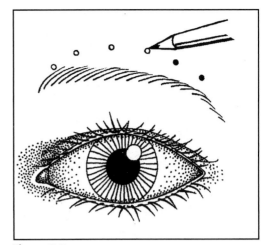

Figure 9-2.

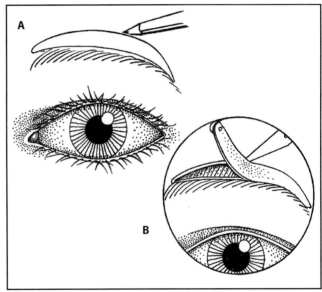

Figure 9-3.

above techniques and have found that the best long-term result with little morbidity, such as alopecia, is suture fixation through a bone tunnel.

Familiarity with the endoscopic view of the forehead and eyebrow anatomy, including key landmarks like the conjoint tendon, deep temporalis fascia, Yassergil's fat pad, lateral canthal tendon, supraorbital neurovascular complex, supratrochlear neurovascular complex, and eyebrow depressor muscles, requires experience. Most complications with this procedure are related to incorrect identification of anatomic structures and planes.

Surgical Procedures

DIRECT EYEBROW LIFT

Step 1

With the patient in the sitting position, the proposed incision site is marked just above the most superior eyebrow hairs. The eyebrow is digitally elevated to the desired level, and the marking pen is placed near, but not touching, the superior brow border (Figure 9-1). When the brow is released, the point beneath the pen tip represents a point on the superior incision line (Figure 9-2). This marking technique is repeated along the entire incision line above the brow (Figure 9-3A).

Step 2

The brow region is infiltrated with 2% lidocaine with 1:100,000 epinephrine and hyaluronidase (Wydase). Fifteen minutes are allowed to pass for adequate vasoconstriction to develop. The incision is carried out using a #15 Bard-Parker blade along the previously demarcated lines. The blade should be held perpendicular to the skin surface (Figure 9-3B). It is not necessary to bevel the incision, as some have suggested in the past. The depth of the incision is carried to a plane just superficial to the frontalis muscle in the region of the supraorbital nerve to avoid forehead anesthesia. In patients with extreme lateral brow ptosis, the excised ellipse of tissue can extend more laterally than the lateral brow. However, the depth of the incision in the lateral portion is just through skin to avoid damage to the temporal branch of the seventh nerve. A scissors is used to remove the ellipse of tissue. Hemostasis is achieved with the unipolar cautery.

Step 3

The wound is closed with a deep layer of buried, interrupted 4-0 polyglactin (Vicryl) suture on a P-3 needle (Figure 9-4A).

Step 4

Multiple, interrupted, vertical mattress sutures of 4-0 nylon or polypropylene (Prolene) are then used to approximate the wound edges (Figure 9-4B). Eversion of the wound edge is important to avoid a depressed scar. Finally, a running 6-0 nylon or Prolene suture on a P-1 needle is used to close and

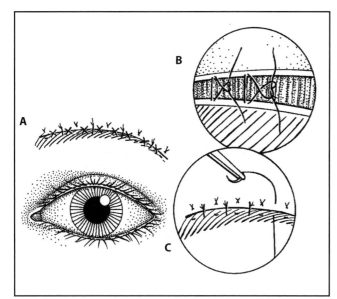

Figure 9-4.

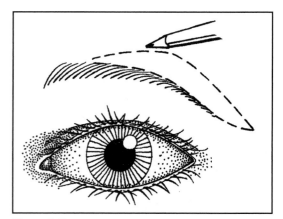

Figure 9-5.

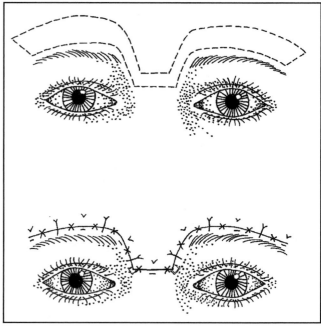

Figure 9-6.

evert the skin edges (Figure 9-4C). The wound is dressed with antibiotic ointment, and ice compresses are applied 4 times a day for 2 to 3 days. The running 6-0 suture is removed in 5 to 7 days, and the vertical mattress sutures are removed in 10 to 14 days. If only lateral brow ptosis is evident, a segmental direct brow lift can be performed (Figure 9-5). The brow elevation is marked, incised, and closed in a similar manner.

PARALYTIC EYEBROW LIFT

Step 1

The patient is examined in the sitting position to determine the preoperative level of the eyebrow. A crescent-shaped area above the brow is demarcated with the marking pen. The paralytic brow should be ovecorrected, for the brow falls with time.

Step 2

After the brow area is infiltrated with 2% lidocaine with 1:100,000 epinephrine and hyaluronidase, the previously demarcated crescent of skin is excised, as described for the direct brow lift (see Figure 9-3).

Step 3

Permanently buried 4-0 Prolene sutures are then placed between the elevated brow tissue and the periosteum of the frontal bone. Then, 5-0 Vicryl sutures are used in a buried subcuticular fashion to approximate the subcutaneous and muscular layers (see Figure 9-4). The skin is closed in the same fashion as described for the direct brow lift.

GULL-WING DIRECT EYEBROW LIFT

Step 1

With the patient in a sitting position, the proposed incision site is marked just above the superior eye-

brow hairs. At the medial aspect of the brow, the marking continues in an almost vertical orientation until the procerus fold is reached. A horizontal mark in the fold is then drawn. A mirror image of the vertical mark is performed on the other side. The superior brow incision line is marked in a manner similar to that for a standard direct eyebrow lift. In the glabellar region, the glabella is digitally elevated, and the marking pen is placed near, but not touching, the previously demarcated procerus fold. When the glabella is released, the point beneath the pen represents a point on the glabellar incision line. This horizontal line should be several millimeters shorter than its inferior counterpart. The superomedial, vertically oriented lines are then drawn. These lines must parallel the inferior lines after the tissues are excised (Figure 9-6).

Step 2

The brow region is infiltrated with 2% lidocaine with 1:100,000 epinephrine and hyaluronidase. Fifteen minutes are allowed to pass for adequate

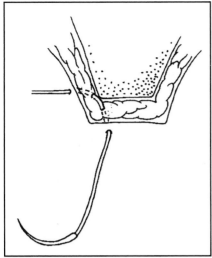

Figure 9-7.

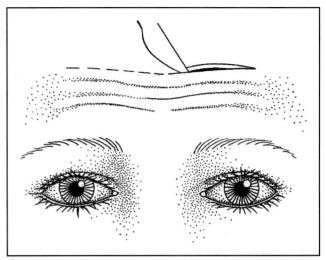

Figure 9-8.

vasoconstriction to occur. The incision is carried out using a #15 Bard-Parker blade along the previously demarcated lines. The blade should be held perpendicular to the skin surface. The depth of the incision is carried to a plane just superficial to the frontalis muscle in the region of the supraorbital nerve to avoid damage to the nerve.

Step 3

The wound is closed with a deep layer of buried, interrupted 4-0 Vicryl sutures on a P-3 needle (see Figure 9-4A). In the glabellar region, the corners are closed with 4-0 Vicryl half-buried horizontal mattress sutures (Figure 9-7).

Step 4

Multiple, interrupted, vertical mattress sutures of 4-0 nylon or Prolene are then used to approximate the wound edges (see Figure 9-4B). Eversion of the wound edge is important to avoid a depressed scar. Finally, a running 6-0 nylon or Prolene suture on a P-l needle is used to close and evert the skin edges (see Figure 9-7). The wound is dressed with antibiotic ointment, and ice compresses are applied 4 times a day for 2 to 3 days. The running 6-0 suture is removed in 5 to 7 days, and the vertical mattress sutures are removed in 10 to 14 days.

ORBICULARIS PLICATION

Step 1

With the patient sitting, the incision site is marked in a rhytid 1- to 1.5-cm above the lateral one half of the brow. Lidocaine 2% with epinephrine 1:100,000 is injected in the region. After 15 minutes to allow for adequate vasoconstriction, the incision is made using a #15 Bard-Parker blade. The depth is just posterior under the subcutaneous fat. Blunt dissection is carried out with tenotomy scissors proceeding inferiorly in the plane just deep to the eyebrow follicles and extending inferiorly in the plane posterior to the orbicularis as far inferior as 5-mm inferior to the inferior-most eyebrow hairs.

The orbicularis muscle becomes evident, and vertical spreading will avoid injury to the muscle and prevent excessive bleeding.

Step 2

The superior-most margin of the orbicularis muscle is grasped and pulled superiorly. Often, the vector of pull is superior and medial, which helps in elevation of the lateral-most aspect of the brow. One or 2 5-0 PDS mattress sutures are placed, attaching the orbicularis to the periosteum.

Step 3

A small amount of skin is removed from the central portion of the wound. The skin is closed in layers with deep buried sutures and a subcuticular suture, making sure not to have tension on the wound edges. Antibiotic ointment is applied 4 times a day for 3 to 5 days. If a nonabsorbable suture is used to close the skin, this can be removed in 5 to 7 days.

MID-FOREHEAD EYEBROW LIFT

Step 1

A prominent brow furrow is selected for the superior incision line and is marked with a surgical marker (Figure 9-8). The incision line can also be broken up by placing the incision in 2 separate brow furrows (Figure 9-9). If a large resection is anticipated in severe brow ptosis, the incision line should be carried across most of the forehead to permit adequate closure. If significant lateral eyebrow ptosis exists, the incision can be carried temporally, following the inferiorly curved eyebrow furrow.

Step 2

It is often difficult to determine preoperatively the amount of tissue to be resected; however, this is often the distance between 2 prominent eyebrow furrows.

Step 3

A bilateral supraorbital nerve block is produced with injection of 2% lidocaine with 1:100,000

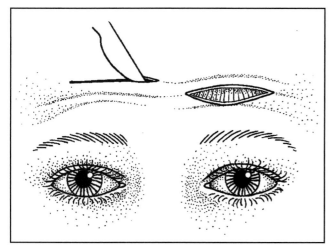

Figure 9-9.

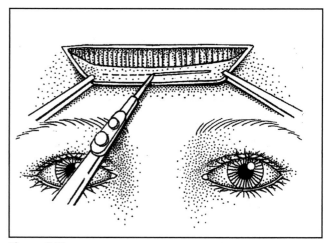

Figure 9-11.

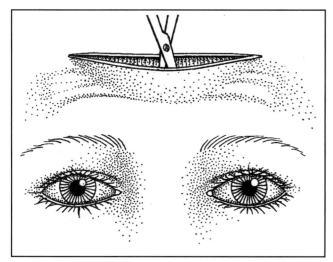

Figure 9-10.

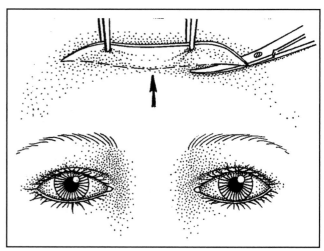

Figure 9-12.

epinephrine and hyaluronidase. The incision site, superior brow, and glabellar region are infiltrated with 1% lidocaine with 1:200,000 epinephrine and hyaluronidase. Fifteen minutes are allowed to elapse for adequate vasoconstriction to develop.

Step 4

A #15 Bard-Parker blade is used to make a full-thickness incision in the previously demarcated lines. The incision is carried down to the level of the galea. In the temporal region beyond the lateral extent of the frontalis muscle, the depth of the incision includes skin only. Blunt and sharp dissection is performed in the loose aponeurotic layer inferior to the superior orbital rims (Figure 9-10). Dissection of the corrugator and procerus muscles may be performed as indicated to eliminate glabellar furrows.

Step 5

Posterior lamella horizontal relaxing incisions can be performed with cutting cautery through the frontalis muscle (Figure 9-11). A strip of untouched frontalis muscle is left at the first forehead crease to permit animation of the brow postoperatively.

Step 6

The flap is then elevated to the desired height. The redundant forehead tissue is then excised full-thickness, as appropriate, to eliminate eyebrow ptosis (Figure 9-12). The tissue can be excised in an asymmetric fashion to correct asymmetric brow ptosis or medial or lateral brow ptosis.

Step 7

The wound is closed in 2 layers, as described for the direct brow lift (Figure 9-13). Antibiotic ointment is applied, and a Telfa dressing is placed over the wound for 48 hours. Ice compresses are used 4 times a day for 4 days to reduce swelling and ecchymosis. Sutures should be removed within 7 to 10 days.

TEMPORAL EYEBROW LIFT

Patients are asked to wash their hair with antibacterial shampoo the evening before surgery. They are also advised that clothing worn on the day of surgery should not require removal over the head.

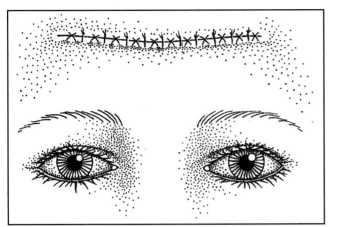

Figure 9-13.

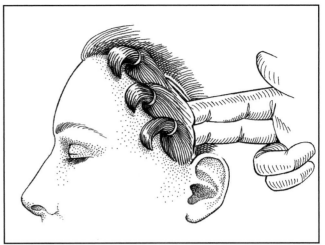

Figure 9-15.

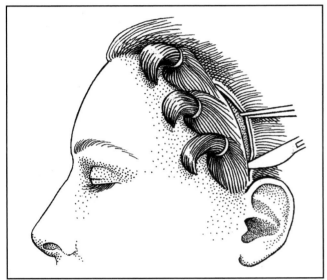

Figure 9-14.

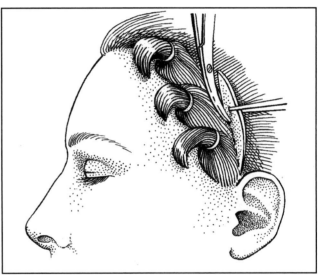

Figure 9-16.

Step 1

With intravenous sedation, several milliliters of 2% lidocaine with 1:200,000 epinephrine and hyaluronidase are given as a supraorbital nerve block. Ten mL of 0.5% lidocaine with 1:200,000 epinephrine and hyaluronidase is infiltrated along the proposed incision line. Fifteen minutes are allowed to elapse for maximal vasoconstriction to develop.

Step 2

The hair is parted, and a #15 Bard-Parker blade is used to make a vertical incision approximately 12-cm long above each ear to the level of the deep temporalis fascia (Figure 9-14).

Step 3

Blunt dissection with the finger or a large blunt scissors is carried along the plane of the deep temporalis fascia toward the eyebrow. The finger may be wrapped with a single layer of gauze to facilitate the blunt dissection (Figure 9-15). The temporal branch of the facial nerve is located in the superficial temporalis fascia, which is in the flap. Damage to the nerve is avoided if the dissection is carried deep to the nerve, along the deep temporalis fascia. The temporal flap is undermined to the level of the brow and lateral canthus. Gentle blunt dissection with the finger wrapped in gauze is least traumatic to the facial nerves incorporated in the flap. To prevent damage to the facial nerve, the use of cautery is avoided.

Step 4

After the flap is developed, it is advanced and rotated slightly. Redundant tissue is then excised (Figure 9-16).

Step 5

The wound is closed in a single layer with wide skin staples (Figure 9-17). No drains are used. Antibiotic ointment is placed on the wound, and fluffs are placed over the flap. Kling and Kerlix are placed as a head wrap. Ice compresses are placed over the eyes and forehead 4 times a day for 4 days. The staples are removed in 10 to 14 days.

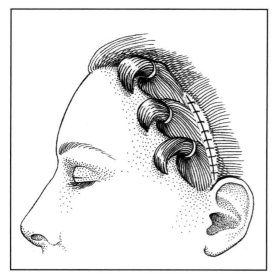

Figure 9-17.

CORONAL FOREHEAD AND EYEBROW LIFT

Patients are asked to wash their hair with antibacterial shampoo the evening before surgery. They are also advised that clothing worn the day of surgery should not require removal over the head.

Step 1

In the operating room, the hair is parted and braided along the proposed coronal incision site with the help of K-Y Jelly. Strips of aluminum foil or dental rubber bands may be used to braid the hair. The incision line extends from the superior point where the ear touches the scalp, from ear to ear. In the midline, the incision is placed 6 to 7 cm posterior to the hairline. The incision line is marked with a marking pen (Figure 9-18A).

Step 2

With a marking pen, a line is marked from the midline (middle of the nose) to the incision line (Figure 9-18B, line N-N). Another line is drawn from the lateral brow just above the position of the lateral limbus to the incision line (see Figure 9-18B, line H-L). This is generally 4 cm from the midline (measured along the coronal line). A line is then drawn from the ala of the nose through the lateral canthus and extended until it intersects the incision line (see Figure 9-18C, line B). This line generally intersects the incision line 10 cm from the midline (measured along the incision line; see Figure 9-18B, dotted line N-T). The hair may then be clipped just anterior to the incision line for 1 to 2 cm.

Step 3

We prefer performing the procedure under local anesthesia with intravenous sedation. General anesthesia causes vasodilatation and more bleeding. Forty mL of 0.5% lidocaine with 1:200,000 epinephrine and hyaluronidase is given as a "vascular tourniquet" along the incision line and across the brows. This is divided into aliquots of 10 mL along the incision line from the top of the ear to the mid-

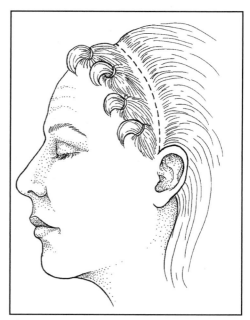

Figure 9-18A.

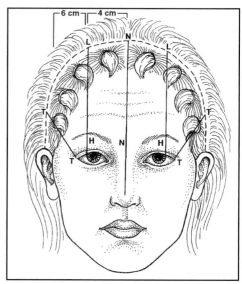

Figure 9-18B.

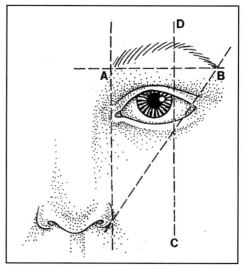

Figure 9-18C.

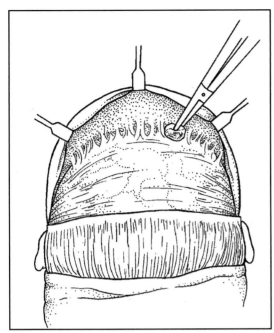

Figure 9-19.

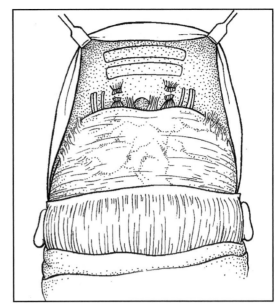

Figure 9-20.

line and from the top of the ear to the center of the forehead, and is repeated on the opposite side. Four mL of 0.5% bupivacaine hydrochloride (Marcaine) with 1:200,000 epinephrine and hyaluronidase is given as a supraorbital block bilaterally. It is also helpful to give several milliliters of the bupivacaine hydrochloride solution above each ear. Excellent hemostasis is generally obtained, and the need for reinjection is rare. Raney clips usually are not necessary.

Step 4

A #15 Bard-Parker blade is used to make an incision through the galea to the level of the periosteum. Dissection between the periosteum and loose aponeurotic tissue is performed with the fingers or with scissors. The forehead flap is elevated down to the level of the superior orbital rims (Figure 9-19). Because the temporal branch of the facial nerve lies within the flap, dissection is carefully performed along the temporalis fascia, and blunt dissection with the finger wrapped in gauze is performed in these areas. Cautery is avoided in the temporal portion of the flap.

Step 5

A subperiosteal plane is established with a Freer elevator 1 to 2 cm superior to the superior orbital rims. This allows maximal elevation of the brows and preservation of the supraorbital neurovascular bundle.

Step 6

At this point, superior traction of the scalp lifts the brows but does not smooth the creases and furrows of the glabella or forehead. The procerus-corragator muscle complex must be cut with scissors or dissected with cutting electrocautery (Figure 9-20).

Step 7

To obliterate forehead furrows, one or more horizontal relaxing incisions are made in the posterior muscle lamella of the forehead flap above the first forehead crease (see Figure 9-20). This allows the posterior lamella to relax and the anterior skin layer to be stretched. The cautery is carried through frontalis muscle to subcutaneous tissue. However, cautery is avoided in the hair-bearing scalp to avoid follicle loss. Inferiorly, a thin strip of frontalis muscle is preserved at the first forehead crease to allow natural animation of the brows.

Step 8

Using a D'Assumpcao clamp, the posterior scalp is advanced in the midline and marked with a satellite incision created with a #11 blade. This procedure is repeated along the previously demarcated lines of tension (Figure 9-21). Redundant scalp is then excised with scissors. A gradual tapering of the incision is performed in the temporal segment, as little lift is gained in this area. Tension on the forehead flap can be adjusted to correct asymmetric brow ptosis and to achieve the desired eyebrow arch.

Step 9

A single closure is performed with wide skin staples (Figure 9-22). No drains are used.

Step 10

The hair may be rinsed with 1.5% hydrogen peroxide to remove blood and then rinsed with saline to avoid bleaching the hair. The hair is dried with a towel, and antibiotic ointment is applied to the wound.

Step 11

Fluffs are placed across the flap, and a head wrap is made with Kling and Kerlix gauze roll anchored with short pieces of tape. Ice compresses are

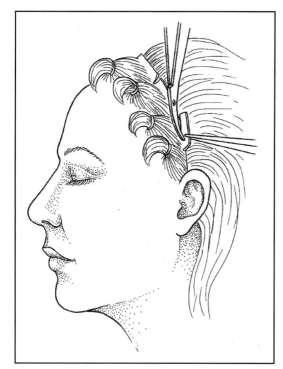

Figure 9-21.

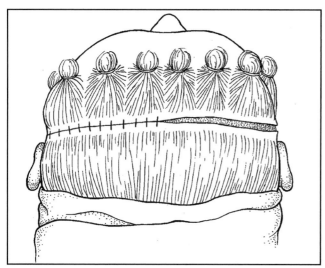

Figure 9-22.

applied to the eyes and forehead constantly for the first postoperative day and continued 3 or 4 times a day for the following 4 days to minimize edema. The head is kept elevated, and the head wrap is removed in 2 to 3 days. Patients are then instructed to shampoo the hair gently for several minutes a day to remove crusts. Staples are removed in 10 to 14 days. Blepharoplasty may be performed after coronal eyebrow lift at the same sitting. However, because of the volume of anesthetic injected and the presence of intraoperative edema, blepharoplasty may be more easily performed as a separate procedure.

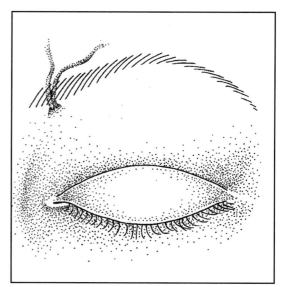

Figure 9-23.

INTERNAL EYEBROWPEXY AND TRANSEYELID EYEBROW LIFT

Step 1

The amount of eyebrow lift desired is determined with the patient in a sitting position. The supraorbital notch is palpated and demarcated to localize the supraorbital nerve and vessels. The upper lid crease is then demarcated as well (Figure 9-23).

Step 2

After the eyebrow and upper lid regions are infiltrated with 2% lidocaine with 1:100,000 epinephrine and hyaluronidase, a lid crease incision is made. A standard upper blepharoplasty can be performed at this time, if so desired.

Step 3

Blunt dissection with scissors is extended superiorly in the submuscular plane toward the eyebrow. The dissection is carried 1.0- to 1.5-cm above the superior orbital rim. The dissection is limited to the central and lateral aspect of the eyebrow to avoid injury to the medial supraorbital neurovascular complex (Figure 9-24).

Step 4

A 4-0 Prolene suture is passed through periosteum approximately 1.0 to 1.5 cm above the orbital rim. The suture is then passed in the sub-brow muscular tissue at the level of the lower edge of the brow cilia (Figure 9-25). A needle can be inserted transcutaneously to facilitate identification of this level. Sutures are placed both laterally and centrally. The brow height and contour are adjusted by replacement of sutures until proper position and symmetry are achieved. The upper blepharoplasty incision is closed with a 6-0 nylon or Prolene suture.

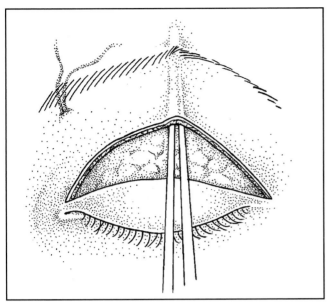

Figure 9-24.

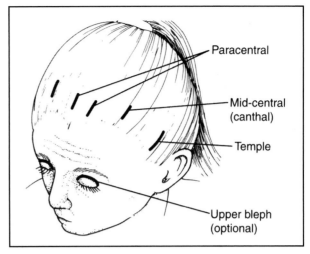

Figure 9-26.

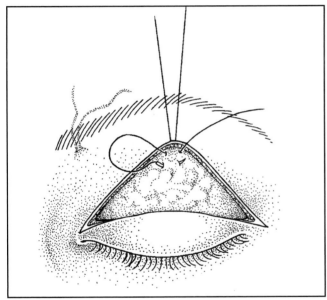

Figure 9-25.

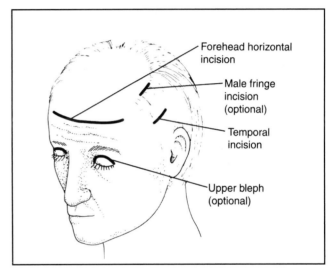

Figure 9-27.

ENDOSCOPIC EYEBROW LIFT

Patients are evaluated during the week before surgery, and the eyebrow depressor muscles are injected with botulinum toxin. Patients are asked to wash their hair with antibacterial shampoo the evening before surgery. They are also advised that clothing worn the day of surgery should not require removal over the head.

Step 1

With the patient in the seated position, a permanent skin marker is used to mark important anatomic landmarks including the hairline, the palpable anterior border of the temporalis fossa, the supraorbital notch, the course of the temporal branch of the facial nerve, and the zygomatic arch. Next, the appropriate forehead and eyebrow vector of elevation is determined by manual and voluntary elevation. This vector usually corresponds to a line connecting the lateral oral commissure and the lateral canthal angle. A mark corresponding to this vector measuring 3 cm is made on the skin 2.5 cm inside the hairline over the temporalis muscle. An identical procedure is performed on the opposite side. Additional marks are made 2.5 cm inside the hairline, marked parallel 2.5 cm and 7.0 cm from the right and left of midline (Figure 9-26). In patients with male pattern baldness, the position of the central incisions can be marked in prominent forehead rhytides and along the temporal fringe of hair (Figure 9-27).

Step 2

In the operating room, the procedure begins under local anesthesia with intravenous sedation. Two milliliters of 0.5% bupivacaine hydrochloride with 1:50,000 epinephrine is given as a supraorbital nerve block bilaterally and under each marked incision site. Three hundred milliliters of Klein's solution (1,000 mL normal saline, 1 ampule 1:1,000 epinephrine, 50 mL 1% lidocaine, 12 mEq sodium bicarbonate) is given as a "vascular tourniquet" throughout the scalp and forehead. Excellent hemostasis is generally obtained, and the need for reinjection is rare. The hair is parted and braided along the proposed incision sites with the help of K-Y Jelly. Strips of aluminum foil or dental rubber bands may be used to braid the hair.

Step 3

The skin is incised using the skin marks with a #15 Bard-Parker blade. Temporally, the tissue is incised down to the deep temporalis fascia; the more medial 4 incisions are made down to the periosteum. Beginning through the temporal incisions, the dissection is carried out between the superficial and deep temporalis fascia, moving toward the midline. The plane is easily sustained with a combination of sharp dissection with a caudal periosteal elevator and blunt finger dissection. Initially, the endoscope is not necessary, but, as the conjoint tendon is approached, it should be used to visualize this landmark. Before releasing the conjoint tendon, dissection is carried out through the medial incisions. A caudal periosteal elevator is used without the endoscope to elevate the periosteum off of the underlying calvarial bone from the occiput to supraorbital ridges.

Step 4

With endoscopic visualization through the temporal incision, the conjoint tendon is dissected beginning superiorly and moving inferiorly. In the area of the lateral eyebrow, 1 to 2 cm superior to the superior orbital rim, the deep temporalis fascia splits into the intermediate and deep temporalis fascia separated by Yassergil's fat pad. This is observed diverging as a "swirl" as it bifurcates. In close, lateral proximity to the "swirl" is the sentinel vessel. The vessel is identified and cauterized. The swirl and the vessel are then safely divided on the deep temporalis fascia, and the dissection is carried down following the lateral orbital rim onto the body of the zygoma in the subperiosteal plane.

Step 5

With endoscopic visualization, the subperiosteal dissection is carried inferiorly to the orbital rims and onto the nasal radix with a rim periosteal elevator. The assistant provides guidance and protects the globe by palpating inside the orbital rim in the area of dissection. The arcus marginalis is selectively released. Great care is taken in the medial third of the brow to identify and preserve the supraorbital and supratrochlear neurovascular bundles. The corrugator, procerus, and depressor supercilii muscles are identified and selectively weakened with blunt and sharp dissection.

Step 6

Skin hooks are then placed in the temporal incisions, and appropriate tension is achieved. While maintaining the tension, a 2-0 Vicryl suture is placed through the deep temporalis fascia, through the overlying scalp in the apex of the skin incision, and back through the deep temporalis fascia in a vertical mattress fashion. The suture is tied

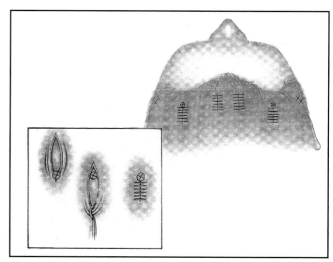

Figure 9-28. (This figure was published in *Cosmetic Oculoplastic Surgery: Eyelid, Forehead, and Facial Techniques,* 3rd ed, Putterman AM, ed, 319, © Elsevier, 1993.)

permanently, and the skin hook is withdrawn while observing for scalp migration. If migration is observed, the suture is replaced.

Step 7

Skin hooks are then placed in the remaining incisions, and the brow height and contour are adjusted by variable tension until proper position and symmetry are achieved. A drill with a 2-mm diameter guarded bit is used to make an appropriate number of holes in the frontal bone. Then, 14-mm screws are positioned, and again the brow height and contour are adjusted by variable tension until proper position and symmetry are achieved. At the appropriate tension and position, skin staples are placed posterior to the screws to maintain forehead and eyebrow suspension. The remaining skin incisions are closed with skin staples. No drains are placed (Figure 9-28).

Step 8

The elastic bands are removed, and the hair may be rinsed with 1.5% hydrogen peroxide to remove blood and then rinsed with saline to avoid bleaching the hair. The hair is dried with a towel, and antibiotic ointment is applied to the wound. Ice compresses are applied to the eyes and forehead constantly for the first postoperative day and continued 3 or 4 times a day for the following 4 days to minimize edema. The head is kept elevated, and the head wrap is removed in 2 to 3 days. Patients are then instructed to shampoo the hair gently for several minutes a day to remove crusts. Staples are removed in 10 to 14 days and the screws in 21 days. This routine can be varied to adjust the height and contour of the eyebrows.

Complications

Complications of brow lifts are few but notable. Proper preoperative evaluation and determination of the patient's specific anatomic abnormalities cannot be overemphasized. The following is a list of the more common complications encountered:

* Nerve damage: Damage to the temporal branches of the seventh nerve (motor), supratrochlear, or supraorbital nerves (sensory) can occur if the dissection is in the wrong surgical plane. Hypesthesia of the forehead can also result when the relaxing incisions of the posterior lamella of the coronal or temporal flaps are extended into the path of the supraorbital nerves. Overuse of cautery in the location of the nerves may also cause damage.

* Scarring: The eyebrow and forehead are areas that are quite visible. Although the incisions are "hidden" above the eyebrow cilia, in the procerus fold, or in a prominent forehead furrow, a visible scar may result. Improper closure and poor eversion of the wound edges may also result in a depressed scar. The patient must be made aware of this potential complication before surgery. Management of facial scarring is beyond the scope of this chapter; however, the surgeon should be familiar with the use of chemoexfoliative agents and dermabrasion.

* Hematoma: If careful hemostasis is not achieved, large hematomas can accumulate under the temporal or coronal flaps and potentially lead to necrosis of the flap. If a scalp hematoma forms and continues to expand, the wound must be opened and the bleeding vessel cauterized.

* Alopecia: Hair loss can occur at the coronal or temporal incision sites. If the plane of dissection is too superficial, the hair follicles are damaged. Overuse of cautery in the region of the hair follicles also results in alopecia.

* Others: Other potential complications include brow asymmetry, scar depigmentation, incision pruritus, and neuralgias.

CHAPTER 10

BLEPHAROPLASTY

John B. Holds, MD, FACS

Blepharoplasty is the cornerstone of eyelid rehabilitation surgery. Surgery is performed for cosmetic or medically necessary reasons on the upper eyelid to re-drape and define the lid crease and to decrease overhanging skin and fullness. In the lower eyelid, blepharoplasty is performed on a cosmetic basis to re-contour the lower lid, diminishing the appearance of "bags" and smooth the skin. Blepharoplasty is often combined with brow lift surgery, ptosis repair, or other facial aesthetic procedures to enhance or achieve a harmonious surgical result.

Preoperative Evaluation

In assessing the patient for upper blepharoplasty, it is important to first assess the motivation and goals of the patient. The older (>70 years) patient with visual obstruction symptoms and no cosmetic desires is a very different patient than the patient (old or young) with specific cosmetic goals. Eyebrow position is particularly relevant to this discussion, as virtually all patients interested in upper blepharoplasty surgery have some degree of brow ptosis and would conceivably benefit from a brow lifting procedure. Many patients will suffer some exacerbation of apparent brow ptosis following blepharoplasty surgery, and even if the patient does not want to pursue concomitant brow lift, it is important to proceed with appropriate understanding and acknowledgment from the patient of the expected outcome. Ptosis is a major confounding factor in blepharoplasty and generally requires concomitant repair. A careful evaluation and discussion of the implications of ptosis repair is essential, and surgeons not comfortable with addressing the patient's ptosis should refer the patient to a more skilled surgeon.

Dry eye complaints seldom present an absolute contraindication to blepharoplasty surgery, but require additional assessment, counseling, and modification of surgical technique. All patients should be queried regarding dry eye symptoms as well as other ocular history and complaints. Routine evaluation should include a slit-lamp examination, if possible. A basic Schirmer's secretion test (after anesthetic) may be worthwhile to document. In preoperative examination and counseling, it is helpful to demonstrate to the patient with a mirror the degree to which the surgeon believes overhanging skin will be improved with surgery and to note and point to fat pads that can be reduced. The limits of upper blepharoplasty are stressed, especially in regard to medial and lateral skin redundancy, which often is noted postoperatively and commonly requires a brow lift to improve. Patients undergoing surgery for medical indications require specific documentation of visual complaints, a desire for surgery, and reversible superior visual field loss on standardized perimetry. All patients require facial photography with multiple views.

Lower blepharoplasty surgery is virtually always cosmetic in nature and inevitably requires an evaluation and discussion of midface aesthetics. Examination must note eyelid position and laxity, snap-back test, and the extent and prominence of the "tear trough," defined by the nasojugal and orbitomalar folds and apparent anterior lamella (skin and muscle) redundancy. Secondary or "malar bags" (festoons) are common aging changes that will increase in prominence during the postoperative period with virtually any upper facial procedure and may be increased in dysthyroid states or any condition predisposing the patient to fluid retention. Preoperative counseling must realistically inform the patient of the ability of surgery to modify all of these features as well as the risk of more common complications.

Levine MR.
Manual of Oculoplastic Surgery, Fourth Edition (pp 75-82).
© 2010 SLACK Incorporated

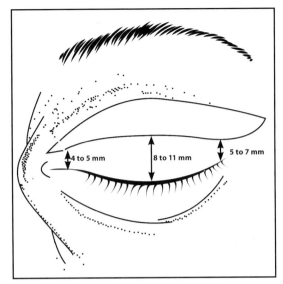

Figure 10-1.

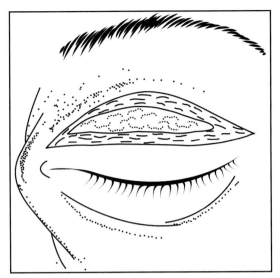

Figure 10-2.

Surgical Technique

Patients should discontinue aspirin and similar blood thinners, herbal medications, and anti-platelet agents 3 to 7 days preoperatively. This is best done in consultation with the patient's general physician and offers an excellent opportunity to ensure no acute or chronic medical condition poses an issue with surgery. The vast majority of patients undergoing upper and/or lower eyelid blepharoplasty surgery can undergo surgery under a local or sedated-local anesthetic. Four-lid blepharoplasty or additional procedures, such as brow or face-lift, may necessitate a general anesthetic.

Upper Blepharoplasty

Step 1

It is preferable to mark the patient in the upright position with a fine-tipped surgical marker before entering the operating room. First marking the eyelid crease, an appropriate amount of skin for excision is then marked. Asymmetries in either overhanging skin or the amount of upper eyelid skin are readily apparent and can be appropriately compensated for. When brow lift surgery is performed simultaneously, it is wise to first perform the brow lift, and then recheck the blepharoplasty excision to ensure excessive lagophthalmos is not induced.

The patient's natural eyelid crease is an excellent guide to appropriate positioning of the lid crease incision. The highest point in the central eyelid is generally aligned with the nasal aspect of the pupil, viewed in a sagittal plane, at 8- to 11-mm height (Figure 10-1). Women generally prefer a slightly higher lid crease than men, but the natural crease and patient's desires will guide this. After marking the central eyelid crease, a smooth downward curve is made medially and laterally, to a low point 4- to 5 mm above the upper punctum and to a temporal low point 5 to 7 mm above the lateral canthal angle. A smooth upward curve is made medially, never extending medial to the canthal angle, while, laterally, the incision ends 12 to 16 mm lateral to the canthal angle and never beyond the orbital rim where the skin thickens. Superiorly, marks are made 10- to 15-mm inferior to the inferior aspect of the brow laterally, smoothly tapering toward the medial and lateral ends of the lid crease incision. It is reasonable to use a smooth forceps to gently pinch together the skin proposed for excision. A slight degree of induced lagophthalmos and eversion of the lashes is generally desirable, and a significant degree of lagophthalmos suggests an overly aggressive excision.

Step 2

After entering the operating suite and providing anesthesia or sedation as requested, it is helpful to inject the patient with 1 mL/eyelid of lidocaine 2% with epinephrine 1:100,000 that is diluted 1:5 with normal saline (final epinephrine concentration 1:600,000). This dilute injection is painless, except for the initial needle stick and will give complete anesthesia of the skin and orbicularis muscle with excellent vasoconstriction while the patient is being sterilely prepped. After carefully draping to ensure the drapes do not induce a brow malposition, distorting the surgical effect, the patient is reinfiltrated with 2% lidocaine with epinephrine 1:100,000. The addition of 8.4% sodium bicarbonate in a 1:10 proportion with the lidocaine further lessens any discomfort. The instillation of topical anesthetic and placement of metallic eye shields that completely cover the anterior bulbar surface protects the eyes and will prevent startling the patient with bright surgical lights.

Step 3

A #15 or preferably 15c Bard-Parker blade is used to incise the skin. Westcott or Kaye scissors are used to remove skin only beginning temporally and working medially until the lateral canthus is reached (Figure 10-2). It is helpful to also remove

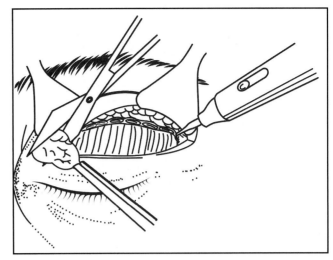

Figure 10-4.

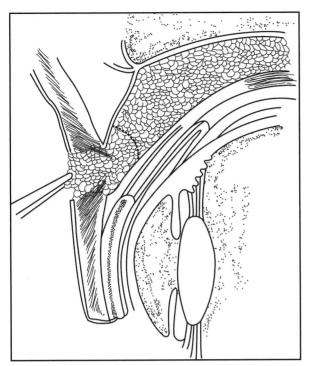

Figure 10-3.

skin only for the first 5 to 6 mm laterally from the most medial aspect of the incision. A skin-only excision lateral to the lateral canthus and medial to the upper punctum will limit cautery and the depth of the excision in these areas and minimize scar formation at the medial and lateral extent of the incision where it is most noticeable postoperatively.

Over the central eyelid, orbicularis muscle is excised, exposing the orbital septum. Patients requiring more debulking may have orbicularis muscle excised almost to the cut skin edge. Elderly or dry eye patients benefit from preservation of the orbicularis muscle and require no muscle or only a small central strip of muscle to be excised.

Step 4

After cautery for hemostasis, additional anesthetic mixture is given beneath the orbital septum centrally (if it is to be opened) and directly into the medial fat pad. Gentle pressure on the globe will cause the preaponeurotic fat to bulge, allowing the orbital septum to be opened medially and centrally. Freeing the fat from the orbital septum and levator aponeurosis that borders it allows the fat to prolapse anteriorly. It is then cauterized, paralleling the incision, leaving a cuff of undisturbed fat anterior to the orbital rim (Figure 10-3). Bipolar cautery or CO_2 laser are most comfortable, with monopolar (Bovie) cautery requiring significant sedation. Surgical indications and individual preferences and variations will determine whether the septum is left intact or fat is excised almost flush with the orbital rim. Fat is excised evenly across the width of the eyelid, avoiding the temptation to excise more fat centrally where it is most accessible. Laterally,

the lacrimal gland is avoided, pre-emptively cauterizing vessels previously disturbed in the surgical exposure.

Medially, the medial fat pad often requires a carefully directed exposure as it lies inferior and medial to the most medial extent of the central (preaponeurotic) fat. Retracting over the medial fat pad with fine skin rakes, pressure is applied, and the capsule of the fat pad is incised while avoiding blood vessels that encircle the base of the medial fat pad. After freeing up the medial fat, pressure is applied, and prolapsing fat is cauterized and excised in a graded fashion (Figure 10-4). In the lateral sub-brow area, cautery shrinkage or a graded excision of the most inferior brow fat may lighten the lateral brow and enhance the result in this area.

Step 5

After achieving meticulous hemostasis, the incision is closed. A simple skin closure is most efficient, and a running closure with 7-0 polypropylene suture is generally sufficient. With large excisions, it is sometimes helpful to place an interrupted suture laterally at the point where the lid crease incision angles upward toward the orbital rim. Centrally, it is helpful to create supratarsal fixation of the pretarsal skin and lid crease (Figure 10-5). This can be created with interrupted sutures or as part of the running suture. Although women may be more discerning regarding the lid crease definition, it is beneficial in most patients to place a few fixation sutures to ensure the final position of the eyelid crease. Concomitant aponeurotic ptosis surgery or aggressive orbicularis muscle excision further destabilizes the pretarsal orbicularis muscle, making appropriate eyelid crease fixation more important. A loose closure centrally is "tightened" with more frequent sutures laterally where the thicker skin is under more tension and tends to gape. At the end of surgery, antibiotic ointment is instilled into the eyes and over the incisions. Head elevation and icing of the eyelids as tolerated for 24 to 48 hours is beneficial in limiting

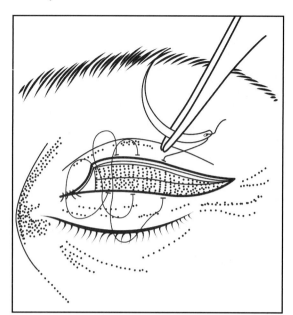

Figure 10-5.

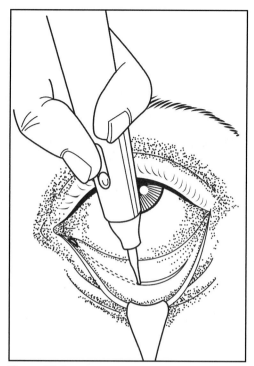

Figure 10-6.

postoperative discomfort and ecchymosis. A mild analgesic, such as acetaminophen/propoxyphene combination (Darvocet), is helpful in the first few hours or days postoperatively.

VARIATIONS

Excess redundancy of skin medially along the upper incision may require a W-plasty excision of an additional triangle of tissue at a 60° angle superior to the medial tip of the excision. It is possible to perform internal lifting of the eyebrow through the blepharoplasty incision. Both suture and Endotine (Coapt Systems, Palo Alto, CA) fixation are performed. Most surgeons find the results of these internal brow lift techniques to be temporary and unreliable. Asian upper blepharoplasty is a separate topic that requires a studied approach beyond the scope of this chapter (see Chapter 12).

Lower Blepharoplasty

Lower blepharoplasty surgery is generally acknowledged to be more difficult and fraught with greater hazards than upper blepharoplasty surgery. There is less agreement among surgeons on the goals of surgery, general treatment paradigm, and surgical approach. Concurrent goals in treatment include reducing fat bulging in the preseptal area, lessening the prominence of the tear trough, reducing apparently redundant skin and photoaging changes of the skin, and addressing eyelid and cheek laxity. Different patients require these issues to be dealt with in different ways, depending on their age, anatomy, expectations, skin pigment type, and concurrent procedures. As such, there is no single lower blepharoplasty procedure that is appropriate for every patient. This chapter describes a transconjunctival fat repositioning technique with skin resurfacing or direct skin excision and canthopexy. Points at which departure in technique may be considered to pursue other techniques are discussed.

Step 1
The patient is marked in the upright position, marking fat pads, the tear trough, and other features requiring special attention. Topical anesthetic is instilled into the eyes, and a pledget of anesthetic is placed in the inferior fornix. Prior to the prep and drape, dilute local anesthetic is injected subconjunctivally in the inferior fornix. If a transconjunctival fat repositioning technique is performed, the needle is very slowly advanced inferiorly over the orbital rim into the premalar area to achieve an infraorbital nerve block.

Step 2
Following a sterile prep and drape, the lower eyelid is reinfiltrated with anesthetic mixture. In 4-lid blepharoplasty performed under local or sedated-local anesthetic, 0.75% bupivacaine with epinephrine 1:100,000 is infiltrated into the upper and lower eyelids at this point. In 2-lid blepharoplasty, 2% lidocaine with epinephrine will suffice. Metallic eye shields are placed. The lower lid is everted, and the conjunctiva is incised 3 mm below the lower edge of the tarsus. The incision extends medially to the caruncle and laterally almost to the lateral canthus (Figure 10-6). The conjunctiva is incised as finely as possible with a CO_2 laser or Colorado needle on a cutting monopolar cautery. The monopolar cautery is associated with considerably more discomfort and will require either moderately deep intravenous sedation or a general anesthetic. A 4-0 silk traction suture is passed through the conjunctiva, and the cutting cautery is used to dissect anterior to the orbital septum down to the orbital rim, exposing the periosteum at the arcus marginalis (Figure 10-7).

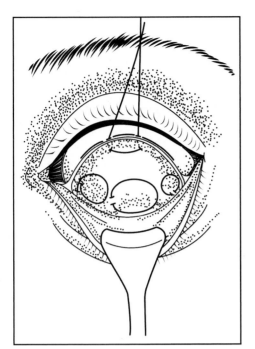

Figure 10-7.

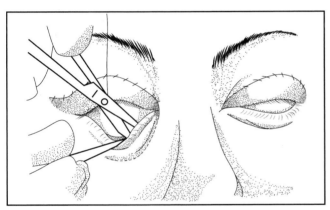

Figure 10-8.

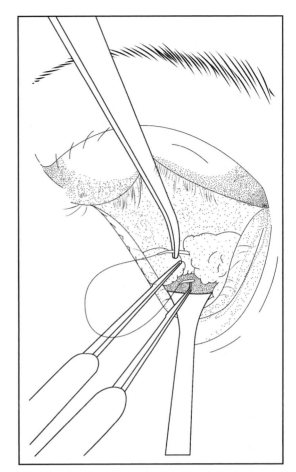

Figure 10-9.

Step 3

Careful blunt dissection is completed in the plane of the suborbicularis oculi fat (SOOF) from the orbital rim just anterior to the arcus marginalis to a level 8 to 12 mm below the orbital rim (Figure 10-8). Medially, the SOOF thins with the muscle lying directly on the periosteum. It is this junction in the central-medial orbital rim where the SOOF ends that generally has the greatest volume loss and skeletonization of the orbital rim and that benefits the most volumetrically from fat repositioning. Each orbital fat pad is opened, and the fat is allowed to prolapse.

A pedicle is developed in any fat to be repositioned, circumferentially releasing the fat to allow advancement. Fat sculpting is done as necessary, most commonly only in the temporal fat pad and minimally of the medial and central fat pads.

Step 4

One to 2 mattress sutures of 5-0 polypropylene are passed from the cheek into the dissected intra-SOOF pocket. A robust bite is taken, weaving through the fat pedicle (Figure 10-9), and the fat pads are each repositioned into the intra-SOOF pocket (Figure 10-10). The polypropylene sutures are passed through the cheek tissues and a foam bolster and tied. In older patients with more eyelid laxity, it is often possible to avoid the externalized bolsters and pass a small half-circle needle (5-0 Vicryl, P-2 needle), suturing the fat pads into the depth of the intra-SOOF pocket previously dissected.

Step 5

The fat repositioning decreases the submuscular volume in the preseptal part of the eyelid. This modest deflation of eyelid volume increases the tendency for skin wrinkling in the preseptal and pretarsal eyelid. In suitable patients, it is desirable to tighten the skin at the end of the procedure, either with a direct excision of skin or with a skin resurfacing technique, such as a medium-depth chemical peel or CO_2 or erbium-YAG laser skin resurfacing.

Lateral canthopexy and direct excision of excess skin via a subciliary incision are performed as clinically

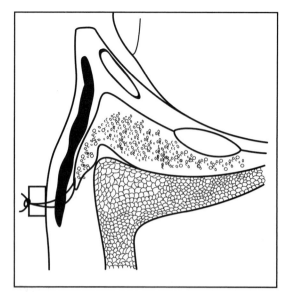

Figure 10-10.

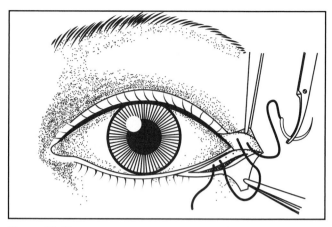

Figure 10-12.

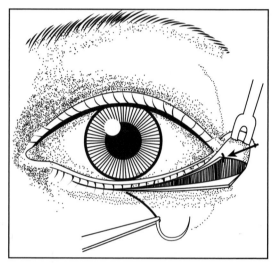

Figure 10-13.

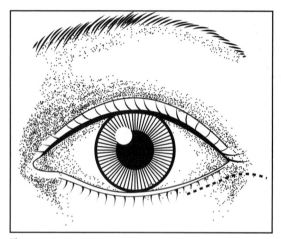

Figure 10-11.

ically indicated. Lateral canthopexy is performed in all cases with significant lid laxity or with skin excision. The canthopexy is accomplished by exposing the canthal angle and lateral orbital rim through a lateral subciliary incision (Figure 10-11). A 5-0 Vicryl suture on a P-2 needle is passed between the lower lid at the canthal angle and the periosteum above and lateral to it (Figure 10-12). Skin is excised as a small ellipse centered in the lateral lid, generally leaving the orbicularis muscle intact. It is rare that it is appropriate to excise more than 3 vertical mm of lower lid skin. With skin excision, it may be appropriate to additionally vertically support the orbicularis muscle laterally with a suture from the orbicularis muscle to the periosteum (Figure 10-13). Undermining in the suborbicularis plane and vertically supporting the anterior lamella laterally in this fashion will also help to blunt the sagging associated with a malar triangle or small lateral festoon. A running skin closure with 6-0 plain gut or 7-0 polypropylene suture is appropriate.

Patients are treated postoperatively with antibiotic ointment and a skin dressing if skin resurfacing was performed. Mild analgesics are prescribed. An oral antibiotic or antiviral medication is not needed unless there is a specific indication. Sutures and bolsters are removed in 6 days.

VARIATIONS

The simplest version of the transconjunctival lower blepharoplasty involves a subtractive technique with fat removal only. Fat is cauterized and sculpted from the medial, central, and lateral fat pads. Under no circumstances is fat sculpted beyond the orbital rim in a coronal plane. In the lateral fat pad, the fat septae are opened to allow prolapse with gentle pressure on the globe. Care is taken to adequately address the medial and lateral fat pads and not oversculpt the central fat pad, which is most readily exposed.

For most patients, a purely subtractive blepharoplasty is not the optimal procedure as it skeletonizes the orbital rim, discarding fat that would otherwise be useful in filling the tear trough, and leaves the anterior lamella unsupported, further increasing wrinkling. A subtractive transconjunctival lower blepharoplasty may be reasonable

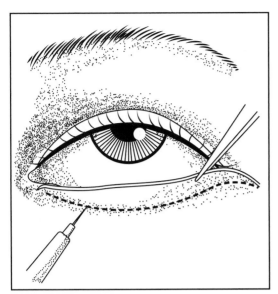

Figure 10-14.

Complications

The most common issues after upper blepharoplasty are early minor asymmetries and concerns postoperatively relating to edema, generally mild hypertrophic scarring, and a relative anesthesia of the lashes and pretarsal skin. Minor asymmetries often relate to brow asymmetry and, with appropriately planned surgery, are generally less severe than in preoperative photographs. A preoperative discussion of asymmetry, especially relating to brow position, and reference postoperatively to photographs is helpful.

Normal wound healing induces a mild hypertrophy and contracture of surgical wounds, generally most apparent 4 to 6 weeks postoperatively. As this resolves over weeks to months, reassurance and temporizing is generally curative. The injection of 0.05 to 0.2 mL of diluted triamcinolone acetonide (Kenalog 10) along the incision will speed resolution of this thickening. A mild anesthesia apparent on placing eyeliner or mascara is normal and will resolve within a few months.

Dry eye complaints are generally mild in patients under good control preoperatively and who respond well to topical tear drops and punctal plugs or other treatment as needed. Severely overdone blepharoplasty may require skin grafting to the eyelid or fat- or dermis-fat grafting to the superior sulcus or lower eyelids. Careful preoperative counseling and attention to surgical technique are essential in treating these cases.

Ptosis is an uncommon complication of blepharoplasty surgery and generally resolves over weeks to months. Review of preoperative photographs may reveal a ptosis missed on preoperative examination, now apparent with the lid margin visible.

In the lower eyelid, ectropion seen early postoperatively may respond to temporizing, with steri-stripping of the eyelid and later a tarsal-strip style canthoplasty, full-thickness skin graft, or other treatment being performed as needed.

Visual loss is a rare complication of bleeding and orbital hematoma. Attention preoperatively to control of blood pressure and avoidance of herbals and medications with anticoagulant properties generally prevents this. Appropriate surgical technique with meticulous cautery of bleeding or potential bleeding vessels and avoidance of higher risk surgical planes prevents this complication. The development of visual loss is an ophthalmic emergency requiring immediate evaluation and relief of orbital pressure via canthotomy and cantholysis. Medical therapy with methylprednisolone sodium succinate (Solu-Medrol) 1000 mg IV stat may offer some protection.

Infection is a rare complication of blepharoplasty. Most cases are superficial and limited infections along the upper eyelid incision. Methicillin-resistant *Staphylococcus aureus* is common in both hospital- and community-acquired infections, requiring appropriate evaluation and therapy.

in the young patient with a congenitally increased lower fat pad and good soft tissue support or in a revision situation.

The subciliary technique of lower blepharoplasty is also time-honored, even if it has faded from the armamentarium of many surgeons. The external approach to lower blepharoplasty is simply visualized by omitting the transconjunctival incision described previously and elevating a skin-muscle flap via a subciliary incision (extending step 5 described previously). The fat pads are exposed, opened, and sculpted via this approach. A canthopexy and cautious and conservative excision of skin and muscle along the subciliary incision (Figure 10-14) is indicated. Fat repositioning into an intra-SOOF or subperiosteal pocket may even be performed via this approach.

The transconjunctival approach to the lower eyelid provides a number of advantages over the external approach. By avoiding a skin incision in many cases, and an external incision that opens the orbital septum in all cases, the "middle-lamella" scarring that may cause intractable lower eyelid retraction and rounding of the lateral canthus is avoided. The transconjunctival incision also releases the lower eyelid retractors. Although this may cause a slightly bothersome "reverse ptosis" in which the lower eyelid rides upward from the corneal limbus early postoperatively in some patients, the effect is something like leaving a traction suture in place for several weeks in combating lower eyelid retraction. The fat repositioning technique not only uses fat that would otherwise be discarded in smoothly transitioning an area of consistent aesthetic concern, but releases the orbicularis muscle at the orbital rim, helping to move the eyelid-cheek transition to a more youthful level.

CHAPTER 11

CHEEK-MIDFACE LIFT

Allen M. Putterman, MD

With age, the cheek migrates inferiorly and nasally (Figure 11-1). This contributes to inferior orbital rim hollowing, a circle effect of the lower eyelids and cheek, a flattening of the cheek, cheek bags (festoons), and a nasolabial fold. In the past, these problems have been treated with face-lifts, excision of cheek bags, and cheek implants.

Hester and colleagues and McCord[1,2] popularized the cheek-midface lift through an external lower blepharoplasty approach. This procedure originally was done by reattaching the suborbicularis orbital fat (SOOF) in a more normal position along with a full-thickness resection of the lower eyelid to stabilize the lid. The procedure has been modified multiple times, and, at present, I perform the procedure by suspending an orbicularis muscle flap along with tarsal strip and skin flap procedures. The operation places the ptotic cheek in a more normal position, relieves cheek bags, fills in the hollow inferior orbital rim with cheek fat, makes the midface more convex, and decreases the nasolabial fold depression. It also gives the effect of cheek implantation, adds skin to the lower eyelids for the treatment of cicatricial ectropion, and reduces the hollowing of the lower eyelid that sometimes occurs secondary to overzealous fat removal in lower blepharoplasty.

At times, the procedure is performed with lower eyelid fat excision, and, at times, it is done with repositioning of the nasal and central lower eyelid fat pads into the inferior orbital rim hollowing area along with temporal fat resection. The tarsal strip procedure is performed to stabilize the lower eyelid and to prevent retraction and ectropion of the lower lid.

Preparation for Surgery

The patient's entire face is prepared with povidone-iodine (Betadine), soap, and paint. The patient is draped so that the entire face is exposed. Topical tetracaine is applied over each eye. A scleral contact lens is placed over the eyes and under the eyelids to protect the eyes from foreign objects, to prevent the operating lights from bothering the patient, and to avoid causing the patient stress from seeing the procedure being performed. A marking pen is used to create a lateral canthal line, which begins at the lateral canthus and extends in a horizontal direction for approximately 1 to 1.5 cm.

Anesthesia

A mixture of 40 mL of 0.5% lidocaine (Xylocaine) with 1:200,000 epinephrine and 4 mL of 0.5% plain bupivacaine (Marcaine) is prepared. Several milliliters of the mixture are injected subcutaneously and diffusely across the lower eyelids. A 25-gauge 1.5-cm needle is passed through the nasal lower eyelid just above the inferior orbital rim and then over the inferior orbital rim slightly in a downward direction to avoid penetrating the eye. The needle is inserted for approximately 1 cm and 0.5 to 1 mL of the anesthetic mixture is injected. This is repeated centrally and temporally.

A mark is applied with a blue marking pen to the area of the infraorbital foramen, and several milliliters of the same anesthetic mixture are injected around the exit of the infraorbital nerve. Approximately 20 mL of the solution is injected subperiosteally over the cheek down to the upper gum and nasolabial fold areas. Approximately 0.5 cc of the anesthetic is also injected subcutaneously at the center of the upper eyelid just above the lid margin.

Surgical Technique

Step 1

A 4-0 black silk suture is passed through skin, orbicularis, and superficial tarsus at the center of the upper eyelids, and the sutures are left long so that

Levine MR.
Manual of Oculoplastic Surgery, Fourth Edition (pp 83-96).
© 2010 SLACK Incorporated

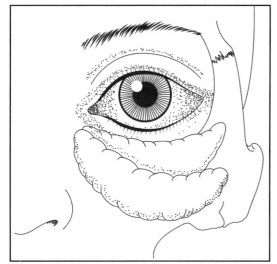

Figure 11-1.

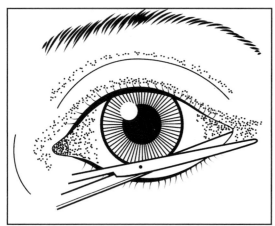

Figure 11-2.

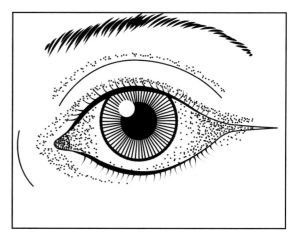

Figure 11-3.

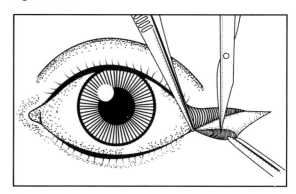

Figure 11-4.

they can be attached to the drape with hemostats to lift the upper lid upward. A similar 4-0 black silk suture is placed through skin, orbicularis, and superficial tarsus of the center of the lower eyelid just adjacent to the lid margin and again is left long for traction.

Step 2

A #15 Bard-Parker blade is then used to make an incision through skin over the lateral canthal mark from the lateral canthus temporally in a horizontal direction for 1 to 1.5 cm. A Westcott scissors is then used to sever the lateral canthus (Figure 11-2). A Colorado needle then incises the orbicularis muscle from the lateral canthus throughout the length of the skin incision (Figure 11-3). The lower limb of the lateral canthal tendon is severed (Figure 11-4). A small Desmarres retractor everts the lower eyelid. One to 2 cubic centimeters of the anesthetic

mixture is then injected subconjunctivally from the inferior tarsal border to the inferior fornix across the eyelid. The Colorado needle is then used to cut conjunctiva from the caruncle to the temporal aspect of the eyelid midway between the inferior tarsal border and the inferior fornix (Figure 11-5). The surgeon grasps the central inferior edge of the severed palpebral conjunctiva while the assistant grasps the adjacent, more superior edge with another forceps. The 2 forceps are pulled apart, and then the Colorado needle is applied across the eyelid between the 2 severed conjunctival layers through Müller's muscle and capsulopalpebral fascia until fat is seen (Figure 11-6).

Step 3

A 4-0 double-arm black silk suture is passed through the inferior edge of conjunctiva, Müller's muscle, and capsulopalpebral fascia with each suture arm. The sutures are then drawn upward and attached to the drape with a hemostat (Figure 11-7). A small piece of tape is applied over any exposed needle to avoid needle sticks and to allow the suture to be reused, if needed.[3] Usually, the needle is cut and removed from the operating field.

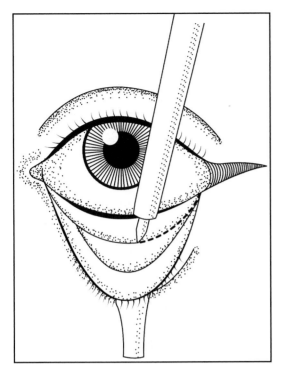

Figure 11-5.

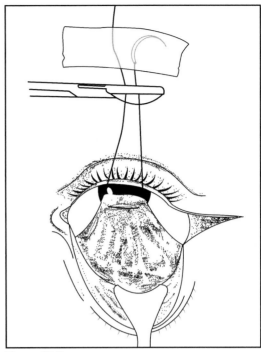

Figure 11-7.

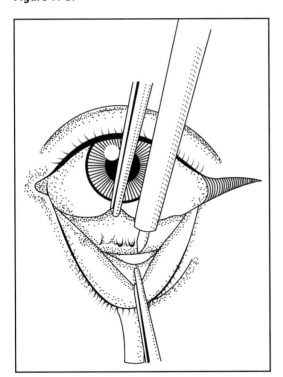

Figure 11-6.

Step 4

A small Desmarres retractor is placed over the superior edge of conjunctiva, Müller's muscle, and capsulopalpebral fascia and is pulled downward and outward to expose the orbital fat. With the use of cotton-tipped applicators and Westcott scissors, blunt dissection is carried out to isolate the 3 orbital fat pads. The central and nasal fat pads are divided by the inferior oblique muscle, which can easily be seen through the internal approach and should be identified to avoid injury to this structure. Also, the nasal and central fat pads are found in a slightly more temporal position than when they are isolated through an external approach.

Step 5

The temporal herniated orbital fat is isolated, and the fat that prolapses with general pressure on the eye is clamped with a hemostat and cut along the hemostat with a #15 Bard-Parker blade (Figure 11-8). Then, cotton-tipped applicators are placed under the hemostat, and a Bovie cautery is applied over the fat stump. The surgeon grasps the fat with the forceps before it is allowed to slide back into the orbit to make sure there is no residual bleeding that might cause a retrobulbar hemorrhage. After the first temporal fat pad is removed, the surgeon applies additional pressure to the eye to determine whether there is a second temporal fat pad.[4] If found, it is removed in a similar manner.

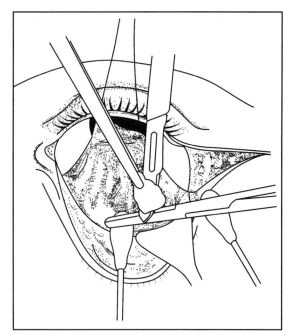

Figure 11-8.

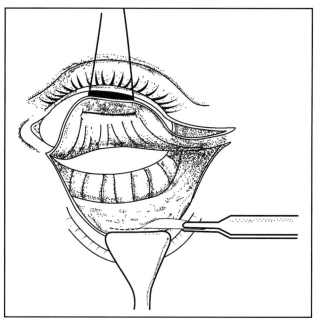

Figure 11-9.

At times, the central and nasal fat pads are removed, and, sometimes, they are repositioned into the inferior orbital rim hollowing. This is a surgical judgment that is made depending on the severity and amount of orbital fat present preoperatively, as well as how much hollowing there is at the inferior orbital rim and nasal-jugal fold areas. If the decision is made to remove the fat, then the nasal and central orbital fat pads are removed in a similar manner to the description of the removal of the temporal fat pads. If the decision is made to reposition the nasal and central orbital fat pads, this is deferred until later in the procedure to avoid having to deal with the fat and sutures at this stage of the procedure.

DISSECTION OF CHEEK PERIOSTEUM

Step 1

A medium-sized Desmarres retractor is used to retract conjunctiva, Müller's muscle, and capsulopalpebral fascia over the inferior orbital rim. Using blunt dissection with the smooth end of a Tenzel periosteal elevator, the periosteum over the inferior orbital rim and lateral orbital rim is isolated. A Colorado needle or #15 Bard-Parker blade is used to incise periosteum several millimeters beneath the orbital rim from the nasal inferior orbital rim all the way across the orbit, sweeping up into the lateral orbital rim (Figure 11-9).

Step 2

The sharp edge of the Tenzel periosteal elevator is used to reflect periosteum from the incision in a downward direction over the cheekbone (Figures 11-10 and 11-11). The surgeon should take care to avoid the area of the infraorbital foramen and nerve

by palpating the inferior orbital foramen, which was previously marked with a marking pen, and by dissecting inferior to this position.

Most of the time, it is unnecessary to dissect periosteum nasal to the infraorbital canal; leaving periosteum nasal to the infraorbital nerve allows the nasal area to act as a fulcrum for the cheek lift. However, if the purpose of the surgery is to add skin to the lower eyelid in the treatment of cicatricial ectropion or to reposition the nasal and central lower eyelid orbital fat pads, then dissection nasal to the infraorbital nerve is performed (Figure 11-12).

During the periosteal dissection, small blood vessels such as the temporal zygomatic artery are commonly encountered; these are treated with the Colorado needle to coagulate these areas and thereby avoid bleeding. Also, should there be any bleeding from other areas of the cheekbone, the Colorado needle can be used to coagulate those and to create a dry field.

Step 3

Periosteum is dissected inferiorly to the level where the cheekbone is and dips inward, which should be close to the upper gum. Nasally and inferiorly, the periosteal dissection extends into the nasolabial fold, with the surgeon taking care not to penetrate into the nasal cavity. Palpation of the periosteal elevator through the external skin and internal nares facilitates the dissection of the nasolabial fold. Also, the dissection in the nasolabial fold area is more superficial to decrease the furrow of the nasolabial fold. The use of an Army-Navy retractor to lift the dissected cheek tissue outward and downward aids in the visualization of the dissection site.

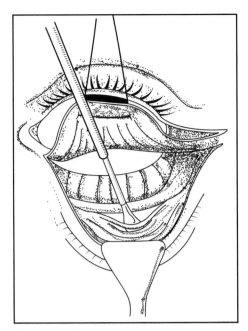

Figure 11-10.

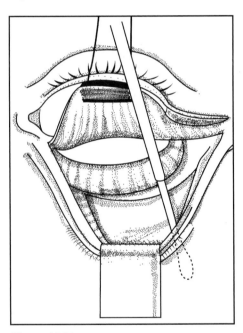

Figure 11-11.

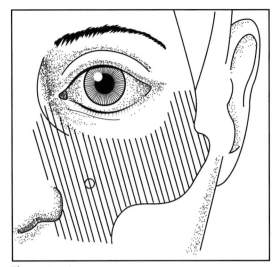

Figure 11-12.

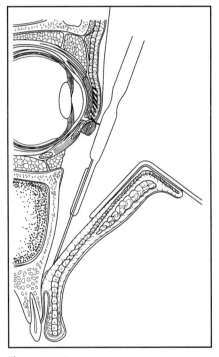

Figure 11-13.

Step 4

A #11 Bard-Parker blade is used to incise the periosteum at the inferior aspect of the dissection, which should be at the area where the cheek bone depresses inward (Figure 11-13). The surgeon should be careful to penetrate only the periosteum and not any of the more superficial tissues. Once the periosteum has been incised over the entire horizontal dimension of the inferior aspect of the flap, the periosteum is reflected superiorly for approximately 1 cm with the Ramirez endoforehead periosteal spreader (Snowden-Pencer 88-5080, No. 7) to sweep the periosteum upward (Figure 11-14). When this is accomplished, the surgeon places his

or her index finger into the subperiosteal space, engages the area of the periosteal incision site, and lifts the periosteum upward and outward (Figure 11-15). With this maneuver, the surgeon should feel a release of tissue that allows the patient's cheek to move upward and outward. The procedure is facilitated by an Adson forceps pulling the lateral canthal orbicularis upward and outward.

Step 5

A 4 x 4 gauze saturated in the anesthetic mixture is wrung out and inserted over the cheek in the subperiosteal plane for hemostasis. During this time, the surgeon begins operating on the opposite lower eyelid and cheek area to allow the anesthetic mixture to control hemostasis over the next 10 to 15 minutes. The gauze is then removed, and, using an

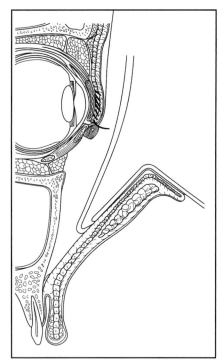

Figure 11-14.

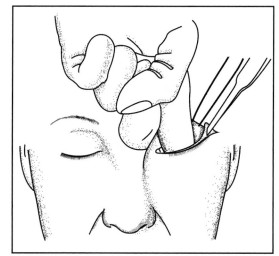

Figure 11-15.

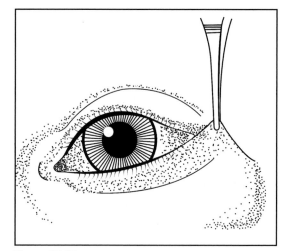

Figure 11-16.

Army-Navy retractor to expose the area of the dissection site, any remaining bleeders are cauterized.

TARSAL STRIP PROCEDURE

Step 1

The protective scleral contact lens is removed. A forceps is used to grasp the temporal aspect of the lower eyelid and to pull it temporally and slightly superior until slight tension of the eyelid is achieved (Figure 11-16). A scratch incision is made with a #11 Bard-Parker blade at the aspect of the lower eyelid margin that is now adjacent to the temporal cut edge of the upper eyelid margin (Figure 11-17). A measurement is made with a ruler from the temporal cut end of the lower eyelid to the scratch incision, which determines the length of the tarsal strip. (It is best to be conservative in the size of the tarsal strip—if it is under too much tension, there is more chance of lateral canthal deformities.)

Step 2

The surgeon then divides the eyelid into 2 lamellae by cutting with a Westcott scissors along the gray line from the temporal end of the eyelid to the scratch incision site (see Figure 11-17). The Westcott scissors is used to remove skin and orbi-

cularis from the anterior aspect of the tarsus of this eyelid segment (Figure 11-18). A disposable cautery is used to cut through conjunctiva, Müller's muscle, and capsulopalpebral fascia at the inferior tarsal edge. Bleeding is controlled with a disposable cautery. The surgeon scrapes the conjunctival epithelium on the posterior surface of the tarsus with a #15 Bard-Parker blade to prevent epithelial inclusion cysts (Figure 11-19).

Step 3

Each arm of a 4-0 polypropylene (Prolene) double-armed suture is passed internally to externally through the tarsal strip at the junction of the strip and eyelid (Figure 11-20). The strip is pulled temporally until the area of the polypropylene suture is adjacent to the lateral orbital wall. The strip is

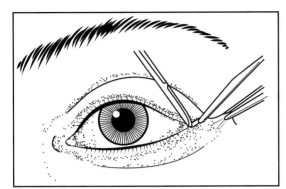

Figure 11-17.

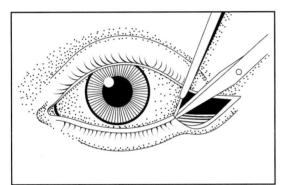

Figure 11-18.

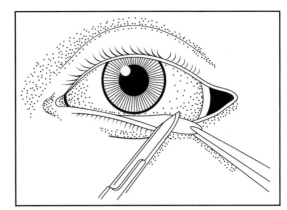

Figure 11-19.

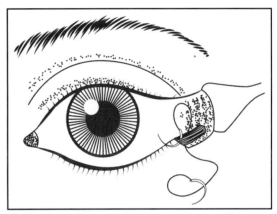

Figure 11-20.

drawn superiorly and internally until it seems to be in an acceptable position. The temporal lower eyelid should also be in contact with the eye, not displaced anterior to the eye. If the patient's eye is proptotic, as in thyroid disease, the tarsal strip should be placed more anteriorly than for a recessed or enophthalmic eye. Once the desired lateral position is determined, each arm of the 4-0 polypropylene suture is passed internally to externally through the lateral orbital periosteum or through the upper limb of the lateral canthal tendon at this position (Figure 11-21).

Step 4

The suture is tied with the first tie of the surgeon's knot over a 4-0 black suture knot-releasing suture (the piece of silk is approximately 5 cm long and does not have a needle attached to it). It is important, in placement of the tarsal strip, that the lower eyelid not retract further from the inferior corneal limbus and pull behind and under the eye. Excessive tension on the eyelid can lead to lower eyelid retraction.

Step 5

The cheek periosteal release and tarsal strip procedure is then performed on the opposite side.

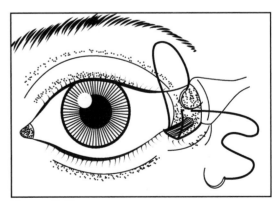

Figure 11-21.

Step 6

The patient is seated on the operating table, and the position of the lateral canthus is compared with the other side. The top of a metal ruler is aligned with each medial canthus, and the level at which the ruler bisects each lateral canthus is noted. The position of the lower eyelid adjacent to the eyes is also judged. If the lateral canthus is too high or low or

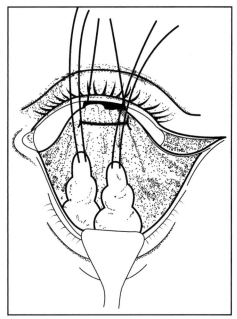

Figure 11-22.

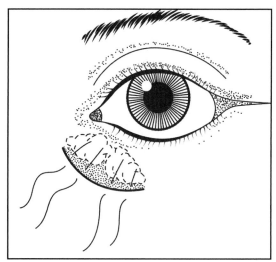

Figure 11-23.

too anterior or posterior, the knot-releasing suture is grasped with a forceps at each end of the 4-0 black silk suture and is pulled outward to release the knot. The suture arms are removed from the lateral wall periosteum or upper lateral canthal tendon and placed in a new position. This procedure is repeated until the desired position of the lateral canthus and lower eyelid is achieved.

REPOSITIONING OF THE NASAL AND CENTRAL LOWER EYELID FAT PADS

Step 7

If the nasal and central orbital fat has been removed, the conjunctiva is closed at this point. However, if there is a relatively deep inferior orbital hollowing or nasal-jugal fold, the nasal and central fat pads are repositioned at this point. The 4-0 knot releasing sutures is grasped with forceps at each end, and the 4-0 polypropylene tarsal strip suture is released. The nasal and central fat pads have their outer capsule opened, and, with blunt dissection with cotton-tipped applicators, a stalk of nasal and central orbital fat pads is formed. Each of these fat pads should easily slide inferiorly into the position of the inferior orbital rim hollowing. A 4-0 polypropylene (Prolene) double-armed suture is passed through the distal end of each of these fat pads (Figure 11-22). This needle passes through multiple bites of distal fat and is threaded so that as much of the distal end of the fat pad is captured with the needle and suture. Each arm of the 4-0 polypropylene suture on the nasal fat pad is passed over the maxillary bone to a position inferior to the hollowed inferior orbital

rim area and then through periosteum orbicularis muscle and out skin. The other 4-0 polypropylene suture that passes through the central fat pad is passed in a similar manner slightly more centrally than the first sutures (Figure 11-23). The needles are taped to the drape at this point.[3]

CONJUNCTIVAL CLOSURE

Step 1

The 4-0 silk suture that attaches conjunctiva, Müller's muscle, and capsulopalpebral fascia to the drape is then severed. Conjunctiva is reapproximated with 3 6-0 plain catgut buried sutures (Figure 11-24). Completion of tarsal strip is accomplished with a 5-0 chromic suture passed from the temporal end of the lower eyelid through the lower gray line several millimeters from the tarsal strip. The suture then is passed through the upper eyelid margin and exits at the cut edge at the temporal upper lid (Figure 11-25). When this suture is drawn up and tied, it reforms the angle of the lateral canthus, and the knot is buried.

Step 2

The polypropylene tarsal strip suture is then tied with approximately 4 knots. A 4-0 polyglactin (Vicryl) suture is passed through periosteum adjacent and temporal to the polypropylene knot. It is then passed through the tarsal strip internally to externally and is tied. This suture further secures the tarsal strip to periosteum and buries the polypropylene suture. The excessive tarsal strip temporal to the polyglactin suture is then severed (see Figure 11-25).

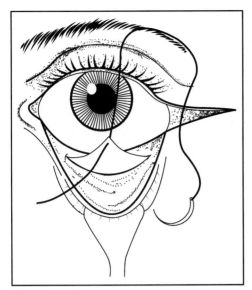

Figure 11-24.

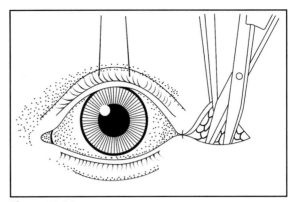

Figure 11-26.

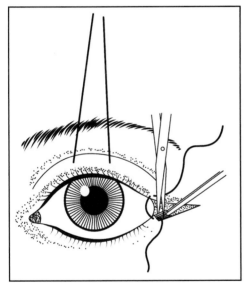

Figure 11-25.

FORMATION OF THE ORBICULARIS FLAP

Step 1

The orbicularis muscle of the lateral canthus is grasped with a forceps and pulled upward. A Westcott scissors is then used to dissect temporal lower eyelid and lateral canthal skin from the orbicularis (Figure 11-26). A small Desmarres retractor is then placed over this skin flap while the orbicularis is still being pulled upward and any bleeding is controlled with a disposable cautery. A 4-0 polypropylene double-armed suture is passed through periosteum over the lateral orbital wall

just temporal to the tarsal strip. A forceps is used to pull the orbicularis flap upward and outward to the point where the cheek and midface are in good position and the inferior orbital rim hollowing is resolved. This will determine the position that the suture will be placed through the orbicularis flap. One arm of the 4-0 polypropylene suture is then passed internally to externally through the orbicularis flap at the site where the flap now meets the lateral canthus. The same arm of the suture is then passed externally to internally (Figure 11-27). The suture is tied with 3 throws over a 4-0 black silk knot-releasing suture that has no needle and is approximately 5 cm long. The procedure is then performed on the opposite side. The patient then sits up on the operating table, and the positions of the cheek and midface are compared with each other. If one side is higher or lower than the other, then the knot-releasing suture is removed, and the suture is replaced until the desired effect is achieved. Once this is accomplished, the knot-releasing suture is removed, and the polypropylene sutures are tied with approximately 4 knots. Another 4-0 polypropylene suture is passed through temporalis fascia and lateral orbital wall just temporal to the first suture. The arm of the suture is then passed internally to externally through the orbicularis flap and then externally to internally so that when that suture is drawn up and tied, it further secures the orbicularis flap (Figure 11-28). If any dimpling occurs in the skin, then further dissection is carried out between the skin and orbicularis muscle until the dimple disappears (Figure 11-29).

Step 2

The part of the orbicularis flap that drapes over the lateral canthal skin is then severed, and bleeding is controlled with a disposable cautery (Figure 11-30). This places the suborbicularis orbital fat (SOOF) back into its normal position (Figure 11-31). A 6-0 Vicryl suture is then passed through orbicularis at the superior aspect of the lateral canthus and then internally to externally through the cut edge of the superior orbicularis flap. The suture is then passed externally to internally so that when the suture is

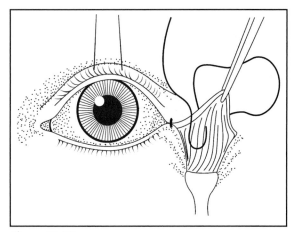

Figure 11-27.

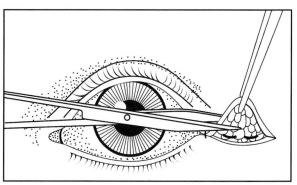

Figure 11-30.

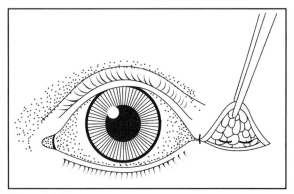

Figure 11-28.

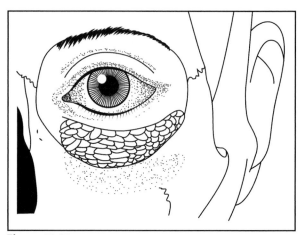

Figure 11-31.

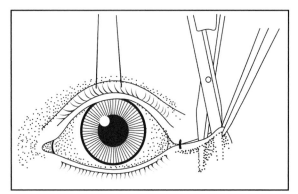

Figure 11-29.

drawn up and tied, it secures orbicularis to orbicularis and covers the polypropylene suture knots (Figure 11-32).

SKIN DISSECTION

Step 1

With a #15 Bard-Parker blade, the skin is incised about 2 mm beneath the cilia beginning 1 to 2 mm temporal to the punctum and extending across the horizontal length of the eyelid to 2 to 3 mm lateral to the lateral canthus (see Figure 11-32). The skin is dissected from orbicularis muscle with Westcott scissors (Figure 11-33). The correct subcutaneous plane is judged by observing the spread scissors blades through the translucent skin. With one blade of the scissors placed beneath the skin and the other at the skin edge, the subcutaneous attachments are severed. The skin usually is undermined from the orbicularis muscle to the level of the inferior orbital rim. If there is tenting of the orbicularis muscle, a small amount of superficial orbicularis is trimmed with Westcott scissors, and bleeding is controlled with a disposable cautery (Figure 11-34) (Solan Accu-Temp). The skin flap is then draped over the incision site while the assistant pushes on the eye by way of the contact lens; this pushes the lower lid upward and simulates its position on upgaze (Figure 11-35). The skin that drapes the incision is excised with a small vertical triangle along the inferior lash line and a larger lateral triangle temporal to the lateral canthus (Figures 11-36 and 11-37). To avoid an ectropion, it is better to tighten the

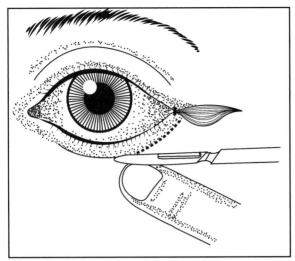

Figure 11-32.

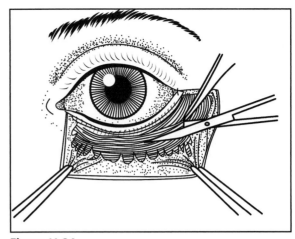

Figure 11-34.

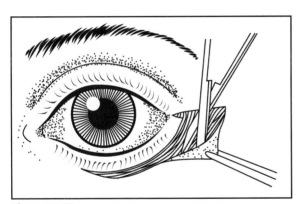

Figure 11-33.

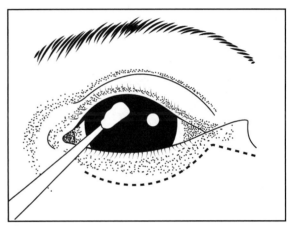

Figure 11-35.

lower eyelid skin with the lateral triangle than the vertical one.

SKIN CLOSURE

Step 2

A 6-0 black silk suture passes through the temporal lower eyelid skin at the lateral canthal angle site and catches a slight amount of orbicularis and tendon, as well. The suture is drawn up and tied with 3 knots, and only one end is cut. A 6-0 Vicryl suture is then passed through the temporal lower eyelid skin edges picking up a slight amount of the inferior tarsal border. When the suture is drawn up and tied, it unites the temporal skin with the inferior tarsal border and prevents over-riding of the lower eyelid skin. Several 6-0 Vicryl sutures are then passed through the skin edges over the area temporal to the lateral canthus. The 6-0 silk suture is then run continuously from lateral canthus to temporal wound edge. Another continuous 6-0 black suture is run continuously across the eyelid in a nasal to temporal direction with fewer bites because this incision site is under minimal tension (Figure 11-38).

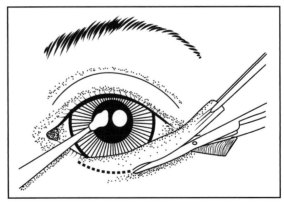

Figure 11-36.

COMPLETION OF FAT REPOSITIONING

If the fat has been repositioned, the 2 4-0 polypropylene sutures that are repositing the nasal and central orbital fat pads are tied with multiple knots over cotton pledgets to secure the fat in the hollowed areas (Figure 11-39).

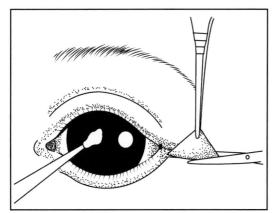

Figure 11-37.

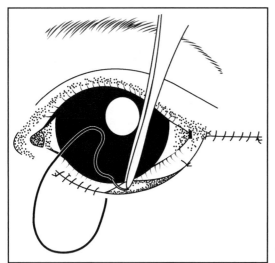

Figure 11-38.

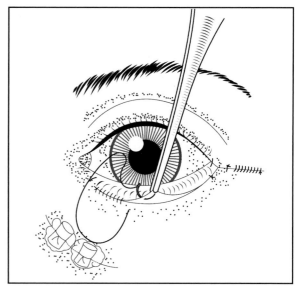

Figure 11-39.

The contact lenses are removed, and Garamycin ointment is applied over the suture sites and eyes. Cold compresses are applied.

Postoperative Care

No dressings are used after surgery. The patient is instructed to apply ice-cold compresses on the eyelids. Pads 4 x 4 inches soaked in a bucket of saline and ice are applied with slight pressure to the lids. When the pads become warm, they are dipped again into the saline and ice and reapplied. This process is repeated for 24 hours. The application should be fairly constant for the first few postoperative hours. After that, the compresses are applied for about 15 minutes with a 15-minute rest period in between until bedtime. The applications are resumed on awakening.

To reduce edema postoperatively, the patient lies in bed with the head approximately 45° higher than the rest of the body. I also routinely use systemic steroids and antibiotics after surgery. Nurses should check for bleeding

associated with proptosis, pain, or loss of vision every 15 minutes for the first 3 hours postoperatively or until the patient leaves the surgical facility. Every hour thereafter until bedtime, the family or patient should monitor the patient's ability to count fingers and should check for unusual proptosis and pain. If the patient cannot count fingers or has proptosis or pain, the family should take him or her to the emergency room. If loss of vision occurs secondary to retrobulbar hemorrhage, it can be detected quickly and treated by opening the incision involved.[5]

The 6-0 black silk sutures are removed 6 days postoperatively. The 4-0 polypropylene sutures that reposition the fat are removed at the same time. The 6-0 polyglactin sutures are removed 3 weeks postoperatively, if they have not dissolved by this point.

Complications

Patients should be aware that they may have an Asian appearance immediately after surgery, which should resolve spontaneously. They should also be told that they may still have a slight puckering or dimpling at the temporal lower eyelid from the polypropylene cheek sutures, which should resolve spontaneously after a few months. If it does not, further skin dissection or removal of sutures can be performed. Occasionally, patients will have discomfort or an inflammatory reaction from the buried polypropylene sutures. If this is the case, they can always be removed. The incision site under the eyelashes usually heals quite well. Should there be any unusual scarring in the lateral canthal area, excision and revision of this can be done.

I have had several patients who have had paresthesia over the cheek area immediately postoperatively, which resolved within 1 month. I have also had several patients who have had webbing or rounding of the lateral canthal area, which has responded to a small lateral canthotomy and suturing of the temporal cut ends of skin and conjunctiva together. I have had one patient with a lower eyelid cicatricial ectropion and retraction from a previous procedure that developed postoperative diplopia. This resolved spontaneously.

In all of the procedures that I have performed, I have not had any long-term complications.

ASIAN BLEPHAROPLASTY
THE ESSENTIAL STEPS

William P. Chen, MD, FACS

The aesthetic procedure of creating an upper eyelid crease in an Asian without a crease has traditionally carried the Chinese term meaning "double eyelid surgery." It has evolved over the past century from using buried suture ligatures into a more anatomically based form of cosmetic blepharoplasty. In Asian countries, it is one of the most frequently performed aesthetic procedures. I first coined the term *Asian blepharoplasty* in 1987[1] while attempting to define the skills and pitfalls necessary for performing primary and revisional surgery in Asians. Various terms like *"double eyelid surgery," inner crease,* and *outer crease* had been used, but lack the precision needed to discuss this topic in a coherent fashion. This chapter will concentrate on the external incision method as it yields more predictable results.[2-5]

Anatomy of the Asian Eyelid, Incidence of Crease, and Crease Shape

On average, within a family, there is approximately a 50% prevalence of upper eyelid crease, and this seems to generalize to Asian populations who are of Han background (Chinese, Korean, Japanese). There are geographical variations in incidence of crease, ranging from 25% to 80% or more, but the overall incidence of 50% seems to hold true in my clinical experience. The vertical height of the upper tarsus is typically between 6.5 and 7.5 mm, with a rare exception of 8 to 9 mm. This is in contrast to the average dimension in non-Asians of 9 to 10.5 mm.

The current consensus on the distinguishing features of an upper eyelid with crease versus one without crease, at least in Asians, seem to be the presence or absence of terminal interdigitations[6] of levator aponeurotic fibers

into the pretarsal orbicularis oculi intermuscular septae and fibers, located in an area just slightly below or along the upper border of the tarsal plate (superior tarsal border) (Figure 12-1).

Asians who possess a natural crease tend to manifest either a nasally tapered crease or a parallel crease. The nasally tapered crease (Figure 12-2) is a natural, low-set crease that runs parallel across the ciliary margin over the central and lateral portion of the upper lid, while over the medial portion it converges inward toward the medial canthus, often blending into a small ethnic medial canthal fold of upper lid skin. The parallel crease (Figure 12-3) runs parallel across the ciliary border, and, over the medial portion, it simply runs independent to and above any residual medial canthal fold.

Both of these crease shapes are different from the semilunar crease typically seen in Occidentals. The latter's upper eyelid typically shows a semilunar crease line on the skin on downgaze, though they may manifest with either a parallel shape or semilunar shape when viewed straight on.

Preoperative Assessment

It is common to see patients with asymmetry of the upper eyelid and its crease, asymmetry of fat and soft tissues (skin and orbicularis) between the 2 sides, asymmetry in shape, with possible presence of latent ptosis, differences in palpebral width and height, and even different degrees of upper lash rotation when comparing the 2 sides.

A detailed history should be taken, going over the goals of the procedure from the patient's view point, as well as a physical exam documenting the various factors mentioned above. I note the shape of the face, its size, the position of the brow, and separation from the upper lid margin. The

Levine MR.
Manual of Oculoplastic Surgery, Fourth Edition (pp 97-102).
© 2010 SLACK Incorporated

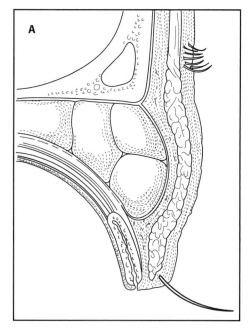

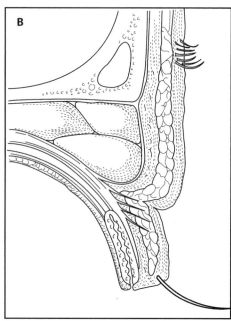

Figure 12-1.

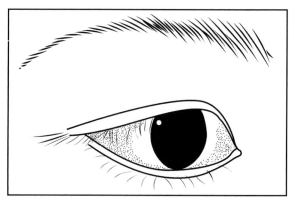

Figure 12-2.

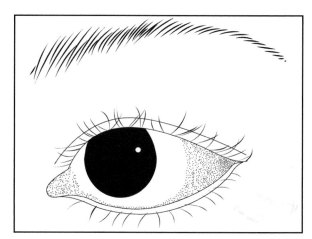

Figure 12-3.

observations are combined into a recommendation for the patient. A surgically constructed crease that does not invaginate as well can result from borderline levator function without the presence of true anatomic ptosis. Patients are shown before-and-after pictures and various stages of the healing process so that their expectations are real. Photos are taken for documentation.

Anesthesia

Local anesthesia is typically used. Preoperative oral medications include a combination of 10 mg of Valium and 1 tablet of Vicodin (or 1000 mg of acetaminophen) given 1 hour before the procedure.

The local anesthetic is 2% Xylocaine with 1:100,000 dilution of epinephrine. A 30-gauge needle is used, and the volume injected is seldom more than 1 mL for each eyelid.

A controlled flow of room air is supplied through a nasal cannula. An intravenous line is inserted in the event that further sedation is necessary.

Surgical Technique

Step 1

Mark the desired eyelid crease—The crease marking involves precise measurement of the vertical height of the central portion of the everted upper eyelid tarsus (Figure 12-4).

Typically, the central tarsal height is between 6.5 and 7.5 mm, with an occasional patient manifesting 8 to 8.5 mm. I decide on the crease height I will use; typically, 7 mm is most often chosen based on patients' stated preference during their initial consultations. A higher or lower crease will be no more than 0.5 mm on either side of this average. This central measurement is then marked on the skin side and determines the overall height of the crease, whether we are planning a "nasally tapered crease" or a "parallel crease." The nasally tapered crease is chosen in more than two thirds of my patients and is easier to mark and execute in my hands. The crease shape is simply merged toward the medial canthus. For a parallel crease shape design, the

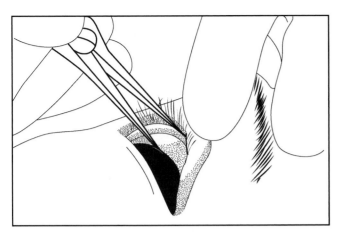

Figure 12-4.

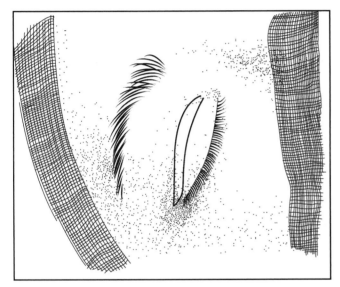

Figure 12-5.

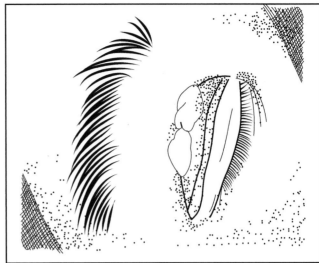

Figure 12-6.

on a monopolar cautery (Bovie), with low setting on the cut mode, to make the transection through orbicularis. The tip is intentionally beveled upward along the orbicularis so that the orbital septum is reached along a higher level from the level of the superior tarsal border (Figure 12-6). The cautery tip is likely to reach the preaponeurotic fat pad rather than injuring the levator aponeurosis with this maneuver, and it allows one to readily identify the preaponeurotic space. This step of beveled transection through preseptal orbicularis oculi constitutes my first vector.[7] The orbicularis typically is the most vascular layer, and it is worthwhile to be meticulous in controlling bleeding here with the bipolar cautery.

Step 4

Approaching and opening of the orbital septum— Preseptal fat is often seen co-mixed with orbicularis fibers plus fascial tissues and can misdirect the surgeon into believing that it is the deeper preaponeurotic fat. The latter fat is distinctly globular, fluctuant, and easily prolapses through small rants in the orbital septum as one reaches it. The septum is opened horizontally with a blunt spring scissors (Westcott), making sure that one is slanting the septal cut upward to avoid cutting blood vessels in the fat pads and not slanting downward and inadvertently injuring vessels of the aponeurosis or the aponeurosis itself (Figure 12-7).

Step 5

Handling of the fat pads—After the septum is opened horizontally, the fragment of tissues bounded by the upper skin incision and transorbicularis first vector can be rotated away from the underlying levator to form a myocutaneous strip. A tissue retractor is applied on the myocutaneous strip to explore the preaponeurotic space. Within the space, one may observe fluctuant preaponeurotic fat, or amorphous, bound-down fatty strands, or smaller "islands" of fat. Depending

surgeon should make a conscious effort to stay parallel to the lash line as one approaches the medial canthus. A segment of redundancy is included in the line of excision, typically a segment of skin measuring about 2 mm centrally, 2.5 mm laterally, and 1 mm medially. Most of the tissue swelling from the local anesthetic's infiltration should have subsided by this point in the procedure.

Step 2

Make a skin incision—The incision is made using a #15 surgical blade along the upper and lower lines of skin marking (Figure 12-5). A dry 4 x 4 dressing is used to stabilize the skin layer during this step. The blade tip cuts through the skin in a full-thickness fashion and stops just when the fascial tissues overlying the orbicularis oculi are reached. The entire length of the incision often requires several positioning and repositioning steps, demanding utmost precision.

Step 3

Transection through orbicularis along the upper edge of skin incision—I use a Colorado needle tip

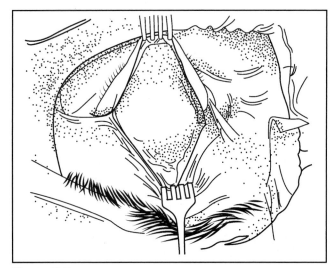

Figure 12-7.

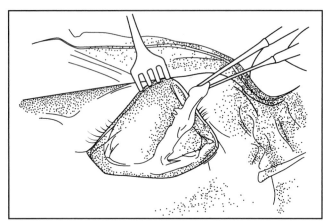

Figure 12-8.

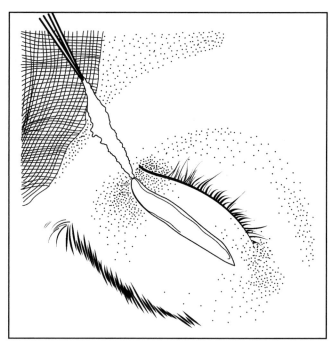

Figure 12-9.

edge of the skin incision, I would trim off some inferior orbicularis fibers so that it will be less likely to interfere with the crease construction (Figure 12-9).

In summary, with skin incision and only 2 additional steps (first vector through the orbicularis and septum, second vector through the orbicularis), one can complete a beveled excision of these layers: skin and orbicularis oculi as a trapezoidal fragment and fragment of orbital septum overlying the distal 4 to 5 mm of the levator aponeurosis. Bleeding is controlled along the 2 planes involving transection through the vascular orbicularis.

Step 7

Resetting of tissue plane—This is an important step in primary as well as revisional Asian blepharoplasty.[9] After the redundant skin and muscle have been appropriately trimmed and the preaponeurotic fat reduced or reposited, it is essential to reset the tissue planes by positioning the anterior skin properly in relation to the underlying aponeurosis. This resetting maneuver avoids lagophthalmos or induction of secondary ptosis. This is because the original operative field may have been isolated using surgical drapes, towels, and adhesive drapes; and, therefore, the surgeon may often end up attaching the skin edges at a higher spatial point of attachment along the aponeurosis rather than just above the superior tarsal border. This results in an overly high crease and a secondary ptosis; an arched eyebrow can then be seen as the frontalis muscles then become overactive. In revisional cases, this resetting allows some skin recruitment and brings in additional soft tissues to partially fill in any prominent sulcus from fat excision associated with aggressive blepharoplasty.

on the preoperative evaluation of the sulcus as well as brow relationship to the upper lid margin, one may decide to (A) reposit all preaponeurotic fat, or (B) partially excise some preaponeurotic fat along the superior tarsal border, creating a clearance along the preaponeurotic platform[7] (Figure 12-8), or (C) when fat strands or islands of fat are observed, it is dissected and allowed to retract upward to fill in the sulcus. This maneuver often seems to greatly facilitate the glide mechanism (glide plane) of the levator relative to the anterior skin lamella, allowing an eyelid crease to indent dynamically against a passively relaxed preseptal skin-muscle layer (the eyelid fold).[8]

Step 6

Excision and debulking of the preaponeurotic platform (myocutaneous strip)—The myocutaneous strip of tissue redundancy (2 mm skin plus a larger fragment of preseptal orbicularis oculi just above the upper tarsus) can be excised along the superior tarsal border using a bovie cautery tip. This cut through the lower edge of the orbicularis strip is named the second vector and completes the trapezoidal debulking of the preaponeurotic platform.[7] If there is some residual fullness along the lower

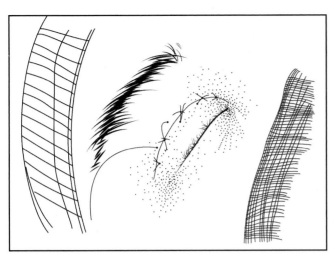

Figure 12-10.

Step 8

Wound closure and crease construction—The crease shape and height are controlled through accurate design as well as meticulous application of crease-forming sutures. I favor the soft texture of 6-0 silk sutures for this purpose. They are applied from the lower skin edge, through the aponeurosis along the superior tarsal border, and through the upper skin edge. Then, they are tied down (Figure 12-10). Six to 9 interrupted sutures are typically used. The rest of the wound can be closed using 7-0 Prolene, nylon, or silk. Topical antibiotic-steroid ointment may be applied for 1 week. Suture removal is usually in 1 week.

During this last step, the crease height is repeatedly measured and compared with the other side to verify symmetry, and adjustment is always made toward the lower measurement of the 2 sides. It is not unusual to find that when one is finishing up on the second side, the crease height on the first side (which has been covered with ice-saline sponges) may measure 0.5-mm lower. I do not use any buried crease fixation suture, even in revisional cases.

Summary

My technique includes the following:

❀ Accurate definition of the crease height and shape determines the visible component of the procedure, as well as outcome and measurable success rate.

❀ A layered and differential debulking of the eyelid tissues makes the completion of these essential steps more efficient and sure-proof. Less hemorrhage and injury of tissues are encountered. It establishes the proper orientation and spatial geometry of the semirigid pretarsal skin and tarsus (posterior lamella, vectored by the levator muscle) relative to the more passive preseptal and periorbital orbicularis (anterior lamella) when the eyelids are opened.

❀ Repositing the preaponeurotic fat and resetting of the eyelid skin and forehead structures relative to the posterior lamella are critical steps in preventing complications associated with this type of aesthetic surgery. It allows for the proper height and crease shape to be achieved as planned. It helps soften the deeper sulcus appearance seen in revisional cases.

❀ Exact anastomosis of levator aponeurosis to lid crease incision along the superior tarsal border. The precise execution of this last point provides a higher probability for a successful outcome.

The proper execution of these 8 steps allows one to create a natural-looking eyelid crease, from an aesthetic as well as anatomic standpoint, without the use of permanent or buried static sutures.

CHAPTER 13

PERIOCULAR REJUVENATION WITH DERMAL FILLERS AND TRICHLOROACETIC ACID

Alan M. Lessner, MD

Dermal fillers offer an adjunctive and sometimes alternative treatment for unwanted contours of a variety of facial regions, including the periorbita. Rather than remove tissue with traditional blepharoplasty and other rhytidectomy methods, volume augmentation can correct tear trough asymmetries and improve the appearance of wrinkles, folds, and depressed scars. Other areas just beyond the periorbita can also be improved by injectable soft tissue agents including atrophy of midface and cheek that contribute to the appearance of an aged upper and midface.

Filler Products

COLLAGEN (ZYDERM/ZYPLAST, COSMODERM/COSMOPLAST, EVOLENCE)

The first used and popularized agents for facial rejuvenation were derivatives of bovine collagen. These products are composed of collagen fibrils made from bovine skin in a mixture of lidocaine. Double skin testing is recommended due to the heterologous nature of these products (bovine is potentially immunogenic). These injectable agents are nonpermanent, bioabsorptive substances that are useful in the treatment of facial lines and scars, as well as lip enhancement. Duration of enhancement varies from 2 to 6 months with the need to repeat maintenance injections. Zyplast (glutaraldehyde cross-linked) is more viscous than Zyderm, with slightly longer duration. Human-derived analogs are currently available that are manufactured identically to these products (Cosmoderm and Cosmoplast) and are also used for fine lines, whereas Cosmoplast (as with Zyplast) is used to treat deeper rhytides and folds. Evolence, a ribose cross-linked porcine collagen, has recently been approved; however, applications,

injection techniques, and longevity are more similar to that of hyaluronans (below).

Procedure

More often, the anesthetic contained within these products is sufficient to reduce pain and deems the procedure more tolerable as injecting proceeds. Those individual patients with a lower pain threshold may benefit from topical or regional anesthetics. Serial puncture technique is a common method of administration (Figure 13-1A) although many other injection techniques are useful, depending on injector preference. The depth of injection should be in the dermal plane to achieve optimal and prolonged results. Although patients can obtain satisfactory results with one treatment, better and more long-lasting results at times can be achieved with 2 treatments administered to a patient within 2 to 6 weeks to compensate for the transient effects of the agent. A very small percentage of patients will be (or become) allergic to the bovine material even after negative skin testing. Adverse reactions may include transient or long-term redness and swelling; intravascular incidents can mostly be avoided with good injection technique and may result in focal tissue necrosis and scarring.

HYALURONIC ACID (INCLUDING JUVEDERM ULTRA, JUVEDERM ULTRA PLUS, RESTYLANE, PERLANE, PREVELLE PLUS, ELEVESSE HYLAFORM, HYLAFORM PLUS)

The family of hyaluronans (ie, hyaluronic acid injectable agents) are biocompatible, natural components of the skin with hydrophilic properties, and they have been shown to be highly effective agents for facial soft tissue augmentation. Early experiences applied these agents more commonly to the nasolabial folds and perioral

Levine MR.
Manual of Oculoplastic Surgery, Fourth Edition (pp 103-106).
© 2010 SLACK Incorporated

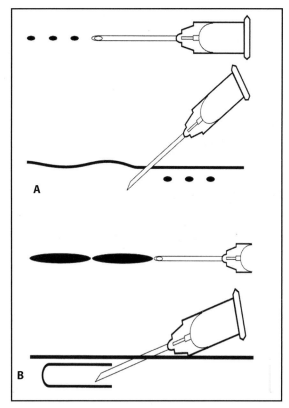

Figure 13-1.

immediate subcutaneous space with sometimes as much as 2 cc (or more) per side.

As always, understanding the regional anatomy and a careful and methodical injection plan with continued awareness of the needle placement to avoid unwanted complications (ie, intravascular injections) will result in safer and more effective treatments.

Chemical Peel of the Eyelid and Periorbital Region

Chemical exfoliation or peeling is a useful adjunct to treatment of lower eyelid rhytides and dyschromia of the eyelid skin. The purpose of this technique is similar to laser resurfacing—to ablate the skin causing a second-degree burn with subsequent collagen remodeling and epithelialization, but in a "gentler," less invasive manner. Recovery of the skin, including normalization of skin pigmentation, is usually in one third the time, when compared to carbon dioxide resurfacing.

Chemical peeling is commonly combined with trans-conjunctival lower eyelid blepharoplasty in lieu of trans-cutaneous resection of lower eyelid skin. Care must be taken to address any laxity of the lower eyelid with pro-phylactic canthoplasty or canthopexy to prevent lower eyelid retraction or ectropion. The risk of hypo- or hyper-pigmentation is relative to the Fitzpatrick skin type of the patient.

The safest peeling agent in the author's opinion is tri-chloroacetic acid (TCA), usually 20% to 40% in concentration. This agent can be compounded at a local pharmacy and is stored in an amber bottle to prevent degradation. It is best to use a fresh bottle, made within several days of the procedure.

TECHNIQUE

The TCA peel can be applied to the eyelids, periocular region, or entire face primarily or in conjunction with blepharoplasty. The blepharoplasty is performed first, relying on the local lidocaine or Marcaine used to keep the skin anesthetized for the peel. Alternatively, TCA peel can be applied directly without local infiltration of anesthetic. Typically, patients describe the peeling sensation as a stinging type of discomfort that is generally well tolerated.

The skin is defatted with acetone applied to the skin prior to applying the TCA peel. Care should be taken to shut off any electrical cautery or oxygen prior to exposing the patient to flammable acetone. After the acetone is applied, it is recommended that it be removed from the operating area to lessen the risk of mistaken application or fire.

Next, protective eye shields are kept over the patient's eyes to protect them during application of the TCA peel. The peel can be placed in a sterile glass medicine bowl and applied with sterile cotton-tipped applicators. Dip the applicator into the TCA bowl, saturating the cotton tip. Touch the saturated tip to a gauze pad or surgical towel to wick up any excess peeling solution to prevent unintend-ed dripping or misapplication. The moistened cotton tip is then gently applied to the eyelid skin in a pattern parallel

crevices; however, they have now been shown to be satisfactory treatments for a variety of aging regions of the upper and lower periorbita and mid- and lower face. Hyaluronans are longer-lasting and less allergenic than animal-derived collagen. No skin testing is required. The currently available agents have unique properties that relate to injectability, gel hardness, concentration, cross-linking, and the accompaniment of local anesthesia. As implied, some agents are better in certain facial regions than others, and duration can be highly variable depending on the agent, region, and injection technique.

Procedure

The injection techniques, although vaguely similar to collagen for the host of facial folds and wrinkles, depend very much on the product used, the region treated, and the injection technique. Although several of these agents have local anesthetic already contained in the syringe, there seems to be a significant advantage to giving regional or local anesthetic blocks prior to treatment that not only is effective in pain management, but that also has a beneficial effect in reducing bruising. Certain areas like the tear trough are best suited to multiple serial puncture injections, approximately 0.5 cc (ranging from 0.2 cc to more than 1 cc) per side to the supraperiosteal inferior orbital rim, and can fill the hollow effectively, creating a smooth transition from eyelid to cheek. The eyebrow region is best treated with a deep dermal injection in a threading technique (either inject as you advance or withdraw to deposit a smooth confluence of product over the region requiring less massage; Figure 13-1B). The midface is best addressed by sufficient inflationary volume to the deep dermis or to the eyelid margin, similar to the way laser resurfacing spots are applied. The malar region is feathered with peeling agent to prevent a stark line of demarcation.

The titrating endpoint for depth of peel is a white frost reaction to the skin. As soon as the skin turns white, Aquaphor ointment is applied to neutralize the reaction of the peel.

Postoperatively, the patient is instructed to apply Aquaphor ointment approximately 8 times a day.

COSMETIC USES OF
BOTULINUM TOXIN

Jill A. Foster, MD, FACS; Wilbur Huang, MD; Julian D. Perry, MD; David E. E. Holck, MD; and Allan E. Wulc, MD, FACS

Botulinum toxin (BoTX) has many applications for treating unwanted facial features that are created by muscle action. These include kinetic facial wrinkle lines, prominent orbicularis in the lower eyelids, depression of the lateral oral commissure, dimpling of the chin, and brow ptosis. BoTX-A is a safe and effective treatment for hyperfunctional glabellar frown lines, crow's feet, and forehead lines. BoTX-A may also be used to soften platysma bands, improve mild eyelid ptosis, diminish migraine headache, and treat palmar and axillary hyperhidrosis. The applications of this medication will continue to expand.

There are several types of facial wrinkling: gravitational redundancy, intrinsic aging with loss of elasticity, sleep creases, and dynamic facial lines. Dynamic lines induced by muscle contraction is the type of wrinkling most amenable to BoTX treatment. These dynamic facial wrinkles occur perpendicular to the force of muscle contraction. It is theorized that repeated creasing of the skin over time induces changes in the dermal structure, resulting in the eventual formation of a crease line at rest as well as deepening of the crease when the muscle is contracted. BoTX works by preventing the expression of impulses from the motor neurons to the neuromuscular junction. Injection of the solution results in a temporary weakening of muscle contractions in the area of the injection.

Muscle weakening diminishes the dynamic wrinkles but also has cosmetic applications for changing facial shape. Brow elevation is accomplished by selectively denervating the depressor muscles of the brow, resulting in unopposed frontalis action. The corners of the lips may be elevated by decreasing the action of the depressor anguli oris. Relaxing the contraction of the lower eyelid orbicularis will soften the prominence of the lower eyelid orbicularis that becomes apparent with smiling and contraction of the muscle. Meticulous knowledge of the actions and interactions of the facial musculature allows the physician to selectively modify facial features dependent on muscle contraction.

Pharmacology

Neurotoxins produced by the gram-positive, anaerobic *Clostridium botulinum* are the most potent toxins known to mankind and are the causative agents of botulism. BoTX acts by blocking the release of acetylcholine from the presynaptic terminal of the neuromuscular junction. Seven distinct antigenic BoTX (BoTX-A, -B, -C, -D, -E, -F, and -G) produced by different strains of *Clostridium botulinum* have been described. The human nervous system is susceptible to 5 toxin serotypes (BoTX-A, -B, -E, -F, and -G) and unaffected by 2 (BoTX-C and -D).

All serotypes act on the peripheral nervous system where they inhibit release of acetylcholine from the presynaptic terminal of the neuromuscular junction. There are 3 steps involved in neurotoxicity. The first step is the irreversible binding of BoTX to presynaptic cholinergic receptors via the H chain's 50-kDa carboxy-terminal. The second step involves internalization of the neurotoxin through a receptor-mediated endocytosis. This process is independent of calcium and is partially dependent on nerve stimulation. After internalization, the disulfide bond is cleaved by an unknown mechanism. The third step is neuromuscular blockade. Within the synapse, isoforms of proteins form a complex platform for docking and fusion of acetylcholine vesicles to the cell membrane before they can be released. With BoTX-A, clinical expression of the effects typically takes 24 to 48 hours, and maximal muscle weakening is not seen for a week. The onset of action for BoTX-B is more rapid, but the duration is shorter.

Levine MR.
Manual of Oculoplastic Surgery, Fourth Edition (pp 107-112).
© 2010 SLACK Incorporated

The dose of BoTX is measured in units (U). The units are a biologic designation related to the lethal dose in similarly sized rodents. The effects of BoTX are species specific, and the units of one toxin do not directly correspond to the units of another. Individual experience with each type of toxin guides dosing.

Preparations

There are currently 3 commercially available BoTX preparations in the United States: 2 types of BoTX type A and one preparation of BoTX type B. BoTX type A made by Allergan is called onabotulinumtoxinA, and Dysport, designated abobotulinumtoxinA, and one preparation of BoTX-B, rimabotulinum B or Myobloc. Because Botox (Allergan, Inc, Irvine, CA) was the first BoTX widely used for treatment in humans, subsequently released BoTX are compared to the dosing levels for Botox. Dysport was recently approved (2009) for use for facial lines, and early experience suggests a 3 to 1 dosing ratio for Dysport as compared to Botox. Comparable dosing for Myobloc and Botox may be in the range of 50 to 100 U of Myobloc to 1 U of Botox. During the next decade, it is likely that other formulations of BoTX-A will become available. Merz and Mentor are actively developing additional formulations of BoTX type A. In clinical use of the BoTX, it is important to remember that while related, different BoTX are all structurally different, and even at what are felt to be comparable dosing levels, results cannot be exactly predicted based on experience with a different toxin molecule.

Each vial of Botox contains 100 MU of *Clostridium* BoTX type A (with 10% variability), 0.5 mg of human albumin, and 0.9 mg of sodium chloride in a sterile, vacuum-dried form without a preservative. The vials are stored in the freezer or are refrigerated before reconstitution for clinical use. The recommended diluent is nonpreserved or preserved normal saline. Preserved saline may diminish injection discomfort. After reconstitution, the product is stored in the refrigerator at 2°C to 8°C, and the manufacturer's labeling recommends use within 4 hours of reconstitution. The concentration of the material is dependent on the volume of added saline and is typically described by how many units are present in 0.1 cc. For cosmetic uses, the reported concentrations of the solution vary from 1 U/0.1 cc to 10 U/0.1 cc. The reported volumes of solutions used for cosmetic indications vary from 0.025 mL to greater than 1.0 mL per site. The effects of BoTX type A are dependent on the location, concentration, and the volume of solution that is injected.

Dysport is available in vials of 300 U of lypholized obotulinum toxin type A that is stabilized with 125 μg of human serum albumin and 2.5 mg lactose. The product is reconstituted with sterile saline. The product insert suggests unpreserved saline, but preserved saline may be used. This preparation also recommends refrigerated storage and use within 4 hours of reconstitution. The concentration is determined by the amount of saline used to reconstitute the material. One common method would be to use 1.5 cc of saline, resulting in a Dysport solution with a concentration of 10 U per 0.05 cc of solution.

Myobloc is the only commercially available preparation of BoTX-B and is supplied as a sterile injectable solution in 3.5-mL glass vials. The vials are available in 2500 U, 5000 U, and 10,000 U volumes. The BoTX-B is in solution with 0.05% human, serum albumin, 0.01 M sodium succinate, and 0.1 M sodium chloride at pH 5.6. The bottles are all ready-to-use solutions and do not require reconstitution. Myobloc is stable for 21 months in refrigerator storage. Myobloc is US Food and Drug Administration approved for use in cervical dystonia. BoTX-B has a faster onset than BoTX-A, but the duration of action is noticeably shorter at 7 to 8 weeks, making its use for cosmetic applications limited.

Treatment Techniques

BoTX is administered by injection. To choose the site of injection to treat wrinkles, the patient is asked to squeeze and relax the muscles in the affected area. The surgeon identifies the location of maximal skin displacement during the contraction of the muscle. The solution is injected at that point and into the muscle rather than into the crease line. Unlike "filler" techniques, the BoTX should be aimed at the muscle rather than the crease to be most effective. The injection should go into the muscle layer or into the subdermal tissue just above the muscle in the areas where the facial skin is thin. The muscles are relaxed before injection to decrease the pain of the injection. The patient experiences the discomfort of the needle stick followed by a localized "stinging" as the solution is injected. There may also be some pressure sensation from the volume of the fluid injected. Some physicians believe that smaller volumes of injection are less painful. The onset of action is variable from patient to patient and different from one injection to another in the same patient, but most notice alteration in muscle contraction within 24 to 48 hours. In research studies, the maximal response in muscle weakness does not occur for 7 days with BoTX-A. The muscle weakening effects of BoTX-A are temporary and typically resolve 3 to 5 months after the injection.

When the patient begins to notice the changes from the BoTX injection, there are 2 phases of the response. The early alteration in the dynamic wrinkle lines comes from a relaxation of the resting tone to the muscle, decreased force of contraction, and perhaps shift in the tissue fluids. The second and more chronic process is remodeling of the dermis that should occur when the mechanical pressure of the contraction is relaxed. In addition to decreasing the wrinkle lines that are present, prolonged use of BoTX should prevent further deepening of the creases. This makes BoTX one of the few preparations that will truly prevent visible signs of aging. The astute observer also notices an aesthetically pleasing change in the skin texture in the area of injection, perhaps initiated by vasodilation. The most dramatic responses to treatment are seen in patients in the age ranges of 30 to 50 years. In these cases, the injections may obliterate the kinetic lines. With deeper wrinkles, treatment with BoTX flattens the edges of the indentation, but additional filler techniques are usually necessary to make the area smooth.

Side effects of BoTX include localized effects of the injection and those that occur when there is inadvertent spread of the BoTX to the surrounding facial neuromuscular junctions. Small hematomas may occur when blood

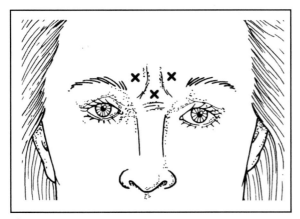

Figure 14-1.

vessels are inadvertently injured by the injection needle. Redness and soft tissue swelling are temporary effects of the injection. The volume of the injection and the location of the injection are planned to minimize unwanted spread to the surrounding muscles. Avoid the levator muscle, the extraocular muscles, excessive weakening of the orbicularis, inadvertent treatment of the depressor labii of the lower lip, and weakening the zygomaticus major/minor complex. When unexpected extension of the paresis does occur, the patient may experience eyelid ptosis, ectropion, corneal exposure, epiphora, brow ptosis, diplopia, decreased strength of oral closure, lip droop, and drooling. Although many of these complications have not yet been reported in cosmetic patients, they have been seen in the patients who receive therapeutic injections. The incidence of unplanned spread of the neurotoxin in the cosmetic patients is low, but postinjection ptosis has been reported.

BoTX has been used to treat glabellar folds, lateral periocular rhytides, lower eyelid orbicularis ridges, brow ptosis, eyelid ptosis, horizontal forehead wrinkles, perioral lines, mouth corner depression, and platysmal bands in the neck. It can be used as a singular therapy or in conjunction with other cosmetic surgical interventions.

BoTX can be used to augment the results of laser resurfacing, chemical peels, collagen injections, other wrinkle "filler" techniques, endoscopic forehead surgery, and lower eyelid blepharoplasty. The treatment techniques discussed in this chapter are starting points and should be modified by the injecting surgeon based on experience and patient response.

Injection Technique for Glabellar Folds

Glabellar folds develop from the repeated contraction of the corrugator, orbicularis, and procerus muscles. The vertical folds are from the corrugators, and the horizontal folds across the bridge of the nose come from the procerus. The patient is asked to squeeze and relax these muscles, and the location of the anterior bulge of the muscles is noted. This is typically approximately 5 mm lateral to the vertical wrinkle lines. The patient may have 2 or more vertical wrinkle lines. The 2 sides of the face may

be asymmetric, and the injection sites may be modified to accommodate for the asymmetry. The procerus is usually injected centrally between the 2 brows just above the bridge of the nose. The corrugators are injected at the site of the bunching of the muscle. Injection sites for the glabellar region are demonstrated in Figure 14-1. In the glabella, the concentration of Botox solution is 5 to 10 U/0.1 cc, and the volume injected is 0.05 to 0.10 cc per site.

Dosing descriptions for the techniques will refer to Botox. Twenty to 30 U of Botox is a typical total injection dose for the glabellar region. To get a starting dose for Dysport, multiply the Botox units used by 2.5 to 3. As the physician's experience with Dysport increases, he or she automatically begins to think in Dysport units rather than having to translate from Botox units. Some references describe a 2.5 to 1 ratio for Dysport dosing. When starting to use Dysport, this more conservative approach may be used. The authors of this chapter have found that sometimes a ratio of 3 to 1 seems to produce better results. Remember that Botox and Dysport are structurally different preparations of BoTX, and these suggested doses are just a starting point. It is not appropriate to expect the different toxins to create the exact same results. The suggested starting dose for Dysport for the glabella is 50 U.

Injection Technique for Horizontal Forehead Wrinkles

Horizontal forehead rhytides may also be treated. These result from repeated contraction of the frontalis muscle. Injecting the frontalis may change brow position. Symmetric treatment for the 2 sides is recommended. This is particularly true for the patient's first injection until the physician can assess the response to the injection locations. The patient is asked to wrinkle up the brow as if surprised, and an alternating pattern above and below the crease lines is injected across the central forehead. Injection sites for the forehead are demonstrated in Figure 14-2. The concentration of the forehead injections is 2.5 to 5 U Botox per 0.1 cc. The volume injected is 0.025 cc per site. Typically, 5 to 15 U total of Botox are used in the central forehead. Occasionally, avoidance of more laterally placed injections (to avoid a brow ptosis) will result in overelevation of the lateral brow (the "Spock" effect), requiring some additional secondary weakening of the frontalis. The suggested starting dose for Dysport for the forehead is 25 U.

Injection Technique for Lateral Periocular Wrinkles (Crow's Feet)

Crow's feet lines are diminished by treating the lateral orbicularis muscles. The concentration of the solution is 5 U/0.1 cc, and the volume per injection site is 0.025 to 0.05 cc per site. The injection sites follow the lateral orbital rim from midline up into the lateral brow (Figure 14-3). Typically, the injections are given in 3 or 4 locations per side and have a total dose of 7 to 15 U of Botox per side. When treating the lateral wrinkles, care is taken to stay lateral along the rim to diminish the chance of

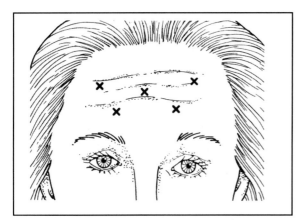

Figure 14-2.

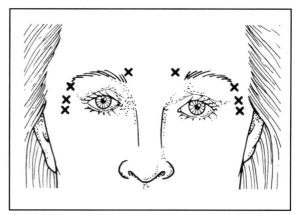

Figure 14-4.

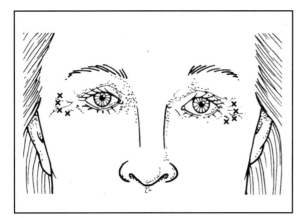

Figure 14-3.

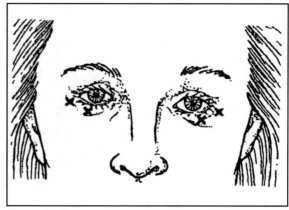

Figure 14-5.

unintended eye muscle weakness and diplopia. The zygomaticus major/minor complex on the maxilla is also avoided to prevent lateral mouth droop. The suggested starting dose of Dysport is 25 U/side.

Injection Technique for Brow Repositioning

When elevation of the brow position is also desired, the lateral injection sites are extended up into the orbicularis below and under the brow (Figure 14-4). The injections are placed superficially to try to avoid deeper penetration into the levator muscle of the eyelid. The concentration of the Botox solution is 2.5 to 5 U/0.1 cc. The volume of the injection is 0.025 to 0.05 cc per site and is given at between 3 to 5 sites per side. Lateral brow repositioning is produced by weakening of the orbicularis muscle. The brow elevation can be contoured, and medial elevation may also be desired. Medial elevation is accomplished by treating the medial depressors of the brow similiarly to the treatment for glabellar wrinkles. Total dose for Botox is 30 to 45 U, and for Dysport 75 to 120 U.

Injection Technique for "Hypertrophic" Orbicularis

Treatment of the lower eyelid orbicularis ridge may be accomplished with treatment of the lower eyelid orbi-

cularis muscle (Figure 14-5). The concentration of Botox solution used in the lower eyelid is 2.5 units/.1 cc. The volume injected is <0.025 cc per site. The injection in the lower eyelid is placed subcutaneously to try to avoid spread beyond the orbital septum to the extraocular muscles. This is a danger area for creation of eye muscle weakness and diplopia. The zygomaticus major/minor complex on the maxilla is also avoided to prevent lateral mouth droop. The total dose for Botox is one unit per site. The Dysport dose would be 2.5 units per site.

Injection Technique for Perioral Wrinkles

In the perioral region, vertical ridges extend above and below the vermilion border on the upper and lower lips. These ridges are produced by contraction of the orbicularis oris. Smoking and sun exposure accentuate the depth of the wrinkles. The patient is asked to contract the lips as if kissing, and the vertical lines are noted. The injections are given just above the vermilion border on the lateral side of the crease. Low concentration and low doses are used. The solution is diluted to 1.0 to 2.5 U BoTX-A per 0.1 cc, and less than 0.025 cc is injected per site. The volume given is just enough to create a bleb in the skin. The total dose is 1 to 5 U per lip. Injection sites are demonstrated in Figure 14-6. In patients with a significant history of oral herpes, preinjection antiviral medications may be given. Symmetric injections between right and left sides are recommended as even small variations in the

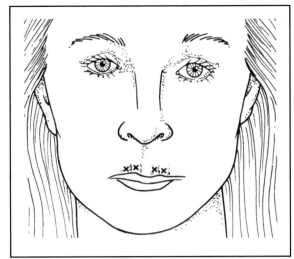

Figure 14-6.

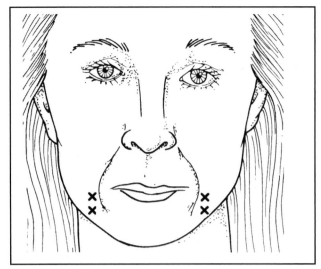

Figure 14-7.

evenness of the dosing may become clinically apparent. The suggested total starting dose for Dysport is 6 to 12 U.

Injection Technique for Melolabial Folds

Lower face treatment with BoTX is more technique dependent and carries more risk for inadvertent spread to adjacent muscles. The lower melolabial folds in the perioral region may be effaced with BoTX treatment to weaken the inferior portion of the depressor anguli oris, but care must be taken not to overtreat this area. The locations for injection are shown in Figure 14-7. The BoTX-A solution concentration in this area is 1.0 to 2.5 U/0.1 cc, and 0.05 cc is injected at one to 2 sites per side. Dosing is 1 to 5 U per side. Keep the injection sites lateral to the oral commissure to avoid the depressor labii muscles. The total dose for both sides for Dysport is 5 to 15 U.

Conclusion

The surge in popularity of BoTX treatments is related to its efficacy, cost, minimal side effects, minimal disruption of life activities, and reversibility. These features are all attractive when compared to other treatment options for facial kinetic lines. The mechanism of action also addresses a feature in the development of facial wrinkles that is not modified by any other therapeutic option. This mechanism of decreasing the muscle contraction is particularly attractive because it should prevent future accentuation of the dynamic lines as well as treating the wrinkles that are present.

SECTION IV

CONGENITAL PTOSIS

ANTERIOR APPROACH TO CORRECTION OF LEVATOR MALDEVELOPMENT PTOSIS

J. Earl Rathbun, MD

When evaluating blepharoptosis, it is best to use a system of classification based on the anatomic defect that caused the ptosis. Treatment can then be directed at the specific anatomic defect. The classifications of Frueh and Beard have been combined here as shown in Table 15-1.

Levator maldevelopment (dysmyogenic) ptosis is the most common type of ptosis seen in children and is caused by a primary dystrophy of the levator muscle. It may be unilateral or bilateral, and it may be mild, giving a slight cosmetic defect, or it may be severe, leading to visual occlusion and amblyopia.

Preoperative Evaluation

The amount of ptosis is measured as the distance between the upper and lower eyelid margins with the brow held in a relaxed position. If the lower eyelid margin is out of normal position just covering the inferior limbus, the measurement can be made from the limbus. An alternative method is to measure the distance of the upper eyelid margin from a midpupil light reflex. This requires the patient to look at a light, which may provoke squinting, which may distort the measurement (Table 15-2).

Levator muscle function is the measurement of upper eyelid excursion from far downgaze to far upgaze with the eyebrow held in a fixed position to eliminate frontalis muscle action (Table 15-3).

The height and contour of the upper eyelid creases are observed to determine the point of action and thus the point of insertion of the levator aponeurosis. The relative positions of the eyelids in downgaze are important because the fibrotic levator muscle in levator maldevelopment ptosis prevents full movement of the upper eyelid in downgaze. Bell's phenomenon, lacrimal secretory function, the presence of synkinetic jaw-winking, strabismus, visual acuity, and the general status of the patient need to be evaluated in the work-up of the ptosis patient.

Choice of Surgical Procedure

If the ptosis is severe (>4 mm) and the levator muscle function poor (<4 mm), the best choice is a frontalis suspension procedure. For other cases, I prefer a levator muscle resection, with the amount of levator aponeurosis and levator muscle resection being determined preoperatively according to Tables 15-4 and 15-5.

An alternative method is levator aponeurosis advancement, with the operative placement of the eyelid on the cornea being determined by the preoperatively determined levator muscle function.

This method has not been as consistently successful for me as has the method outlined earlier, using both the amount of ptosis and the levator muscle function to preoperatively determine the amount of levator muscle resection.

Anesthesia

Most cases of ptosis correction in children require the use of general anesthesia, although some older children may be able to undergo surgery with a combination of local anesthesia and intravenous sedation. The latter method allows evaluation of eyelid contour, height, and lash position intraoperatively. Even if general anesthesia is required, local anesthetic consisting of equal parts 0.75% bupivacaine and 2% lidocaine with 1:100,000 epinephrine is injected for operative hemostasis and postoperative pain control.

Levine MR.
Manual of Oculoplastic Surgery, Fourth Edition (pp 115-120).
© 2010 SLACK Incorporated

Table 15-1

CLASSIFICATION OF PTOSIS

Levator maldevelopment (dysmyogenic) ptosis

- Simple (defect isolated to levator muscle)
- With superior rectus muscle weakness
- Blepharophimosis syndrome
- Congenital fibrosis of the extraocular muscles

Myogenic (myopathic) ptosis

- Oculopharyngeal dystrophy
- Chronic progressive external ophthalmoplegia
- Muscular dystrophy
- Myasthenia gravis
- Trauma to the muscular levator

Neurogenic ptosis

- Oculomotor nerve palsy (third nerve)
- Misdirected oculomotor nerve regeneration
- Marcus-Gunn jaw-winking ptosis
- Horner's syndrome
- Ophthalmoplegic migraine

Aponeurotic ptosis (dehisced or disinserted aponeurosis secondary to the following)

- Age
- Cataract or other ocular surgery
- Local blunt trauma
- Blepharochalasis
- Chronic edema (Graves' disease, allergy, etc)

Mechanical ptosis

- Excess lid weight (lid or orbital mass)
- Scarring

Pseudoptosis

- Due to lack of posterior eyelid support
- Due to hypotropia
- Due to dermatochalasis
- Due to globe malposition

Adapted from Rathbun JE. *Eyelid Surgery.* Boston, MA: Little, Brown; 1990:203.

Table 15-2

AMOUNT OF PTOSIS

AMOUNT OF PTOSIS (MM)	CLASSIFICATION
≤2	Mild
3	Moderate
≥4	Severe

Table 15-3

LEVATOR MUSCLE FUNCTION

LEVATOR MUSCLE FUNCTION (MM)	CLASSIFICATION
15	Normal
≥8	Good
5 to 7	Fair
≤4	Poor

Surgical Procedure

Step 1

After sterile skin preparation and sterile draping, the upper eyelid crease is marked at the desired height so as to be symmetric with the opposite upper eyelid crease.

Step 2

Local anesthesia is injected subcutaneously along the eyelid crease and subconjunctivally along the superior border of the tarsus.

Step 3

The skin is incised along the marked eyelid crease with a blade. The incision is made deeper through the orbicularis muscle to expose the superior border of the tarsus from medial to lateral with scissors (Figure 15-1).

Step 4

A 4-0 silk traction suture is placed centrally in the upper eyelid just above the lash line, and the lid is placed on traction. This is done after the eyelid incision is carried to the tarsus so as to not distort the various layers of the anterior lamella.

Step 5

The orbicularis muscle is dissected inferiorly 3 to 4 mm to expose the superior tarsus and approximately 10 mm superiorly to expose the levator aponeurosis and the orbital septum.

Step 6

At the medial and lateral ends of the tarsus, scissor incisions are made through the remaining eyelid at the edge of the tarsal border (Figure 15-2).

Table 15-4

QUANTITATIVE APPROACH TO CONGENITAL PTOSIS

DESCRIPTION	PROCEDURE
Moderate ptosis (3 mm) with good levator muscle function (≥8 mm)	Moderate muscle resection (14 to 17 mm)
Moderate ptosis (3 mm) with fair levator muscle function (5 to 7 mm)	Large levator resection (18 to 22 mm)
Moderate ptosis (3 mm) with poor levator muscle function (≤4 mm)	Maximum levator muscle resection (≥23 mm)
Severe ptosis (>4 mm) with fair levator muscle function (5 to 7 mm)	Maximum levator muscle resection (≥23 mm)

Adapted from Beard C. The surgical treatment of blepharoptosis: the quantitative approach. *Trans Am Ophthalmol Soc.* 1966;64:401 and Rathbun JE. *Eyelid Surgery.* Boston, MA: Little, Brown; 1990:222.

Table 15-5

LEVATOR RESECTION

LEVATOR FUNCTION 12 TO 15 MM	
Levator Ptosis (mm)	Resection (mm)
2	10
3	12
4	14
LEVATOR FUNCTION 9 TO 11 MM	
Levator Ptosis (mm)	Resection (mm)
2	12
3	14
4	16
LEVATOR FUNCTION 6 TO 8 MM	
Levator Ptosis (mm)	Resection (mm)
2	14
3	16
4	18

Adapted from data courtesy of Mark R. Levine, MD.

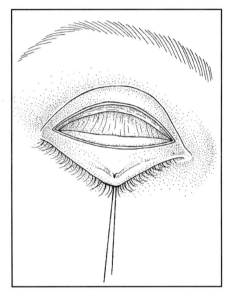

Figure 15-1.

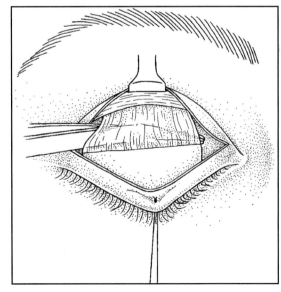

Figure 15-2.

Step 7

A Berke ptosis clamp is placed between the 2 incisions incorporating levator aponeurosis, superior tarsal muscle (Müller's muscle), and conjunctiva (Figure 15-3).

Step 8

The tissue is severed adjacent to the clamp on the tarsal side (Figure 15-4).

Step 9

The conjunctiva is undermined and dissected off the posterior surface of the superior tarsal muscle and is severed at the superior edge of the clamp (Figure 15-5).

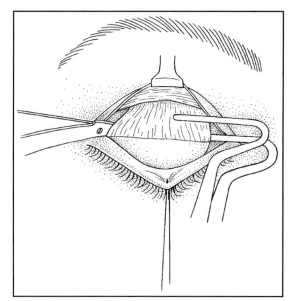

Figure 15-3.

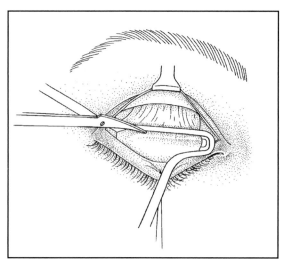

Figure 15-4.

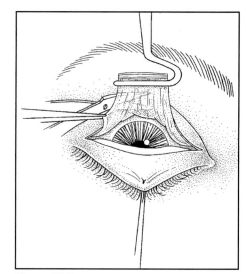

Figure 15-5.

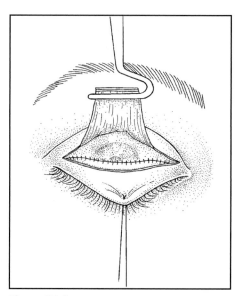

Figure 15-6.

Step 10

The conjunctival edge is sutured to the superior border of the tarsus with 7-0 chromic gut using a running suture (Figure 15-6).

Step 11

With the Berke ptosis clamp rotated downward, dissection is done along the anterior surface of the levator aponeurosis and the muscular levator to separate off the orbital septum. Gentle pressure on the globe prolapses the preaponeurotic fat, aiding in identifying the plane between the levator muscle and the orbital septum (Figure 15-7).

Step 12

Inferior traction is placed on the ptosis clamp, and the medial and lateral horns of the levator are identified both visually and by palpation. The horns are cut only as much as necessary to allow resection of the amount of levator resection desired. The scissors are directed toward the center of the levator so as to avoid damage to the superior oblique muscle

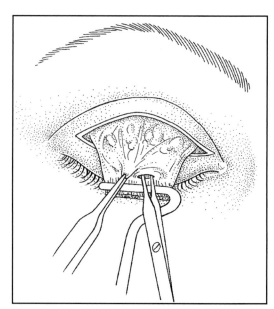

Figure 15-7.

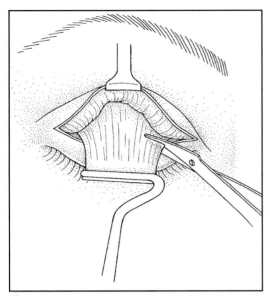

Figure 15-8.

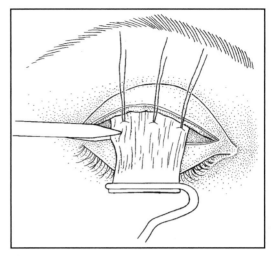

Figure 15-10.

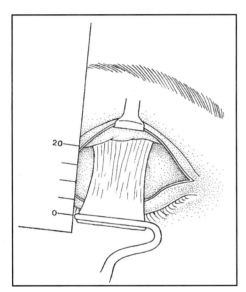

Figure 15-9.

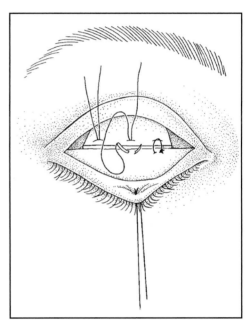

Figure 15-11.

medially and the lacrimal gland laterally (Figure 15-8).

Step 13

The amount of levator resection is measured from the inferior edge of the Berke ptosis clamp to the desired height (Figure 15-9).

Step 14

Three 5-0 chromic gut sutures are placed at the desired amount of resection with the central suture being slightly higher than the medial and lateral sutures. The excess levator and superior tarsal muscles are excised (Figure 15-10).

Step 15

The 3 sutures are placed through the anterior one half to three fourths of the tarsal thickness at the superior tarsal border, or they can be placed 2 to 4 mm below the superior border if additional advancement is desired. The eyelid height and

contour are evaluated, and adjustments are made as necessary (Figure 15-11).

Step 16

Skin may be excised superior to the incision before closure. Usually, 2 to 3 mm of skin is excised in levator maldevelopment ptosis in children and more in older individuals. Lid crease sutures, usually 3 or 4, are placed through the skin and orbicularis muscle inferiorly, then through the edge of the levator and out through the orbicularis muscle and skin superiorly. The remainder of the skin incision is closed with a running 7-0 chromic or silk suture (Figure 15-12).

Step 17

A 4-0 silk traction suture is placed in the lower eyelid margin and taped to the forehead for ocular protection.

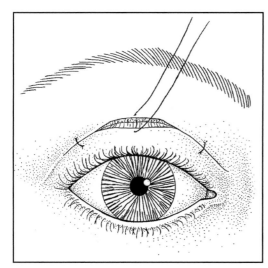

Figure 15-12.

Alternative Step 6

An alternate approach may be considered at Step 6. Instead of buttonholing the lid medially and laterally to the tarsus, the levator aponeurosis may be dissected off Müller's muscle and conjunctiva with a hand-held cautery. This is facilitated by injecting anesthetic between the levator and Müller's muscle, ballooning up a plane. With inferior traction on the pretarsal skin muscle flap, a hand-held cautery is used to dissect levator aponeurosis off the tarsal plate, then carry the dissection superiorly off Müller's muscle and conjunctiva to the desired pre-determined level. This step significantly reduces bleeding and saves the step of resuturing the conjunctiva back to the superior tarsal border.

Postoperative Management

Antibiotic-steroid ophthalmic ointment is applied to the suture line. A full or partial eye pad may be applied. The patient is instructed to keep the head elevated and to apply ice packs for at least 15 minutes every 2 hours. Aspirin and other clot-inhibiting medications are to be avoided. Nonabsorbable skin sutures are removed in 6 to 7 days. Frequent corneal lubrication with artificial tears and lubricating ointment is very important and may be augmented with a plastic bubble or plastic wrap during the day or evening if exposure is a problem.

Complications

Overcorrection or undercorrection may occur. Massage may be used in cases in which there is still overcorrection 2 weeks postoperatively. Further surgical correction may be considered 8 weeks postoperatively if the inflammatory response has resolved. Overcorrection is treated by upper eyelid retractor recession, with possible placement of a spacer between the tarsus and the levator muscle. Undercorrection is treated based on the amount of ptosis and levator muscle function. Conjunctival prolapse is not uncommon in the early postoperative period and usually resolves spontaneously. If it does not resolve, full-thickness sutures to fixate the conjunctiva in the upper fornix may be used.

CHAPTER 16

FRONTALIS SLING FOR CONGENITAL PTOSIS

Robert G. Small, MD

The frontalis sling operation is used for blepharoptosis when there is little or no levator action. The upper eyelid is suspended from the brow with autogenous fascia lata so the patient opens the eye by elevating the brow and closes the eye by contracting the orbicularis. This operation is used for severe unilateral or bilateral ptosis, which cannot be corrected with conventional ptosis surgery on the levator muscle. When properly performed, frontalis suspension provides remarkably good results. This chapter emphasizes the exact method of obtaining a fascia lata autograft. Note that congenital ptosis is seen in adults as well as children.

Preoperative Management

Discuss the following possible complications with the patient and the family before surgery: lagophthalmos, exposure of the cornea with possible eye irritation or ulceration, sleeping with the eye open, and infection or rejection of the fascia or other material used to elevate the eyelid. Mention the unlikely possibility of hemorrhage or bulging at the fascial donor site in the thigh as well as rare problems with general anesthesia. Note that blinking after fascia lata eyelid suspension is not normal. Tell the patient there may be asymmetry between the 2 eyelids.

Selection of Material for Eyelid Suspension

In patients older than 3 years, autogenous fascia from the thigh is the preferred material. The superiority of autogenous over alloplastic material is well documented in the literature. The technique for obtaining fascia lata is described in detail here. For children with legs too small to harvest fascia, one must use alloplastic material or cadaver fascia. When autogenous fascia cannot be obtained, I use nylon cable suture (Supramid) on ski needles.

Anesthesia

General anesthesia is required for adults and children. The operation can be done in an outpatient setting, but it occasionally may be necessary to have the patient stay overnight.

Surgical Procedure

Step 1

Place the patient on the operating table with the donor leg flexed and elevated with a small pillow. This puts the tensor fascia lata muscle on stretch and makes the graft easier to obtain.

Step 2

After general anesthesia, prepare and drape the outer thigh from knee to hip and the upper face and forehead. Palpate the tensor fascia lata muscle to plan the incision. Mark a 3-cm longitudinal incision beginning 2 fingerbreadths above the lateral condyle of the femur in a line from the lateral condyle of the femur to the anterior superior iliac spine (Figure 16-1A).

Step 3

Make a 3.5-cm incision through skin and fat to expose the white glistening fascia lata. Insert 8- or 9-inch curved Metzenbaum scissors into the incision, and create a 10-cm tunnel extending up the thigh. Spread the scissors to separate all the attachments of the subcutaneous tissue to the fascia. Make short parallel facial incisions 8 mm apart in the direction of the fascial fibers. Open the Metzenbaum scissors slightly, and insert one blade of the scissors in the first fascial incision (Figure

Levine MR.
Manual of Oculoplastic Surgery, Fourth Edition (pp 121-124).
© 2010 SLACK Incorporated

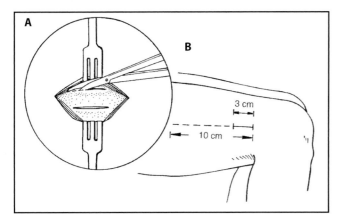

Figure 16-1.

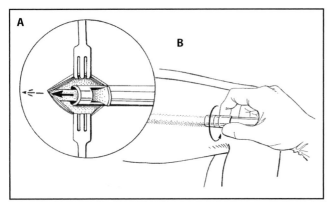

Figure 16-2.

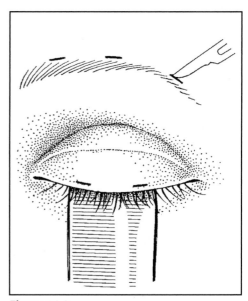

Figure 16-3.

16-1B). Pass the scissors that are engaged in the fascial strip 10 cm upward in the subcutaneous tunnel created by the previous dissection. Repeat this maneuver along the second fascial incision. This isolates a 10-cm fascial strip 8-mm wide medially, laterally, and anteriorly. A little more length can be obtained by extending the fascial incisions a short distance toward the knee. Now, pass the scissors underneath the isolated fascial strip and free the underside of the strip. The fascial strip is now isolated medially, laterally, anteriorly, and posteriorly in situ. Experience shows that, without this complete preliminary fascial dissection, it is difficult to pass fascial strippers up the leg to cut and isolate a fascial strip of adequate length (10 cm).

Step 4

Cut the fascial strip free as far distally as possible (toward the knee joint), and introduce it into the Masson fascial stripper (Figure 16-2A). Grasp the end of the fascia with a small clamp, and pass the stripper proximally up the leg at least 10 cm (Figure 16-2B). Palpate the stripper beneath the tunnel of skin created by the dissection, and measure it to be sure that it extends up the leg the required 10 cm. Unscrew the barrel of the stripper, and move it proximally with a continuous circular motion to sever the fascial strip. I have found that the Masson stripper cuts the fascia more easily than the Crawford stripper.

Step 5

Measure the fascia to be sure that at least 10 cm has been harvested. Place it on a tongue blade, and remove small amounts of fat and connective tissue with Westcott scissors. Cut the fascia in 2 strips, each measuring 3.5 to 4.0 mm in width. Even if only one eyelid is being operated on, an 8-mm wide strip of fascia must be harvested because it is difficult to remove a narrow 4-mm strip of fascia from the leg.

Step 6

Close the dermal layer wound with 5-0 colorless nylon sutures placed below the skin surface with the knots buried in the deep dermis. These nonabsorbable nylon sutures hold the tough dermal layer permanently apposed and prevent a wide scar. Close the skin edge with a running suture of your choice. Apply a pressure dressing to the wound along the fascial donor site but do not completely encircle the thigh with tape. Bed rest with bathroom privileges is recommended the day of surgery. Bleeding from the donor site with a hematoma of the thigh is an infrequent complication.

Step 7

Direct your attention to the eyelid to be elevated. Mark 5 3-mm horizontal incisions in the shape of a pentagon—3 just above the brow and 2 above the edge of the upper eyelid. Place the upper eyelid incisions where the corneal limbus intersects the eyelid with the eye in the primary position as shown in Figure 16-3. Pull up the upper lid with 2 forceps in the direction of the proposed incisions, and observe the curve of the elevated eyelid. If the eyelid incisions are too close, the elevated eyelid will be peaked; if they are too far apart, the lid edge will be flat centrally. All 5 incisions must be placed accurately so that, when the fascial strip is tied, a pleasing lid curve and lid crease result.

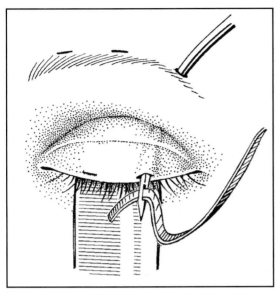

Figure 16-4.

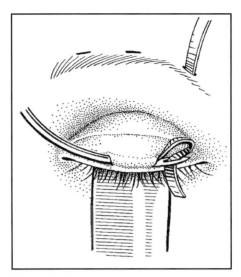

Figure 16-5.

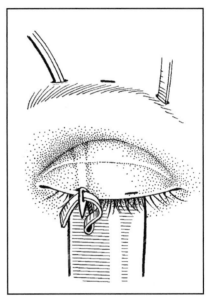

Figure 16-6.

Step 8

Cut down through each brow incision to the frontal bone with a #15 Bard-Parker blade or a mini-dissection bipolar electrocautery (Colorado needle). The Colorado needle inserted deep into the brow incisions provides hemostasis. Firm pressure through gauze placed over each incision also helps control bleeding. Make eyelid incisions through the skin and pretarsal orbicularis muscle to the tarsus. Scissors dissection between the 2 eyelid incisions creates a tunnel that facilitates passage of the Wright needle.

Step 9

Place a Jaeger lid plate under the eyelid, and bring it into contact with the orbital rim to protect the globe during the passage of the Wright fascia lata needle. Pass the Wright needle through the temporal brow incision deep in the tissues of the lid with the point of the needle constantly palpated and directed by your index finger so that the needle exits at a lid incision. If the needle is not placed deep enough, the fascia will bow the skin. To load fascia into the Wright needle, press the fascia with your index finger into the eye of the needle, and pull a 2-cm segment through with a 0.5-mm toothed forceps (Figure 16-4). Pull back the Wright needle to draw the fascia into the lid. The strip is now in position for the next passage of the needle.

Step 10

Pass the Wright needle just above the tarsus, and bring the strip under the pretarsal orbicularis muscle to exit through the nasal eyelid incision (Figure 16-5). Some surgeons suture the fascia to the tarsus at this point. Again, load the fascia into the needle, pass the Wright needle from the nasal brow incision to the nasal eyelid incision, and draw the strip through to the brow (Figure 16-6). Pass the Wright needle deep in the central brow incision, and bring out each fascial strip to complete the pentagon (Figures 16-7 and 16-8).

Step 11

Pull the eyelid up as high as possible with the fascia so that it is overcorrected (Figure 16-9A). Tie the ends of the fascial strip with a single square knot. Pass a 5-0 braided polyester suture back and forth through the fascial knot, and tie the suture to prevent it from unraveling (Figure 16-9B). Place the knot deep in the central brow incision to bring the eyelid in position 1.5-mm below the upper limbus.

Step 12

Close each brow incision with 1 or 2 6-0 mild chromic catgut sutures. No sutures are used in the eyelid incisions.

Step 13

The eye remains open at the end of the procedure. A Frost suture is not used. Antibiotic eye ointment is instilled, and an eye patch is lightly secured with tape.

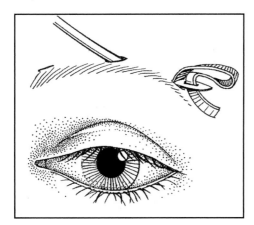

Figure 16-7.

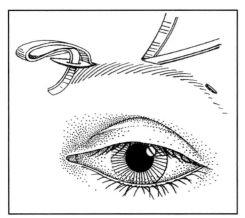

Figure 16-8.

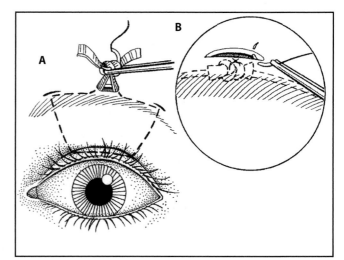

Figure 16-9.

Step 14

Remove the patch as soon as the patient recovers from anesthesia. Instruct the nurse to immediately begin protecting the exposed cornea with artificial tears and lubricating ophthalmic ointment. Teach the corneal protection routine to nurses, patients, and caregivers. Provide a printed sheet with instructions for keeping the cornea moist.

Postoperative Care

Give the patient (or caregivers) verbal and written instructions for treatment of the expected postoperative lagophthalmos. Stress the need for conscious blinking of the eyes 15 times per minute, and explain how to instill lubricating eye drops and ointment often enough to prevent corneal drying. There is no set time schedule for administration of ocular lubricants. Each patient develops his or her own routine for corneal care. The use of prophylactic antibiotics is advisable because infection can lead to failure of the operation.

Complications

Most children and adults adjust rapidly to fascia lata eyelid suspension. They learn to open their eyes with frontalis muscle contraction and to close their eyes with orbicularis muscle contraction. There is usually lagophthalmos while the incisions are tender, but, within a few days, patients usually open and close their eyes in a relatively normal manner and sleep with the eyes closed. Corneal ulceration from exposure keratopathy after fascia lata eyelid suspension is rare. Patients should be observed closely, however, to be sure that this does not occur. Infection or rejection of autogenous fascia is rare and is more likely to occur with cadaver fascia or alloplastic material. The use of alloplastic material in infants and young children is usually successful, but gradual recurrence of ptosis may occur; therefore, autogenous fascia may need to be placed in later childhood.

Bleeding into the leg is occasionally a complication at the fascia donor site. It is best for the patient to be on limited activity for at least 1 week after surgery. Eyelid symmetry is usually excellent after bilateral fascia lata eyelid suspension. After unilateral eyelid suspension, the patient must close the treated eye with voluntary orbicularis contraction, whereas blinking remains normal on the untreated side. After some time, blinking usually appears almost normal. Some surgeons surgically defunctionalize the normal levator muscle and perform bilateral fascia lata eyelid suspension when only one lid is ptotic in an attempt to achieve symmetry. This, however, is at the expense of making a normal lid abnormal. "Symmetry" after fascia lata eyelid suspension is only present in repose because there is always lagophthalmos of the operated eyelid or eyelids. After eyelid suspension for unilateral third nerve paralysis, patients are likely to experience diplopia and squeeze the eye shut. This mars the result. Because there is no way to predict surgical results, tell the patient that there may be undercorrection or eyelid asymmetry after unilateral or bilateral fascia lata eyelid suspension. Overcorrection is rare.

Conclusion

Fascia lata eyelid suspension is a useful ptosis procedure. When properly used, it gives gratifying results in most patients. The technique presented here has evolved over a period of years. Because obtaining a fascial strip of proper length is essential, the details of this part of the procedure are stressed. Other configurations of fascial placement may be used depending on your experience.

SECTION V

ACQUIRED PTOSIS

CHAPTER 17

LEVATOR APONEUROSIS DEHISCENCE

John A. Burns, MD, FACS; Kenneth V. Cahill, MD, FACS; Jill A. Foster, MD, FACS; and Kevin S. Michels, MD

Levator aponeurosis dehiscence is the most frequent cause of acquired ptosis. It can be diagnosed on the basis of characteristic clinical findings: elevated upper lid crease, deep superior lid sulcus, upper lid thinning, transillumination of the lid at the upper edge of the tarsal plate, normal levator function, and the absence of lagophthalmos. The aponeurosis dehiscence may be spontaneous or secondary to other ophthalmic conditions. It may be unilateral or bilateral. If lid thinning is absent or if levator function is abnormal, the diagnosis of levator aponeurosis dehiscence must be questioned.

Preoperative Management

If the patient is satisfied with his or her field of vision and appearance, no ptosis treatment is indicated. Nonsurgical management of ptosis is limited. Wires can be attached to eyeglass frames, serving as ptosis crutches to hold up the upper eyelids. However, the wires tend to lose their hold on the lid tissue as the patient blinks. If they support the lids too securely, they can impair the patient's ability to blink. In general, they are not an effective long-term solution for this form of ptosis. Taping the upper lid has the same disadvantages as ptosis crutches.

The most effective therapy for ptosis is surgical exploration and repair of the defective levator aponeurosis. A variation of external levator resection technique is used. If the patient has bilateral dehiscence, both lids should be corrected at the same time because it has been demonstrated that greater symmetry will be achieved.

Before surgery is recommended, the ophthalmologist must evaluate Bell's phenomenon, corneal sensation, the corneal tear break-up time, and the basic tear test. Any deficiency in these 4 factors increases the patient's risk of postoperative discomfort, corneal damage, and visual loss. No matter how skillful the surgeon, the possibility of over- and undercorrection as well as asymmetry are real. These potential problems must be carefully explained to the patient before a decision is made regarding surgery.

Anesthesia

Local anesthesia is preferable so that upper lid position, contour, and movement can be monitored and adjusted intraoperatively. Some controversy exists as to whether epinephrine should be used. Epinephrine-induced hemostasis certainly facilitates the surgical dissection. However, even weak concentrations of epinephrine may stimulate Müller's muscle, making the final position of the lid less predictable. That said, virtually all surgeons use epinephrine. The injection of anesthetic should be confined to the eyelid and not into the orbit, as with a frontal nerve block. This will avoid the added variable of motor block to the levator muscle.

Operative Procedure

Step 1

A skin marker is used to draw an incision at the position of the desired lid crease. Surgical correction of a patient's ptosis will move the lid margin closer to the lid crease and may result in unacceptable dermatochalasis. If this is anticipated, skin excision (ie, blepharoplasty) should be performed at the same time.

Step 2

A drop of 0.5% tetracaine is instilled into the eyes. Subcutaneous infiltration under the skin marks, using 1.0 mL of 2% lidocaine with epinephrine per eyelid, provides anesthesia with minimal effect on levator function.

Levine MR.
Manual of Oculoplastic Surgery, Fourth Edition (pp 127-130).
© 2010 SLACK Incorporated

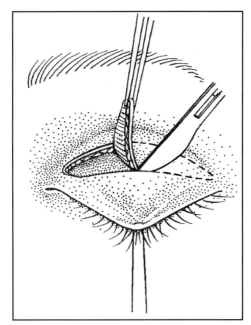

Figure 17-1.

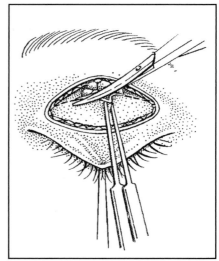

Figure 17-2.

Step 3

The upper face is prepared with povidone-iodine (Betadine) solution. The surgical drape is applied so that both eyes are exposed. A protective rigid corneoscleral contact lens may be placed on the eye to protect it from sharp instruments, needles, and cautery.

Step 4

A 4-0 silk traction suture is placed through the gray line in the central upper lid margin and clamped to the drape below with a hemostat. This puts the upper lid structures on stretch.

Step 5

The lid crease and blepharoplasty skin marks are incised using a #15 Bard-Parker blade (Figure 17-1). The excessive skin is undermined with blunt dissection using blunt-tipped Westcott scissors. It is then excised.

Step 6

The orbicularis muscle is tented anteriorly with toothed forceps immediately superior to the upper margin of the tarsus. It is also important to have simultaneous inferiorly directed tension of the lid margin with the traction suture. The orbicularis muscle is incised centrally by a horizontal snip with scissors. The scissors should enter the avascular fascial plane posterior to the orbicularis muscle. Ordinarily, this is a potential space, but tenting the orbicularis muscle makes it an open space. Blunt dissection both medially and laterally extends this space for the entire width of the lid crease incision. Orbicularis muscle is then cut horizontally for full exposure of this space.

Step 7

The superior edge of the orbicularis incision is retracted superiorly with a rake. Additional blunt dissection may be necessary to separate the orbicularis muscle from the levator aponeurosis. Identification of the levator aponeurosis is facilitated and confirmed by asking the patient to look up and down to activate the levator muscle. Superior to the region of dehiscence, a thicker white edge of the levator aponeurosis may be prominent. However, this is not constant. In some cases, the aponeurosis becomes gradually thicker, making its identification more difficult. In these cases, Müller's muscle should be readily visible and can be followed superiorly until the dehisced edge of the levator aponeurosis is found. Identifying the position of the aponeurosis posterior to the preaponeurotic fat pad if helpful, as is finding the insertion of the orbital septum onto the anterior surface of the aponeurosis.

Step 8

Gentle pressure on the globe causes the preaponeurotic fat pad and the orbital septum to bulge anteriorly. A horizontal buttonhole in the septum should be created with scissors superior to its fusion with the aponeurosis (Figure 17-2). In many cases, the disinserted levator aponeurosis will have retracted back to the site where the orbital septum fuses with it. The orbital septum should be completely separated from the aponeurosis with scissors. This exposes the preaponeurotic fat pad. The vertically oriented fibers of the levator aponeurosis should be clearly identified posterior to the preaponeurotic fat pad (Figure 17-3A).

Step 9

The pretarsal orbicularis muscle covering the superior edge of the tarsal plate should be excised.

Step 10

The dehisced levator aponeurosis is mobilized from the underlying Müller's muscle using blunt and sharp dissection. Müller's muscle is richly vascularized. Care must be taken when cauterizing bleeding sites to avoid damaging the globe.

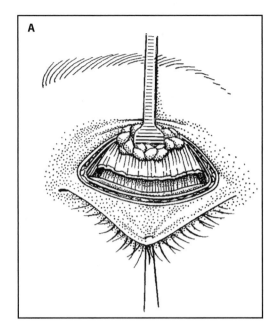

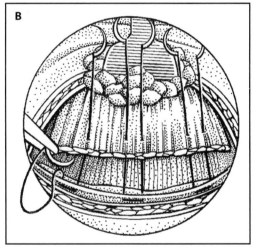

Figure 17-3.

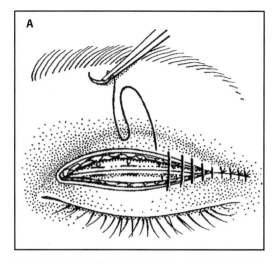

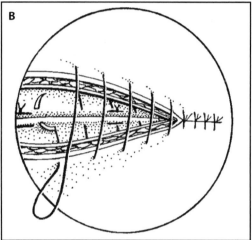

Figure 17-4.

Step 11

The free edge of the levator aponeurosis is attached to the upper edge of the tarsal plate using a 5-0 polyglactin suture (Vicryl, Dexon) double-armed with spatula needles (Figure 17-3B). The tarsal bites should be partial thickness so that the suture will not cause a corneal abrasion. Sutures should be placed centrally at the highest point of the lid curve and also both nasally and temporally. These should be tied temporarily to allow for removal or adjustment.

Step 12

The locally anesthetized patient is elevated to a sitting position so that the eyelid position and contour can be evaluated. If the eyelid is too low, the aponeurosis can be advanced several millimeters down the anterior surface of the tarsus. In some cases, a small resection of levator aponeurosis may also be necessary. Once the desired lid position and contour are achieved, the sutures are tied permanently. If lidocaine with epinephrine is used for anesthesia, the eyelid should be set 1 to 2 mm higher than the normal side to allow for postoperative drop when the anesthesia wears off.

Step 13

The blepharoplasty skin incision is closed with 6-0 or 7-0 monofilament skin sutures. Deep bites to the aponeurosis are taken if a prominent lid crease is desired (Figure 17-4). This will also help eyelash ptosis, if present.

Postoperative Management

Ophthalmic antibiotic ointment is applied to the incision site and globe. Intermittent application of an ice pack is useful in minimizing edema. An eye patch is not usually necessary. Less lagophthalmos will be noted initially after the repair of a levator aponeurosis dehiscence than after a levator resection procedure. Bland ophthalmic ointment will need to be used on the globe at bedtime and, in some cases, during the day until full lid excursion returns and the potential for exposure keratitis has passed. Skin sutures are removed after 6 days.

Management of Postoperative Complications

The most common postoperative complications are over- and undercorrection with each having approximately a 5% incidence. Small amounts of overcorrection (1 to 2 mL) can usually be corrected with inferior traction on the lid margin. The patient should pull down on the lid 10 to 15 times, 4 times daily starting on the second postoperative day. Larger amounts of overcorrection and undercorrection can be improved by reblocking the lid, opening the incision, and moving the levator aponeurosis sutures up or down as indicated by the lid position. For this to be successful, it should be done in the first week. If early postoperative correction is deferred, then additional surgery should be considered at 6 months. At that point, complete re-evaluation is indicated. Almost all scar tissue will have stabilized then, and a repeat of the surgical steps will be possible.

Significant postoperative bleeding is rare, but if a hematoma forms, it should be aggressively managed because the orbital septum has been opened and a compartment syndrome is possible.

Prognosis

Once strong levator aponeurosis tissue is reattached to the tarsus, the chance of recurrent dehiscence is slight. If there is a recurrence, it should be re-evaluated just as carefully as the original ptosis. Repeat external levator aponeurosis surgery can be performed, and, if needed, permanent sutures (silk or nylon) are recommended.

CHAPTER 18

MÜLLER'S MUSCLE-CONJUNCTIVA RESECTION

Allen M. Putterman, MD

The Müller's muscle-conjunctiva resection ptosis procedure is recommended for patients with blepharoptosis whose upper eyelids elevate to a normal level when 10% phenylephrine drops are applied to the upper ocular fornix. Candidates usually have minimal congenital ptosis and varying degrees of acquired ptosis. The advantage over the Fasanella procedure is that Müller's muscle-conjunctiva resection preserves the tarsus, and the advantage over the levator aponeurosis procedure is that it produces predictable results.

Preoperative Management

MARGIN REFLEX DISTANCE 1

Before performing the phenylephrine test, it is important to assess the upper eyelid levels with the margin reflex distance 1 (MRD_1) measurement (Figure 18-1). The surgeon holds a muscle light at eye level and shines it onto the patient's eyes. The distance from the corneal light reflex to the central upper lid margin is the MRD_1, measured in positive millimeters. If the eyelid is below the middle of the pupil, the surgeon elevates the lid until the light reflex is first seen; the estimated number of millimeters the lid is lifted is the MRD, in negative millimeters. The difference in the MRD, on the normal side compared with the ptotic side, indicates the degree of ptosis. The normal MRD is approximately 4.5 mm; this number is used as a reference in bilateral cases. The MRD measurement has the advantage of measuring the ptosis and not the palpebral fissure width. (This is preferred because there is a Müller's muscle in the lower lid that can also respond to the phenylephrine. Measuring the palpebral fissure width would lead to erroneous interpretation of the upper lid level after phenylephrine instillation.)

PHENYLEPHRINE TEST

To avoid precipitating any side effects, such as myocardial infarction, hypertension, and acute glaucoma, it is important to make sure that the patient does not have a cardiac problem or shallow anterior chamber before instilling phenylephrine drops. The patient's head is tilted backward, the upper eyelid is lifted, and the patient is instructed to gaze downward. Several drops of 10% phenylephrine are dropped between the upper eyelid and globe. (The canaliculi are compressed with the examiner's finger for 10 seconds to minimize the excretion of phenylephrine into the nasal cavity and the potential side effect of systemic absorption.) This is repeated immediately 2 more times. One minute later, 2 additional drops are applied.

Three to 5 minutes after instillation of the phenylephrine, the MRD is measured. If the eyelid elevates to a normal level with the phenylephrine test, 8.25 mm of Müller's muscle is resected. A 6.25- to 9.75-mm resection of Müller's muscle is performed if the upper eyelid elevates slightly higher or lower than the opposite lid, respectively.

Anesthesia

General anesthesia is used in children; local anesthesia is preferred in adults.

Surgical Procedure

Step 1

A frontal nerve block is used with local anesthesia to avoid swelling of the upper eyelid by local infiltration, which would make the operation more difficult and inexact. A 23-gauge retrobulbar-type

Levine MR.
Manual of Oculoplastic Surgery, Fourth Edition (pp 131-136).
© 2010 SLACK Incorporated

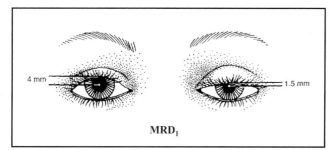

Figure 18-1.

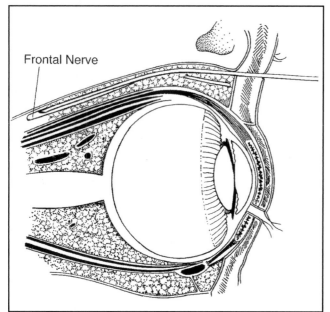

Figure 18-2.

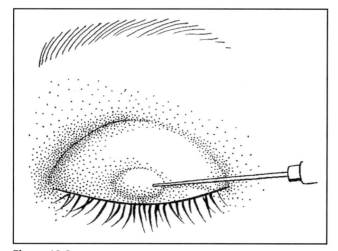

Figure 18-3.

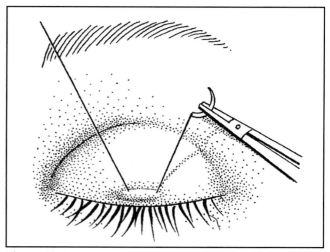

Figure 18-4.

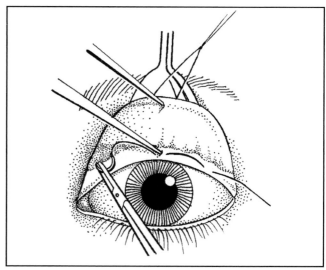

Figure 18-5.

Step 2

A 4-0 black silk traction suture is inserted through skin, orbicularis muscle, and superficial tarsus 2 mm above the eyelashes at the center of the upper eyelid (Figure 18-4). A medium-sized Desmarres retractor everts the upper eyelid and exposes the palpebral conjunctiva from the superior tarsal border to the superior fornix. Topical tetracaine drops are applied over the upper palpebral conjunctiva.

Step 3

A caliper set at 8.25 mm, with one arm at the superior tarsal border, facilitates insertion of a 6-0 black silk suture through the conjunctiva, 8.25 mm above the superior tarsal border (Figure 18-5). One passage centrally and 2 others, approximately 7 mm nasal and temporal to the center, mark the site. (I usually place the suture 8.25 mm above the superior tarsal border, but it may be placed 6.25 to 9.75 mm above it if the response of the upper eyelid level to the phenylephrine test is slightly more or less than desired.)

needle is inserted into the superior orbit, entering just under the middle of the superior orbital rim (Figure 18-2). The needle should hug the roof of the orbit during insertion and is advanced until a depth of 4 cm is reached; 1.5 mL of 2% lidocaine with epinephrine is injected. Another 0.25 mL is injected subcutaneously over the center upper eyelid, just above the eyelid margin (Figure 18-3).

Step 4

A toothed forceps grasps conjunctiva and Müller's muscle between the superior tarsal border and marking suture and separates Müller's muscle from its loose attachment to the levator aponeurosis (Figure 18-6). (This maneuver is possible because Müller's muscle is firmly attached to conjunctiva but only loosely attached to the levator aponeurosis.)

Step 5

One blade of a specially designed clamp (Putterman Müller's muscle-conjunctival resection clamp, STORZ Company, Manchester, MO) is placed at the level of the marking suture. Each tooth of this blade engages each suture bite that passes through the palpebral conjunctiva (Figure 18-7). The Desmarres retractor is then slowly released as the outer blade of the clamp engages conjunctiva and Müller's muscle adjacent to the superior tarsal border (Figure 18-8). Any entrapped tarsus is pulled out of the clamp with the surgeon's finger (Figure 18-9). The clamp is compressed, and the handle is locked, incorporating conjunctiva and Müller's muscle between the superior tarsal border and the marking suture.

Step 6

The upper eyelid skin is then pulled in one direction while the clamp is pulled simultaneously in the opposite direction (Figure 18-10). If the surgeon feels a sense of attachment between the skin and clamp during this maneuver, the levator aponeurosis has been inadvertently trapped in the clamp. If this occurs, the clamp should be released and reapplied in its proper position. (This maneuver is possible because the levator aponeurosis sends extensions to orbicularis muscle and skin to form the lid crease.)

Step 7

With the clamp held straight up, a 5-0 double-armed plain catgut mattress suture is run 1.5 mm below the clamp along its entire width in a temporal to nasal direction, through the upper margin of the tarsus, and through Müller's muscle and conjunctiva on the other side, and vice versa (Figure 18-11). The sutures are placed approximately 2 to 3 mm apart.

Step 8

A #15 surgical blade is used to excise the tissues held in the clamp by cutting between the sutures and the clamp. The knife blade is rotated slightly, with its sharp edge hugging the clamp. As the tissues are sliced from the clamp, the surgeon and assistant watch to ensure that the stitches on each side are not cut (Figure 18-12).

Step 9

The Desmarres retractor again everts the eyelid while gentle traction is applied to the 4-0 black silk centering suture. The nasal end of the suture is then run continuously in a temporal direction; the stitches should be approximately 2 mm apart as they pass through the

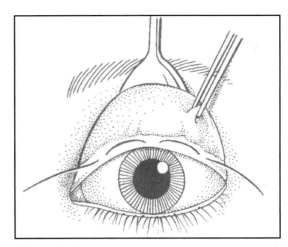

Figure 18-6.

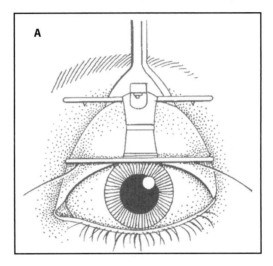

Figure 18-7.

edges of superior tarsal border, Müller's muscle, and conjunctiva (Figure 18-13). The surgeon must be careful to avoid cutting the original mattress suture during this continuous closure. Toward this end, the surgeon uses a small suture needle

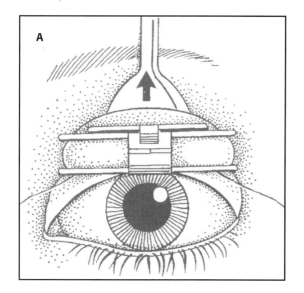

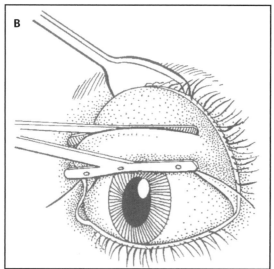

Figure 18-8.

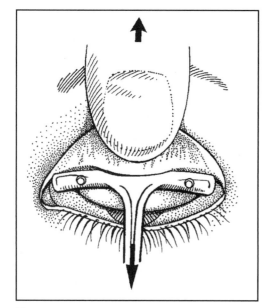

Figure 18-9.

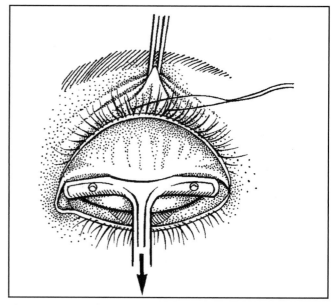

Figure 18-10.

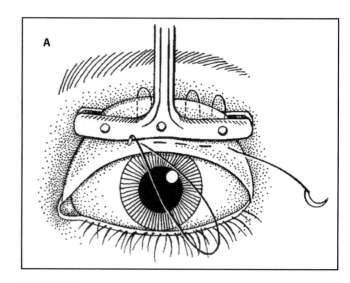

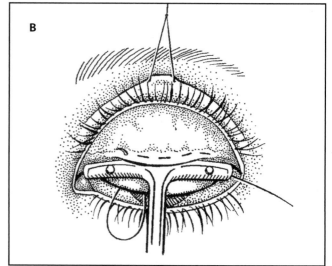

Figure 18-11.

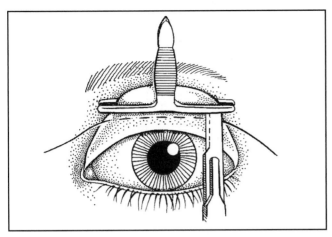

Figure 18-12.

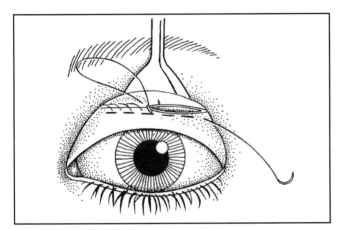

Figure 18-13.

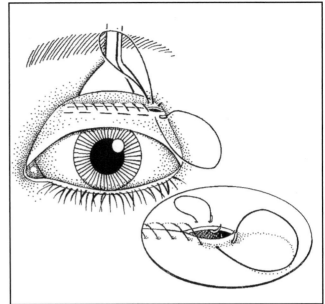

Figure 18-14.

(S-14 spatula), observing the mattress suture position during each bite, and the assistant applies continuous suction along the incision edges.

Step 10

Once each arm of the suture reaches the temporal end of the eyelid, it is passed through each side of the conjunctiva and Müller's muscle before it exits through the temporal end of the incision (Figure 18-14). The suture arms are then tied with approximately 4 to 5 knots, and the ends are cut close to the knot. (In this way, the knot can be buried subconjunctivally, thereby lessening postoperative keratopathy.)

Postoperative Management

A topical antibiotic such as gentamicin (Garamycin) is placed on the eye. Cold compresses are applied to the eyelids for 24 hours. Topical antibiotic ointment is applied to the eyes twice a day for 1 week and once a day for a second week. If the eyelid elevates higher than desired, the eyebrow is held upward while the upper lid is pushed in and downward several times each day. The eyelid usually attains its final level 3 to 6 weeks postoperatively.

Complications

Several complications can occur from a Müller's muscle-conjunctiva resection. One that can occur postoperatively is a corneal abrasion caused by the catgut mattress suture. Placing the suture bites closer together on the tarsal surface and further apart on the conjunctival surface decreases the incidence of this complication.

Should it occur, a soft contact lens can be worn for 2 to 7 days postoperatively until the suture dissolves. There is an approximately 3% to 5% chance of an over- or undercorrection with this procedure. If an overcorrection occurs, downward massage of the eyelid can be used during the immediate postoperative period. Should the overcorrection persist, it can be treated with a levator recession procedure. If an undercorrection occurs, the next line of treatment would be a levator aponeurosis advancement, tuck, and resection ptosis procedure. Exposure keratopathy is still another complication of this procedure, and this can be treated with artificial tears or topical ointments.

CHAPTER 19

TARSAL-CONJUNCTIVAL-MÜLLER'S MUSCLE RESECTION (FASANELLA-SERVAT PROCEDURE)

Randal Pham, MD, FACS

Tarsectomy-Müllerectomy-conjunctivectomy is a procedure used in mild to moderate ptosis with good to excellent levator function (10 to 15 mm) and a good response to phenylephrine hydrochloride (Neo-Synephrine). It can correct 2 mm of congenital ptosis and 2 to 3 mm of acquired ptosis. It is particularly useful in treating patients with Horner's syndrome. Other indications are steroid-induced ptosis, ptosis of pregnancy, chronic progressive external ophthalmoplegia, and myasthenia gravis. It is a quick, reliable, and predictable ptosis correction procedure. The resected upper eyelid graft may be used to elevate a lower eyelid malposition. It may also be used in conjunction with a blepharoplasty.

Preoperative Management

Preoperative photographs should be taken. Phenylephrine hydrochloride 2.5% can be used preoperatively to ascertain whether the ptotic lid will rise with tarsectomy-Müllerectomy-conjunctivectomy.

Anesthesia

Local anesthesia may be used by infiltrating 2% lidocaine (Xylocaine) with epinephrine subcutaneously, approximately 10 mm superior to the eyelid margin. A modified frontal nerve block may also be used. Some surgeons infiltrate along the border of the tarsus subconjunctivally, with the eyelid everted. We find that this tends to distort the tissues and the measurement.

Surgical Procedure

Step 1

Anesthesia is administered subcutaneously with a 30-gauge needle and 2% Xylocaine with 1:100,000 epinephrine below the superior palpebral crease. Several drops of 0.5% proparacaine are instilled on the eye.

Step 2

An Adson forceps is used to fixate the upper lid margin. A 5-0 nylon suture on a P-1 or FS-2 needle is passed at the superior palpebral crease temporally from the skin surface to the conjunctival surface just above the tarsus (Figure 19-1). A plastic corneoscleral protector should be used to protect the globe.

Step 3

The upper eyelid is everted by a Desmarres retractor. Two equally curved hemostats are placed at the superior tarsal margin. The clamps should be placed 3 mm from the superior tarsal margin. The clamp incorporates tarsus, Müller's muscle, and conjunctiva. There is no levator aponeurosis in the clamp. Care must be taken not to clamp more tarsus centrally. This central placement of the clamp will lead to central eyelid peaking. If more than 3 mm of ptosis is present, an additional 4 to 6 mm of conjunctival Müller's muscle may be incorporated into the clamps (Figure 19-2).

Step 4

The suture is placed below the clamps from the temporal to the nasal side. The suture should pass approximately 5 mm below the clamp and at a 45° angle. An effort is made to pass the needle through the same hole the needle made on a previous pass. This brings the suture under the conjunctiva and avoids corneal abrasions.

Step 5

After the needle is passed the whole length of the clamps, it is further passed nasally, from the

Levine MR.
Manual of Oculoplastic Surgery, Fourth Edition (pp 137-140).
© 2010 SLACK Incorporated

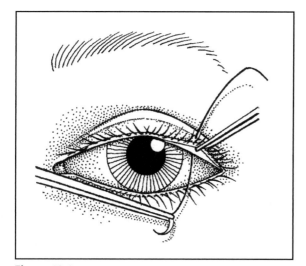

Figure 19-1.

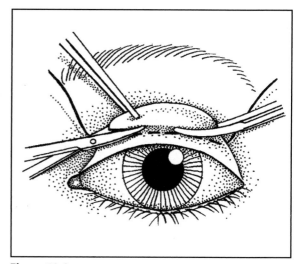

Figure 19-3.

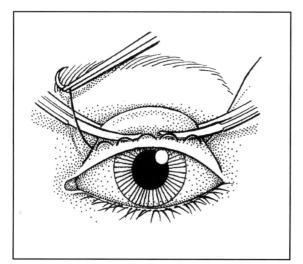

Figure 19-2.

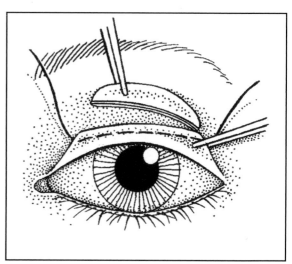

Figure 19-4.

conjunctiva through the full thickness of the eyelid and out the skin at the superior palpebral crease.

Step 6

One clamp is removed. The clamp is then used to hold the eyelid at the inferior tarsal margin. A Westcott spring-handled scissors is then used to cut the conjunctiva-tarsus-Müller's muscle through the crush marks made by the clamps. The other clamp is removed, and a forceps with 0.5-mm teeth is used to hold the excised tissue (Figure 19-3).

Step 7

The tissue may be used as a graft to elevate the lower lid or other reconstructive procedures (Figure 19-4).

Step 8

The smooth side of a #15 Bard-Parker blade handle is used to smooth the inner surface of the conjunctiva to avoid any rough irregularities on the inner surface of the eyelid.

Step 9

Each end of the nylon suture is tied to itself (Figure 19-5).

Step 10

The plastic corneoscleral shield is removed, and an antibiotic ointment is placed on the eye.

Postoperative Management

Ice compresses are used for the first 24 hours. This procedure is usually done on an ambulatory basis, and the patient goes home the same day of the surgery. Systemic antibiotics may be used prophylactically. The suture is removed in 10 days. If the eyelid is too high postoperatively, the suture should be removed earlier than 10 days, and gentle traction should be placed on the eyelid to separate the wound adhesion to the desired level.

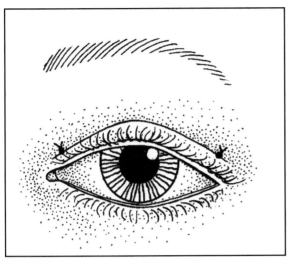

Figure 19-5.

Complications

This procedure is only effective with small amounts of ptosis, good levator function, and a good response to phenylephrine hydrochloride (2.5%). Its advantage is in its simplicity and predictability. Possible complications include a peaked eyelid because of misapplication of the hemostats, corneal abrasion from too much exposed suture material on the tarsus, and occasional duplication of the eyelid crease secondary to tarsus removal. Other complications can include dry eyes or undercorrection. Patients with poor eye protective mechanism or eyelid malposition may benefit from a lower eyelid elevation procedure using the resected tarsus-conjunctiva-Müller's muscle graft to avoid dry eyes. Undercorrection is best treated with an aponeurosis advancement.

In memory of Albert Hornblass, MD, who wrote this chapter in the first three editions of *Manual of Oculoplastic Surgery.*

SECTION VI

EYELID MALPOSITIONS

CHAPTER 20

THYROID EYELID RETRACTION

Richard L. Anderson, MD and David R. Jordan, MD, FRCSC, FACS

The etiology of eyelid retraction in thyroid-associated orbitopathy (TAO) is not fully understood, but several factors appear to contribute. In the upper eyelid, these factors include (1) Müller's muscle contraction caused by adrenergic stimulation, (2) involvement of the levator muscle by the thyroid disease process, and (3) overaction of the levator-superior rectus muscle complex in response to hypophoria produced by fibrosis and retraction of the inferior rectus. In the lower eyelid, stimulation of the sympathetic muscle plays a lesser role; a more important factor seems to be fibrosis of the inferior rectus, which exerts a retracting action on the lower eyelid via its capsulopalpebral head. In many thyroid patients, there is both a true and an apparent eyelid retraction, the latter being the result of proptosis.

Treatment of eyelid retraction may be indicated for a variety of reasons, including significant corneal exposure and lagophthalmos, chronic conjunctival and episcleral injection, and cosmesis. Treatment may be medical or surgical. Steroids and sympatholytic agents, such as guanethidine, bethanidine, and thymoxamine, are examples of medical treatment but play little role in the long-term correction of lid retraction. Botulinum toxin A may be used in the inflammatory phase of thyroid eye disease to reduce upper eyelid retraction. A dose of 2 to 5 units given transconjunctivally just above the superior border of tarsus into the elevator complex (Müller's/levator) of the upper eyelid will drop the eyelid 1 to 3 mm. Each patient reacts differently, and, because of this variability, dosing should be individually titrated. Patients should return in 10 to 14 days after injection for re-evaluation of their lid position.

Surgical intervention is the best mode of treatment. Before contemplating elective surgery, it is essential to determine that the patient's eyelid height and Graves' disease have been stable for at least 6 months to 1 year. If there is active orbital disease or recent changes in eye-lid height, results are unpredictable, and surgery is best deferred.

A number of surgical approaches have been described for thyroid upper eyelid retraction. These can basically be divided into 2 groups: the conjunctival approach and the cutaneous approach. In the conjunctival approach, the surgeon enters the eyelid from the conjunctival side just above the level of the tarsal plate. The goal is to recess Müller's muscle and the levator muscle from their insertions. In some techniques, Müller's muscle is completely removed, whereas in others it is recessed along with the levator.

A cutaneous approach for levator recession has also been advocated by several investigators. Once again, the goal is to identify the levator aponeurosis and Müller's muscles and to disinsert or remove them.

Surgical Technique

GRADED APONEUROTIC APPROACH TO THE UPPER EYELID

The aponeurotic approach for upper eyelid retraction involves an anterior skin approach to the levator and Müller's muscles in the upper eyelid. Once the levator is identified, the lateral horn is transected, and the lateral levator, in conjunction with Müller's muscle, is recessed in a graded fashion. No spacers are used. Eyelid height and contour are predictable and adjusted intraoperatively while the patient is sitting up. This approach facilitates visualization of the anatomy, especially the lateral horn of the aponeurosis, which must be cut to relieve the temporal retraction. This approach also avoids cutting the conjunctiva and the lacrimal gland and its ductules, which may result in a dry eye.

Levine MR.
Manual of Oculoplastic Surgery, Fourth Edition (pp 143-148).
© 2010 SLACK Incorporated

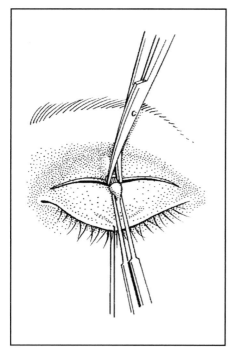

Figure 20-1.

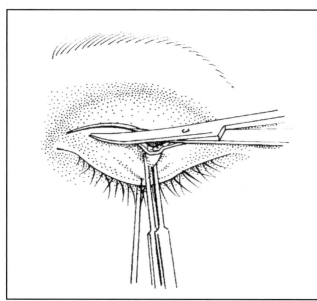

Figure 20-2.

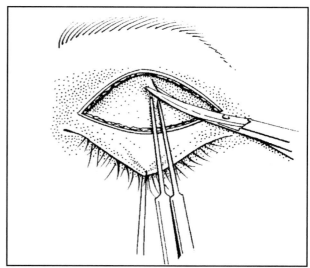

Figure 20-3.

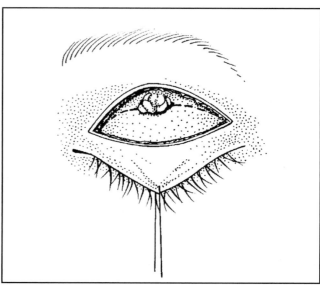

Figure 20-4.

Step 1
The normal skin crease is marked out with gentian violet.

Step 2
Anesthesia is obtained by subcutaneous infiltration of 1.0 to 2.0 mL of 2% lidocaine hydrochloride with 1:100,000 epinephrine along the marked skin crease. Tetracaine hydrochloride 0.5% or 1.0% is used on the cornea and conjunctiva.

Step 3
A 4-0 silk traction suture is placed in the eyelid margin and secured inferiorly. This puts the eyelid structures posterior to the orbicularis on tension while permitting redundant skin and orbicularis anteriorly to be mobilized.

Step 4
The skin is incised along the marked lid creases with a scalpel.

Step 5
The orbicularis muscle is tented anteriorly (Figure 20-1), and a cut is made into the posterior orbicularis fascial plane. Scissors are used to open this plane medially and laterally for the length of the wound (Figure 20-2), so that the underlying levator aponeurosis is exposed.

Step 6
The orbital septal attachments to the aponeurosis are identified. The septum is incised (Figure 20-3), and the key landmark (preaponeurotic fat) is seen (Figure 20-4). The septum is then opened medially and laterally, and the fat is gently teased away from the underlying aponeurosis.

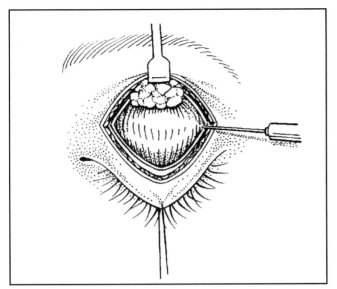

Figure 20-5.

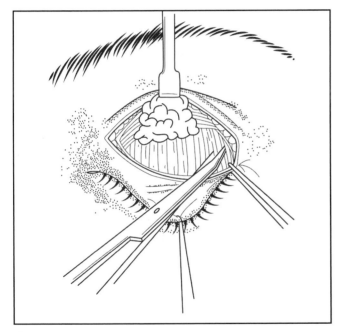

Figure 20-6.

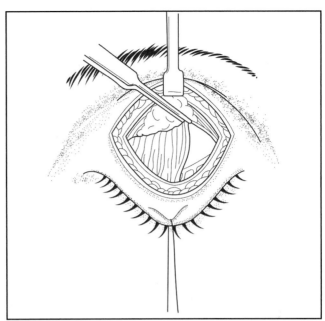

Figure 20-7.

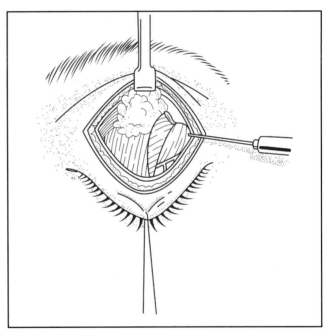

Figure 20-8.

Step 7

Local anesthetic (0.25 mL) is injected under the levator aponeurosis to separate it from underlying Müller's muscle (Figure 20-5).

Step 8

Using blunt and sharp dissection, the lateral aponeurosis is dissected away from Müller's muscle for the lateral 20% of the lid. The lateral horn is cut with care to avoid the lacrimal gland and its ducts (Figure 20-6). As it is cut, one can feel the "give," and the lateral aponeurosis becomes fully mobile. The lateral 20% of aponeurosis, now freed (Figure 20-7), retracts superiorly, exposing Müller's muscle. The peripheral arcade of vessels is seen in Müller's muscle just above the tarsal border. Müller's muscle can be seen as a thin vascular structure with mus-cular fibers running vertically from the superior aspect of the tarsal plate. It is often infiltrated with fat and, therefore, may appear quite yellow.

Step 9

Local anesthetic (0.25 to 0.50 mL) is injected into the plane between Müller's muscle and the conjunctiva to balloon Müller's muscle away from the underlying tissue (Figure 20-8).

Step 10

The lateral 20% of Müller's muscle is then undermined (Figure 20-9). Bleeding into the fornix usually occurs at this stage because of the highly vascular nature of Müller's muscle. Care should be taken not to buttonhole the closely adherent

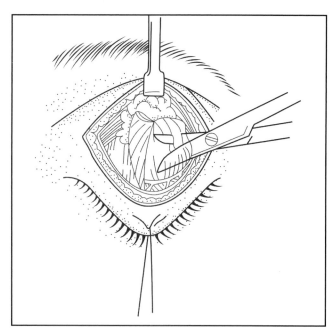

Figure 20-9.

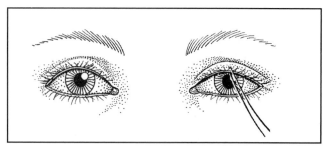

Figure 20-10.

conjunctiva. If rents occur, they are closed with 7-0 chromic catgut suture.

Step 11

The patient is assisted to a sitting position at this step, and the lid heights are compared. The patient is asked to look up and down after being brought to a sitting position. Lid height and contour are assessed (Figure 20-10). If additional lid lowering is required, further dissection of Müller's and levator muscles can be done while the patient is still in the sitting position. Adjustments are made as necessary so that the eyelid is placed at the desired height and contour. The lid height measured intraoperatively should be the expected postoperative height.

Step 12

The levator horn and dissected Müller's muscle are transected, and the remaining aponeurosis and Müller's muscle are then sutured with 6-0 chromic catgut to the conjunctiva where they lay (Figure 20-11).

Step 13

If prolapsing orbital fat is present, it can be excised in the manner of a blepharoplasty.

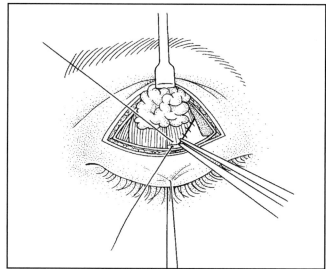

Figure 20-11.

Step 14

Skin is closed with a running 6-0 plain absorbable suture. A steroid antibiotic ointment is instilled in the eye.

APONEUROTIC APPROACH TO THE LOWER EYELID

In the lower eyelid, a similar aponeurotic approach is performed from a posterior (conjunctival) approach. For lower lid retraction of less than 2 mm, retractor disinsertion and extirpation are effective. For lid retraction greater than 2 mm, a spacer is more effective. Either ear cartilage or hard palate mucosa is effective, but the latter is preferred because the hard palate has a mucosa, is less irritating, and is less rigid or board-like than cartilage. The hard palate tends to conform to the shape of the globe better than does the cartilage. The amount of hard palate or cartilage to use is a ratio of 2:1 (ie, 2 mm of graft per 1 mm of lid retraction to be corrected).

In the lower eyelid, a complete extirpation of the retractors is performed. Height and contour adjustment as performed in the upper eyelid is unnecessary. Gravity and facial tension assist in lowering the upper eyelid but work against raising the lower eyelid. Postoperatively, the lower eyelids are elevated using superior traction sutures for several days after surgery.

Step 1

Two percent lidocaine hydrochloride with epinephrine is injected subconjunctivally in the lower lid.

Step 2

A 4-0 silk traction suture is placed in such a manner that it can be left as a modified Frost suture after surgery.

Step 3

The plane between the orbicularis muscle and retractors is isolated by tenting conjunctiva and retractors away from the orbicularis and by making a horizontal snip into the plane (Figure 20-12).

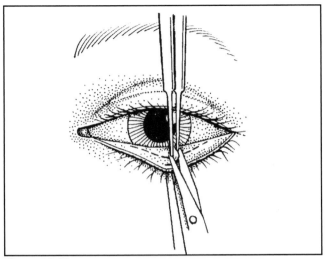

Figure 20-12.

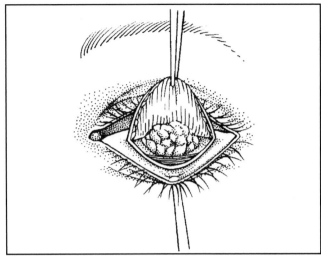

Figure 20-14.

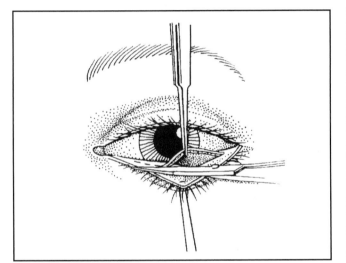

Figure 20-13.

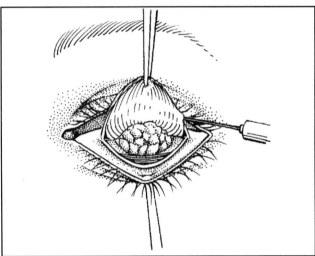

Figure 20-15.

Step 4

With Westcott scissors, this plane is then opened medially and laterally (Figure 20-13).

Step 5

Using blunt and sharp dissection, the aponeurosis of the lower eyelid is separated from the orbital septum and preaponeurotic fat pad (Figure 20-14). The retractor aponeurosis of the lower eyelid lies immediately behind the fat pad as in the upper eyelid. It appears as a white structure, looking thinner but remarkably similar to the aponeurosis of the upper eyelid. The aponeurosis and the sympathetic muscle of the lower eyelid together are referred to as the retractors.

Step 6

The retractors are ballooned away from the conjunctiva with local anesthesia (Figure 20-15).

Step 7

The aponeurosis and sympathetic muscle are undermined together by blunt and sharp dissection from conjunctiva. Care should be taken to preserve the underlying conjunctiva. The dissection is carried inferiorly toward Lockwood's ligament. The inferior oblique and the insertion of the inferior rectus may be seen. The retractors are freed inferiorly as far as possible and then extirpated to permit maximum lid elevation (Figure 20-16).

Step 8

The conjunctiva is reapproximated with 2 or 3 6-0 plain sutures. Two modified Frost sutures are used to place the lower lid on superior tension by taping these sutures to the forehead for a few days.

Step 9

If more than 2 mm of lower lid retraction is present, a spacer, preferably hard palate, is put into position before conjunctival closure. The hard palate should be put in position from the punctum to the lateral end of the tarsus. If it is not long enough to reach this length, the available piece is moved lateral to the punctum. The superior edge of hard palate is sutured to the inferior edge of the tarsus with interrupted 7-0 chromic sutures, whereas the lower edge

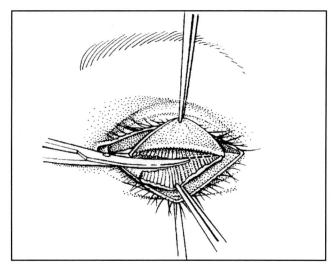

Figure 20-16.

of the hard palate is sutured to the conjunctival edge in the lower fornix area (Figure 20-17).

Step 10

Postoperatively, antibiotic ointment is applied at night, and antibiotic drops are used during the day.

Complications

The graded aponeurotic-Müller's approach to upper lid retraction offers a high degree of reliability. The most common complication, which occurs infrequently, is a mild temporal droop, indicating that too much of the levator and Müller's muscles have been transected. This can be readily corrected with a lateral levator advancement through an external crease approach or small lateral Fasanella-Servat procedure. Undercorrection or recurrence of retraction is seen infrequently.

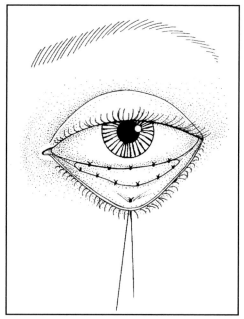

Figure 20-17.

Residual temporal eyelid flare is the most common problem reported with other techniques. With the technique described here, the surgeon can clearly see the lateral horn running between the orbital and palpebral lobes of the lacrimal gland and cut it completely without damaging these structures. This step is of paramount importance to achieve adequate lowering of the lateral portion of the retracted eyelid. A blind cut of the horn is to be avoided at all costs. The aponeurotic approach also enables the surgeon to avoid the palpebral lobe of the lacrimal gland and its ducts to the fornix, which are difficult to avoid from the posterior approach.

CHAPTER 21

INVOLUTIONAL LOWER EYELID ENTROPION

James Karesh, MD, FACS

Entropion is defined as an inward rotation of the eyelid margin and eyelashes toward the globe. While the lower eyelid is most commonly affected, this condition can also involve the upper eyelid. It can be unilateral or bilateral and may affect only a segment of an eyelid. It has many etiologies including inflammation, autoimmune disease, congenital abnormalities, and trauma. However, it is most commonly caused by involutional changes associated with aging and subsequent disruption of the normal eyelid anatomy. It is not known to what extent other factors such as sun exposure, chronic blepharitis and meibomitis, irritation-induced eyelid spasm, chronic eyelid manipulation associated with ocular allergy, contact lens insertion, the instillation of ocular medications, or conditions such as floppy-eyelid syndrome are also involved.

The discussion that follows will be limited to an understanding of the changes associated with involutional lower eyelid entropion and the surgical management of this condition and will include a description of the lower eyelid anatomy, the various pathologic changes that occur within the eyelid due to aging, and the mechanisms by which these changes destabilize the eyelid, resulting in entropion. This is followed by a discussion of a variety of nonsurgical and surgical approaches for managing this problem. No attempt will be made to comprehensively discuss all management options. Instead, the focus will be on those nonsurgical and surgical options that can be used in a variety of situations and have a proven track record of success.

Anatomy and Pathophysiology

The lower eyelid maintains its position and function through the delicate balance of its relationships with internal anatomic structures, external attachments to the bony orbit, and contiguous structures such as the globe. With aging, blinking, eye rubbing, and other factors, these relationships tend to stretch, tear, and break down, destabilizing the eyelid and resulting in various pathologic conditions, one of which is involutional entropion.

The 3 major anatomic structures responsible for the eyelid's position are the canthal tendons (MCL, LCL, Figure 21-1), orbicularis muscle (OOM, Figures 21-1 and 21-2), and capsulopalpebral fascia. In the horizontal dimension, the eyelids are attached medially to the anterior and posterior lacrimal crest (ALC and PLC, Figure 21-1) by the deep and superficial heads of the preseptal and pretarsal portions of the orbicularis muscle (MCL, Figure 21-1). Laterally the orbicularis muscle fibers interdigitate and form a raphe, commonly called the lateral canthal tendon. This structure is attached to the periosteum of the lateral orbital rim several millimeters posterior to its most anterior edge. There are also additional septal attachments both medially and laterally (S, Figures 21-1 and 21-2). Over a period of years, aging, genetics, eyelid manipulation, and other factors result in variable amounts of canthal tendon stretching and laxity. Most often these affect the lateral canthal tendon. As an isolated phenomenon, eyelid laxity is most often associated with involutional ectropion or tearing secondary to a failure of the lacrimal pump mechanism. It is variably present in involutional entropion where it is partnered with other anatomic abnormalities.

In addition to being responsible for the eyelid's horizontal attachments, the orbicularis muscle (OOM, Figures 21-1 and 21-2) exerts vertical and anterior-posterior forces on the lid during both eyelid closure and blinking. With contraction, the muscle pushes the lower eyelid upward and, with relaxation, the eyelid moves downward. Additionally, as the lower eyelid moves upward, it is also pushed posteriorly against the globe. Involutional changes, including muscle atrophy or hypertrophy, intramuscular collagen or fat deposition, and muscle fiber microtears, variably affect orbicularis muscle anatomy and function. These can cause the preseptal portion of

Levine MR.
Manual of Oculoplastic Surgery, Fourth Edition (pp 149-156).
© 2010 SLACK Incorporated

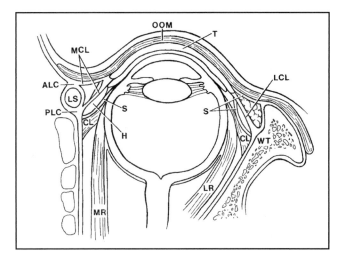

Figure 21-1.

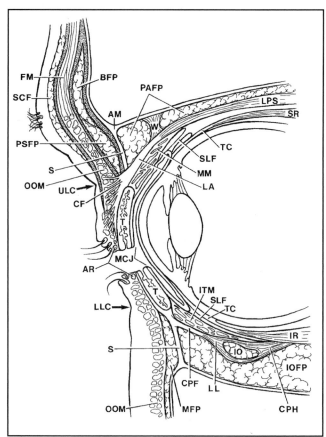

Figure 21-2.

the muscle to move upward and over the pretarsal portion with subsequent entropion formation during blinking and lid closure.

The capsulopalpebral fascia (CPF, Figure 21-2; the retractor of the lower eyelid) is the final structure that helps to maintain normal eyelid position and function. This structure is analogous to the levator aponeurosis and Müller's muscle complex in the upper eyelid. It extends from Lockwood's ligament (LL, Figure 21-2, horizontal transverse) to the inferior and anterior face of the lower eyelid tarsus (T, Figure 21-2). It functions to stabilize the tarsus and upper eyelid by opposing the posterior and superior forces exerted by the orbicularis muscle as it contracts. Additionally, its insertion along the inferior and anterior face of the tarsus helps keep the lower border of the tarsus slightly posterior to its superior border. This also acts to prevent the eyelid from inturning.

A final factor that helps maintain the normal position of the eyelid is the anterior projection of the globe, which acts to oppose any tendency of the eyelid to rotate inwardly. However, with aging, there may be orbital fat atrophy with a subsequent loss of orbital volume and enophthalmos. This change in globe position weakens its countering effect and can be a contributing factor to subsequent entropion formation.

Diagnosis

Tearing, ocular irritation, and conjunctival injection are the most common symptoms associated with entropion. These can be either constant or intermittent and are caused by eyelashes and keratinized eyelid skin rubbing the cornea and bulbar conjunctiva. Superficial punctate keratopathy and a fine papillary conjunctivitis are commonly present. Corneal ulceration and scarring are uncommon as normal lashes are long and pliable. While it is often tempting to cut or pull the lashes that are abrading the cornea, such action is contraindicated as short lash stubble is stiff and causes more significant corneal irritation and epithelial injury than long lashes. While usually unilateral, entropion can present simultaneously in both lower eyelids or present unilaterally and then present at a later date in an opposite lid.

A simple external examination with a penlight is usually sufficient for demonstrating the presence of an entropion. Sometimes a patient will present with the eyelid taped to keep it from turning inward. Occasionally, the entire margin is rolled inwardly, making it appear to be absent. Pulling the lower eyelid skin downward will reveal the actual problem as the margin and lashes are exposed. In such cases, when the patient blinks or forcibly closes the lids, the entropion will recur. This is also a helpful observation when the condition is intermittent.

There are several simple tests for demonstrating the involutional changes associated with entropion. Eyelid laxity and canthal tendon weakness can be demonstrated by the "snap-back" test and the eyelid distraction test. The former is performed by pulling the lower eyelid downward with a finger and then slowly releasing it. Normally, the eyelid will "snap-back" to its normal position almost immediately. Any delay in this indicates eyelid laxity. Severe laxity is evident when the eyelid completely fails to return to its resting position. A similar test is the eyelid distraction test. In this test, the eyelid is pulled away from the globe. Normally, the maximum distance the eyelid can be distracted is only 2 or 3 mm. More than this amount indicates the presence of eyelid laxity. In extreme cases, the eyelid can be distracted as much as 2 cm.

Medial and lateral canthal tendon integrity can also be assessed using the horizontal eyelid distraction test. The medial and lateral aspects of the eyelid are normally firmly attached to the periosteum. Involutional changes can cause these to weaken and stretch. This can be

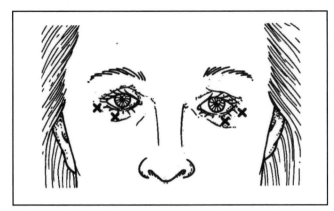

Figure 21-3.

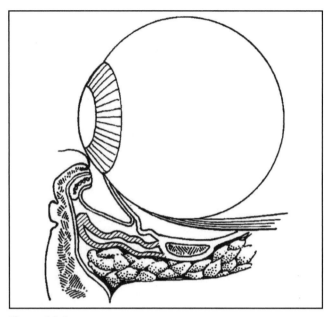

Figure 21-4.

demonstrated by moving the eyelid either medially or laterally. When the medial canthal tendon is lax, it is often possible to pull the eyelid laterally to such an extent that the punctum can be moved past the medial limbus. When the lateral canthal tendon is lax, it is often possible to move the entire lateral canthal angle medially 1 cm or more.

Nonsurgical Management

Options for the nonsurgical management of entropion include lubrication to protect the cornea and various procedures to stabilize the eyelid margin. These are usually temporizing until surgical intervention can be arranged. Copious application of artificial tear ointment to the affected eye is a basic management option. This should be done at bedtime, upon awakening, and as many times during the waking hours as necessary to control the patient's symptoms.

Another option is to tape the lower eyelid either at a downward angle or horizontally to prevent the margin from rotating inwardly and to reduce horizontal laxity. A problem with this technique is that artificial tear ointment can interfere with the ability of tape to adhere to the skin. Tincture of benzoin, cyanoacrylate, and other surgical adhesives and cements as well as various surgical tapes may be useful for extending the length of time an eyelid can be successfully taped in an acceptable position. A problem with the long-term use of tape and adhesives is their association with an inflammatory dermatitis. This necessitates their discontinuance.

Nonincisional Entropion Correction

TEMPORARY DRUG-INDUCED ENTROPION CORRECTION

Focal injections of botulinum toxin into the lower eyelid orbicularis muscle will temporarily alleviate an entropion's spastic component. This effect can last 4 to 6 months and may be helpful for delaying surgical intervention. Two or 3 subcutaneous injections of 2.5 to 5.0 units each are adequate for paralyzing the orbicularis muscle. These should be given at the level of the inferior tarsus medial to the medial limbus, lateral to the lateral limbus, and, if necessary, approximately 10 mm beyond the lateral canthus (Figure 21-3). The technique for injection is discussed elsewhere in this volume and will not be further discussed here.

ROTATIONAL SUTURES

Eyelid rotation sutures create a scar barrier that prevents the preseptal segment of the orbicularis muscle from moving superiorly over the pretarsal segment during blinking or eyelid closure (Figure 21-4). Additionally, these sutures will plicate and possibly reattach the capsulopalpebral fascia to the anterior and inferior aspect of the tarsus thereby stabilizing this structure. The use of a reactive absorbable double-armed suture such as a 4-0 chromic gut helps greatly in titrating the amount of eyelid eversion, creating an adequate scar barrier, and in suture placement. While this procedure is easily performed in the office or at the bedside under local anesthesia, it is only a temporary fix and frequently the entropion will recur after several weeks.

Step 1

After instilling a topical anesthetic, local anesthesia is achieved by injecting 2% lidocaine with 1:100,000 epinephrine across the entire eyelid either transcutaneously or transconjunctivally. Approximately 3 mL of anesthesia is usually sufficient.

Step 2

Three or 4 double-armed 4-0 or 5-0 chromic gut sutures with relatively large cutting needles attached are placed as horizontal mattress sutures. These sutures are equally spaced across the eyelid. Each suture arm is placed deeply into the palpebral conjunctiva and the lower eyelid retractors are placed several millimeters below the inferior border of the tarsus. The distance between each arm of the suture should be approximately 4 or 5 mm (Figure 21-5).

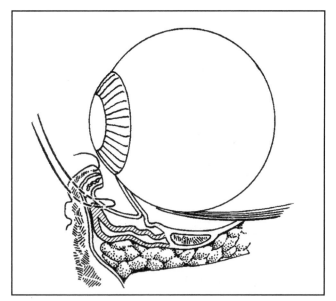

Figure 21-5.

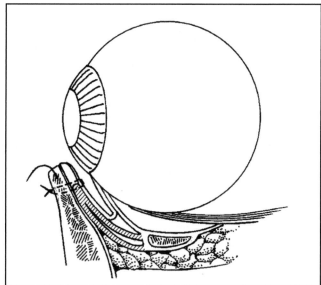

Figure 21-6.

Step 3

The sutures are passed just inferior to the inferior tarsal border and enter the orbicularis muscle to finally exit from the eyelid skin 3 or 4 mm below the cilia of the lower eyelid (Figure 21-6).

Step 4

The sutures are tied and tightened sufficiently to create a small amount of ectropion. This will resolve over several weeks as the sutures are absorbed. No bolsters are required. Ophthalmic antibiotic ointment is instilled onto the sutures twice daily for a week.

Surgical Management

In general, the surgical correction of involution entropion attempts to correct the 3 anatomic abnormalities underlying its occurrence, namely, eyelid laxity, overaction of the orbicularis muscle, and dehisced or weakened lower eyelid retractors. The procedure to accomplish these goals is usually performed transconjunctivally. However, there may be occasions when a transcutaneous approach is appropriate, such as when there is no obvious lower eyelid or lateral canthal tendon laxity or when the surgeon feels more comfortable with visualizing the eyelid structures using this type of incision. For this reason, a transcutaneous approach to retractor plication and excision of hyperactive orbicularis muscle is also described in addition to the transconjunctival approach. The transcutaneous approach can be easily combined with a tarsal strip procedure for correcting eyelid and tendon laxity if this problem is also present.

TRANSCUTANEOUS RETRACTOR PLICATION/ REINSERTION

Step 1

After the instillation of a topical anesthetic, 2% lidocaine with 1:100,000 epinephrine is diffusely injected either transconjunctivally or subcutaneously across the lower eyelid extending from the eyelid margin to the level of the inferior orbital rim. Approximately 3 to 6 mL of anesthetic is required to achieve adequate pain control and hemostasis.

Step 2

Using either cutting cautery or a scalpel blade, a subciliary incision is made across the lower eyelid from approximately the punctum to the lateral canthus. It is preferable that this incision be approximately 3 or 4 mm below the lid margin to facilitate entry into the suborbicularis plane. A 4-0 silk suture for upward traction on the eyelid is placed approximately 2 mm below the eyelid margin. This suture should be placed through the anterior superficial portion of the tarsus to prevent tear-out during dissection.

Step 3

With upward traction on the 4-0 silk suture, the orbicularis muscle is button-holed with scissors centrally and immediately inferior to the lower border of the tarsus. It is helpful to tent up the orbicularis by lifting the skin inferior to the incision when attempting to enter the suborbicularis space. The 4-0 silk traction suture can be attached to the surgical drapes superiorly, enabling the surgeon to use one hand to incise the muscle and the other to lift up the skin. The opening is extended across the entire eyelid, severing the preseptal orbicularis fibers from the pretarsal orbicularis fibers (Figure 21-7).

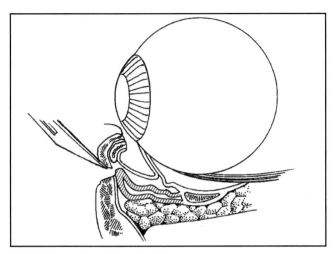

Figure 21-7.

Step 4

Blunt dissection with either scissors or cotton-tipped applicators is then used to expose the vertical extent of the eyelid retractors to the level of the orbital septum and orbital fat. If desired, the orbital septum may be incised and orbital fat excised as is done during a transcutaneous blepharoplasty.

Step 5

A horizontal sliver of orbicularis muscle 3 or 4 mm in height is excised across the entire horizontal extent of the skin muscle flap created by entering the suborbicularis space. It is usually not necessary to remove any skin in addition to the muscle.

Step 6

The lower eyelid retractors appear as a whitish colored layer of tissue the extends from the septum to the inferior tarsal border. When a patient looks up and down, this layer of tissue can be seen to move in the same direction as the globe. The retractors are plicated or reattached using either interrupted single or double armed 5-0 or 6-0 polyglactin suture passed through the lower eyelid skin inferior to the skin incision, the superior edge of the retractors, and the inferior edge of the skin immediately superior to the skin incision. Tying the suture closes the skin incision, plicates or reattaches the retractors, and rotates the eyelid margin outward. Three or 4 sutures evenly spaced across the eyelid are usually sufficient to achieve the desired amount of lid correction. The tightness with which these sutures are tied will modify the amount of correction that is achieved (Figure 21-8). It is best to combine a lateral tarsal strip (further described next) with this procedure to avoid a postoperative ectropion if any degree of lid laxity is also present. Another variation is to advance and suture the inferior retractors directly to the inferior tarsal border followed by a running 6-0 plain gut suture to close the skin.

Step 7

At the end of the procedure, the 4-0 silk traction suture is removed and ophthalmic antibiotic

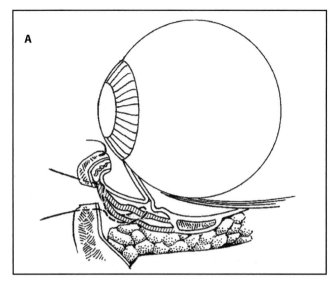

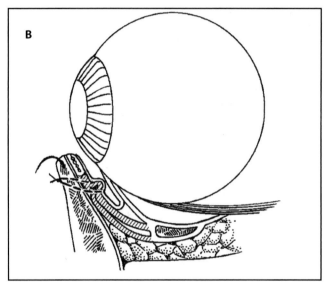

Figure 21-8.

ointment is placed on the incision twice daily for 1 week. The eyelid is not patched after surgery.

TRANSCONJUNCTIVAL ENTROPION CORRECTION

Transconjunctival entropion repair can be performed either in the office with local anesthesia or in the operating suite with local anesthesia and sedation. An experienced surgeon can perform the surgery in approximately 30 minutes or less. There are 3 parts to the procedure: a tarsal strip horizontal eyelid shortening to correct eyelid and tendon laxity, an excision of a horizontal portion of the preseptal orbicularis muscle to correct the overriding or hyperactivity of this portion of the orbicularis muscle, and a reattachment of the capsulopalpebral fascia to the anterior and inferior portion of the tarsus to vertically stabilize the tarsus and help reform the lower eyelid subciliary crease. These basic pieces of the procedure can be augmented with a transconjunctival removal of lower eyelid fat as well as a modified cheek lift if either are required.

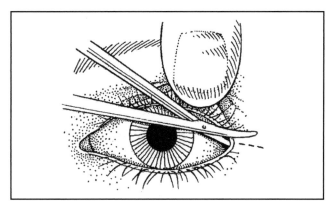

Figure 21-9.

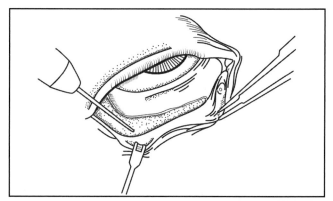

Figure 21-11.

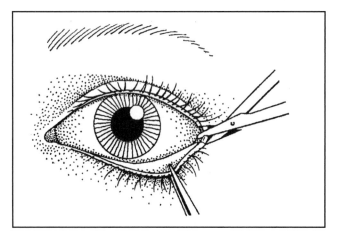

Figure 21-10.

Step 1

After topical anesthetic drops are instilled into the inferior conjunctival cul-de-sac, 2% lidocaine with 1:100,000 epinephrine is diffusely injected either subcutaneously or transconjunctivally across the lower eyelid from the lid margin to the inferior orbital rim. The 3 fat pockets in the lower lid are also injected if fat removal is anticipated. Approximately 3 to 6 mL are required for this. An additional 3 mL of anesthesia are injected into the lateral canthal area, the inner surface of the lateral orbital rim, and the lateral upper eyelid.

Step 2

Using either cutting electrocautery with a needle tip or scissors, a full-thickness lateral canthotomy incision is made extending approximately 10 mm horizontally from the canthus (Figure 21-9).

Step 3

The inferior limb of the lateral canthal tendon is incised by pulling the lateral lower eyelid upward with a toothed forceps and cutting through the tendon with the scissors directed medially and inferiorly (in the direction of the tip of the nose). It is helpful to "strum" the tendon with the cutting instrument to identify its extent and to demonstrate that all of its attachments have been incised (Figure 21-10).

Step 4

The surgical incision is extended across the palpebral conjunctiva just below the inferior tarsal border. This will divide the conjunctiva and lower eyelid retractors from the tarsus. This will allow visualization of the suborbicularis space. Blunt and sharp dissection is then employed to completely expose this area to the level of the orbital septum and fat. At this point, the septum can be incised and fat excised if necessary (Figure 21-11).

Step 5

Using scissors, a strip of hyperactive preseptal orbicularis muscle is carefully excised across the entire eyelid, making sure that the skin is not accidentally button-holed. Undermining the muscle with scissors separating it from the overlying skin facilitates this excision. Cautery is necessary to control bleeding as the orbicularis muscle is quite vascular.

Step 6

The eyelid retractors and conjunctiva are reattached to the anterior inferior surface of the lower eyelid tarsus with 3 or 4 double armed 4-0 or 5-0 chromic gut sutures as was described above for rotation sutures. Each arm of the suture is placed though the palpebral conjunctiva and, with direct visualization, through the eyelid retractors. The suture arms are spaced approximately 4 or 5 mm from each other and the individual sutures should be evenly spaced across the eyelid. No additional conjunctival sutures are necessary (Figure 21-12).

Step 7

The sutures are then passed backhand through the pretarsal orbicularis attached to the anterior and inferior surface of the tarsus. They are brought out through the skin 3 or 4 mm inferior to the lashes. The sutures are tied and adjusted until the eyelid is mildly ectropic but not retracted. The ectropion will be managed by performing a tarsal strip procedure.

Step 8

The final step is to horizontally tighten the lid and reattach it to the lateral orbital rim periosteum. This is carried out by forming a tarsal strip as already described elsewhere in Chapter 24. To avoid redundancy, the steps for this will only be summarized.

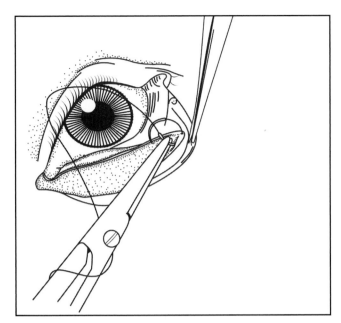

Figure 21-12.

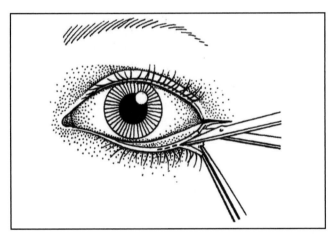

Figure 21-13.

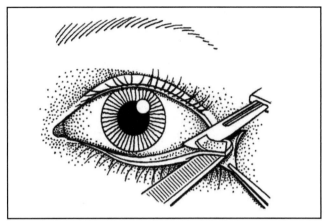

Figure 21-14.

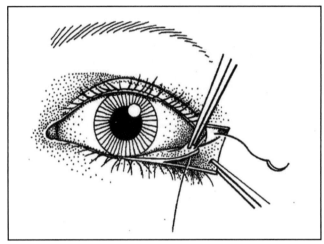

Figure 21-15.

Step 8a

The lower eyelid is pulled laterally and a mark is made near the lash line where the lower lid crosses the upper lid. This will be the new lateral extent of the lower lid. At this point, merely pulling the eyelid laterally should correct any ectropion that is present. If it does not, it may be necessary to adjust the sutures used to reattach the lower eyelid retractors.

Step 8b

Pretarsal skin and orbicularis muscle are excised with scissors up to the mark made in the previous step. It is better to err on the side of less eyelid shortening than more. The inferior border of the excision should be the inferior border of the tarsus and the superior border should be the eyelid margin.

Step 8c

Using scissors, excise the eyelid margin and eyelashes up to the previously made mark. It is important to completely remove all lashes and follicles to avoid postoperative trichiasis (Figure 21-13).

Step 8d

Excise and eyelid retractors are attached to this lateral tarsal strip and using a #15 Bard-Parker blade, scrape all palpebral conjunctiva from the strip. This will prevent cyst formation. Shorten the strip as needed to keep it approximately 5 mm in length (Figure 21-14).

Step 8e

Reattaching the strip to the lateral orbital rim periosteum is the most difficult part of the procedure. The strip needs to be sutured on the inner surface of the lateral orbital rim and as far superior as possible to ensure that the lateral canthal angle is symmetrical with the opposite side and higher than the medial canthal angle. Two single-armed 5-0 nylon, polypropylene, or polyglactin sutures or a single double-armed suture of similar material is passed through the tarsal strip (Figure 21-15).

Step 8f

Using a cotton-tipped applicator or an instrument (usually a forceps), the inner surface of the orbital rim is exposed. Each suture needle in the tarsal strip is then passed through the periosteum of the inner surface of the rim at least 5 mm posterior to the rim and slightly more superior than the point at which the lateral upper eyelid is attached. The

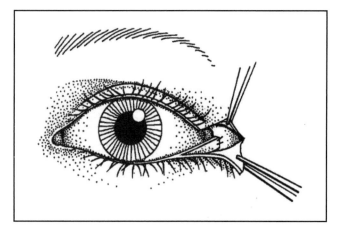

Figure 21-16.

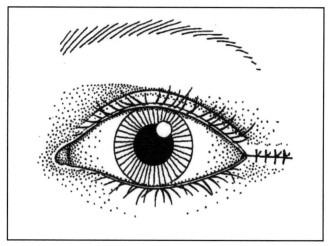

Figure 21-17.

needle needs to scrape the bone as it is passed to ensure that the periosteum is caught by the needle. The needle exits from the canthal soft tissue slightly above the level of the upper eyelid's lateral attachment (Figure 21-16).

Step 8g

The tarsal strip sutures are adjusted and tied, making sure that there is no residual ectropion or entropion and that the canthus is at approximately the same level as the opposite side. Finally, a 5-0 or 6-0 polyglactin or fast-absorbing polyglactin suture is used to attach the upper eyelid lateral canthus to the new lateral lower eyelid and to reform the lateral canthal angle. This suture is passed laterally through the orbicularis muscle of one lid and exits from the most lateral aspect of that lid at approximately the point where the eyelid margin ends. The needle is then passed through the most lateral aspect of the other lid and exits from the orbicularis of that eyelid. When the suture is tied, the lateral canthal angle is reformed.

Step 8h

Skin closure should be with an absorbable material such as 6-0 gut, chromic gut, or polyglactin as it can be difficult to remove sutures postoperatively when there is swelling. Ophthalmic antibiotic drops should be instilled 4 times daily for 1 week and ophthalmic antibiotic ointment should be placed on the skin incision twice daily for 1 week. No dressing is required, although some surgeons may feel the need to place Steri-Strips over the skin incision (Figure 21-17).

Complications

Complications of transconjunctival entropion repair include overcorrection resulting in an ectropion, recurrent entropion, and vertical lower eyelid retraction. Overcorrection may occur when the lower eyelid retractors are advanced without doing a lateral tarsal strip procedure when there is significant coexisting horizontal eyelid laxity. This problem is easily managed by taking the patient back to surgery and performing a tarsal strip procedure. Recurrent entropion results from inadequate advancement of the lower eyelid retractors onto the inferior anterior aspect of the lower eyelid tarsus. Correction of this problem requires that the retractors be advanced. Finally, a too aggressive advancement of the retractors may result in lower eyelid retraction and lagophthalmos. This is particularly apt to occur in association with a lower eyelid that is particularly tight following a tarsal strip procedure or when the globe is prominent. Initial management includes upward massage of the lower eyelid and tincture of time. If the problem continues, surgery to release the retractors or release of the lateral canthal tendon may be necessary.

CHAPTER 22

CICATRICIAL ENTROPION

Ralph E. Wesley, MD and Kimberly A. Klippenstein, MD

Cicatricial entropion results from a scarring process that causes the tarsus and conjunctiva to shrink. Considerable force is required to pull the tarsal plate inward. Common causes include chemical burns, trachoma, chronic eyelid infections, trauma, and conjunctival shrinkage diseases, such as cicatricial pemphigoid or Stevens-Johnson syndrome. Unlike involutional entropion, correction of cicatricial entropion requires incision of some scar tissue. Cicatricial forces are redirected by sutures or placement of a graft such as mucous membrane or hard palate. The surgeon must decide whether the entropion is severe enough to require placement of a graft. Differentiating cicatricial from spastic, involutional entropion is of prime importance.

Lower Eyelid Cicatricial Entropion

The Wies procedure is used to correct mild to moderate lower lid cicatricial entropion. This transmarginal rotation procedure uses horizontal fracturing of the tarsal plate so the eyelid margin can be rotated outward with everting sutures.

SURGICAL PROCEDURE

Step 1

Local infiltration with 1% lidocaine (Xylocaine) with epinephrine and hyaluronidase (Wydase) several minutes before the procedure provides good anesthesia and helps with hemostasis. The use of hyaluronidase in the anesthetic mixture causes the mixture to diffuse through the tissues more readily. A topical anesthetic is applied to the cornea.

Step 2

A horizontal incision is marked with methylene blue approximately 3 mm below the eyelash margin, avoiding the marginal artery to prevent a lid margin slough. The incision starts a few millimeters temporal to the inferior punctum and extends nearly to the lateral canthus (Figure 22-1).

Step 3

A scleral protective lens is inserted into the cul-de-sac, or a shoehorn protector is inserted.

Step 4

A 4-0 black silk suture is passed through the gray line in the center of the lower lid margin. The suture is attached to the surgical head drape with a hemostat.

Step 5

An incision is made with a #15 blade through the skin and orbicularis muscle as marked in Step 2.

Step 6

The superior traction suture is released, and the lower eyelid is inverted. An incision on the inside of the lower lid is made through the conjunctiva to connect to the skin incision. Blunt-tipped Westcott scissors can be used for a full-thickness incision. When completed, the tarsal and skin incisions coincide so that the lid margin is separated from the inferior portion of the eyelid but is still connected to the lower portion of the lid medially and laterally.

Step 7

The rotation is accomplished with 3 4-0 double-armed silk mattress sutures passed from the tarsus and conjunctiva internally out and up to the upper outer wound edge of skin and orbicularis muscle of the lid 2 to 3 mm from the eyelid margin (Figure 22-2). The amount of rotation depends on how close the sutures are placed to the eyelashes. The sutures are evenly spaced along the lid margin (see Figure 22-2).

Levine MR.
Manual of Oculoplastic Surgery, Fourth Edition (pp 157-162).
© 2010 SLACK Incorporated

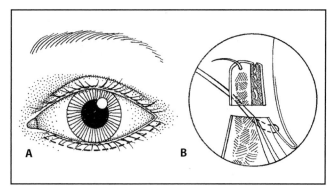

Figure 22-1.

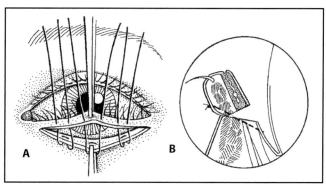

Figure 22-2.

Step 8

Before the mattress suture is tied, the skin incision is closed with a running 6-0 plain gut suture.

Step 9

The protective lens is removed, and the sutures are tied over small cotton bolsters, which can be fashioned by rolling cotton from a cotton applicator. The bolsters help maintain the lid rotation and direct the eyelashes outward.

Step 10

Antibiotic ointment is applied to the incision and lower fornix. Antibiotic ointment should be applied 2 or 3 times daily around the sutures.

Step 11

Cold wet compresses can be applied postoperatively to reduce swelling, pain, and bruising. Eye pads are unnecessary and may counteract the eversion produced by the sutures.

Step 12

The everting sutures are removed in 10 days. The 6-0 plain gut sutures are removed if they have not already sloughed. The scar produced by the horizontal mattress suture and the fixation of the superficial lid margin tissue to the deep tissue of the lower portion of the incision rotates the lid margin into proper position.

The primary complication of the Wies procedure is overcorrection. This, in effect, produces a cicatricial ectropion. Overcorrection is secondary to maximizing the potential rotation of the lid margin. This is seen when the incision is placed more than 3 to 4 mm from the lid margin or the sutures exit too close to the lid margin. Mild overcorrection usually resolves and is even desirable in the early postoperative period. Moderate overcorrection is handled by early cutting of sutures. The more severe cases are treated by severing the cicatricial bands and placing stabilization sutures. Other potential complications include eyelid necrosis caused by improperly placed sutures and eyelid fistula with epiphora.

This procedure works well for mild or moderate lower lid cicatricial entropion. More severe scarring requires the placement of mucous membrane grafts. Lower eyelid cicatricial entropion can be managed more successfully than upper eyelid entropion without grafts because the lower

eyelid does not constantly blink over the cornea. Rolling the eyelashes out away from the cornea with this procedure is frequently all that is needed for relief of cicatricial entropion in the lower eyelid.

Cicatricial Entropion of the Lower Eyelid Requiring Mucous Membrane Graft

Mucous membrane grafts must be placed into the inside of the lower eyelid when scarring and shortening of the inside surface are severe. Full-thickness grafts of mucous membrane contract less and provide better long-term results than thinner material. Full-thickness buccal mucosal or lower lip mucosal grafts provide a simple and effective method for correcting moderate or severe cicatricial entropion of the lower eyelid. Other materials, such as ear cartilage and nasal septal cartilage mucosal grafts, can be effective despite their stiffness and the increased difficulty of harvesting them. Eye-bank sclera or free conjunctival grafts work well initially but fail to resist contracting forces of cicatricial entropion, generally giving poor long-term results. Hard palate grafts work well in the lower eyelid but can cause painful corneal irritation as the squamous surface in the upper eyelid moves up and down over the corneal surface.

SURGICAL PROCEDURE: LOWER EYELID CICATRICIAL ENTROPION WITH FULL-THICKNESS LOWER LIP GRAFT

Step 1

The lower eyelid is anesthetized with 1% Xylocaine with epinephrine and hyaluronidase for anesthesia and hemostasis. Hyaluronidase facilitates spreading of the mixture through the tissue. Topical anesthesia should be applied to the cornea.

Step 2

A protective lens is inserted.

Step 3

An Erhardt clamp is applied to rotate the lower lid outward.

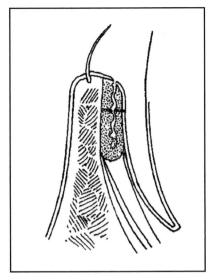

Figure 22-3.

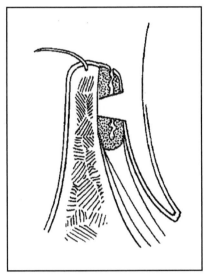

Figure 22-4.

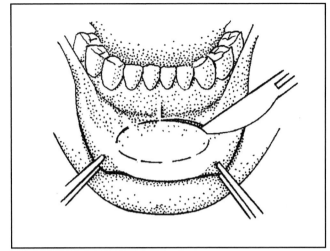

Figure 22-5.

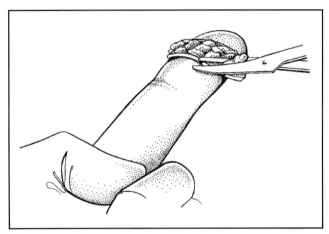

Figure 22-6.

Step 4

A horizontal incision is made inside the eyelid from the medial portion over to the lateral canthus (Figure 22-3). The incision should be approximately in the middle portion of the tarsal plate. The incision must be full-thickness through the tarsal plate to permit the lid margin to roll outward to a normal position (Figure 22-4).

Step 5a

The length and height of the defect are measured. An ellipse is then drawn with methylene blue inside the lower lip on the basis of 3 dimensions.

Step 6a

The lower lip is injected with the anesthetic mixture. The injection is used even if the patient is under general anesthesia because it provides better hemostasis. The mixture should balloon the mucous membrane for ease of dissection.

Step 7a

After 5 to 7 minutes have elapsed to allow the epinephrine to constrict the local blood vessels, 2 towel clips are applied to the lip for use as retractors.

Step 8a

A #15 blade is used to incise the mucosa on the lower lip as the assistant retracts the lip outward (Figure 22-5).

Step 9a

Westcott scissors and forceps are used to excise the graft. The dissection is performed carefully to avoid taking submucosal tissue with the graft.

Step 10a

After the graft has been excised, a small piece of Gelfoam should be pressed against the bare surface for hemostasis. The area may ooze somewhat throughout the remainder of the procedure. Cautery should be avoided to lessen the chance of soreness and contraction.

Step 11

The graft is draped backward over the finger, and any subcutaneous tissue is excised (Figure 22-6).

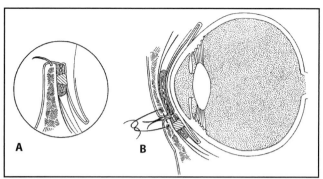

Figure 22-7.

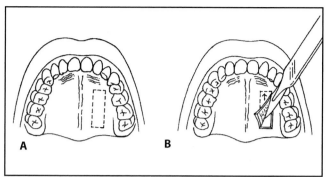

Figure 22-8.

Step 12

The graft is draped into the defect (Figure 22-7A).

Step 13

The graft is sewn into position with running 6-0 plain gut sutures.

Step 14

Antibiotic ointment is applied to the graft. The clamp and protective lens are removed.

Step 15

The eyelids are sewn together for 1 week with intermarginal sutures to keep the graft on stretch. Three stitches of 5-0 polyglactin (Vicryl) are passed through the upper and lower eyelids such that they exit at the margin (Figure 22-7B). (Full-thickness stitches would seriously damage the cornea.)

Step 16

Antibiotic ointment is applied to the Vicryl sutures twice daily until they are removed 1 week later. The 6-0 plain gut sutures do not require removal.

The procedure provides a simple, effective method for correction of lower eyelid entropion. In cases in which the lower fornix has been obliterated by conjunctival shrinkage, as with cicatricial pemphigoid, surgery is unnecessary unless the lid margin has scarred inward against the cornea. The donor site requires no treatment on the lower lip, although a soft diet may cause less irritation. Frequently, the patient does not experience discomfort from the donor site until approximately 3 to 4 days after surgery. Viscous lidocaine applied to the donor site provides considerable relief when pain does occur. The donor site forms a fibrin covering in a few days and undergoes complete re-epithelialization in 7 to 10 days. There have been reported complications of buccal or lip mucosal membrane donor sites, including submucosal scarring with contracture. This can be asymptomatic or result in web formation, which can potentially restrict mandible or lip mobility. This is corrected by resection of fibrotic tissue with reconstruction using Z-plasty to minimize tension. Rarely does the patient end up with too much graft. Even full-thickness grafts undergo some shrinkage. A generous-sized graft combined with sewing the lid together for 1 week helps to allow for late shrinkage. Another source of mucosal graft is the hard palate. This graft provides replacement of the posterior lamella via its dual composition of collagen and mucous membrane, yielding structural support

with an appropriate surface. The superficial collagen is loosely arranged; however, the deep collagen consists of thick bundles aligned in a parallel fashion. This graft affords minimal shrinkage compared with other sources of mucous membrane; estimates of shrinkage are on the order of less than 10%. These grafts maintain their firm support, are readily available, and have low morbidity.

SURGICAL PROCEDURE: LOWER EYELID CICATRICIAL ENTROPION WITH HARD PALATE GRAFT

Step 5b

After following steps 1 to 4, a bite block is placed to keep the mouth open. The length and height of the defect are measured, and 1 to 2 mm is added to allow for shrinkage. The graft is marked with methylene blue pen on the hard palate directly, or after a template is fashioned from surgical glove wrapper. The graft is positioned between the gingiva and the palatine raphe, avoiding the midline.

Step 6b

The mucosa is injected with the anesthetic mixture diffusely or via a greater palatine block.

Step 7b

After 5 to 7 minutes have elapsed, a #15 blade is used to incise the mucosa on the hard palate (Figure 22-8).

Step 8b

Westcott scissors and forceps are used to harvest the graft while the periosteum is left intact. Only briskly bleeding vessels are cauterized.

Step 9b

A piece of oxidized regenerated cellulose is placed on the palate defect. The bite block is removed, and the patient is asked to bite down.

Step 10b

The graft size averages 7 to 10 mm wide, 25 to 30 mm long, and 2 to 4 mm thick. The graft is trimmed to the appropriate size, if needed. The procedure continues as in steps 11 to 16. The mild discomfort at the donor site, which lasts approximately 1 week, is usually well tolerated. Postoperative care includes rinses with 0.5% hydrogen peroxide twice daily. The donor site usually re-epithelializes in 3 weeks. Noted complications of the hard palate mucosal graft include mild shrinkage, hemorrhage, keratinization, and, rarely, graft necrosis. These methods should be used for severe cicatricial entropion and moderate entropion that is likely to be progressive.

CHAPTER 23

EYELID RETRACTION

Roger A. Dailey, MD, FACS and Mauricio R. Chavez, MD

Vertical eyelid shortening has numerous and varied causes. Upper eyelid retraction commonly occurs with thyroid-related orbitopathy and can occur with overcorrection of ptosis, aggressive blepharoplasty, trauma, and cicatricial inflammatory conditions of the eyelids. Lower eyelid shortening most commonly occurs after lower eyelid blepharoplasty via an external approach. It also can occur secondary to thyroid-related orbitopathy, postsurgical and traumatic contracture, and cicatricial-inflammatory changes.

The upper eyelid margin usually covers 1 to 2 mm of the superior cornea. The eyelid is composed of an anterior lamella (skin and orbicularis) and a posterior lamella (tarsus, conjunctiva, levator, and Müller's muscle). The lower eyelid margin is usually tangential to the inferior limbus. The lower eyelid is composed of 3 separate lamellae: anterior (skin and orbicularis), middle (orbital septum), and posterior (conjunctiva, tarsus, and lid retractors). Any shortening or retraction of the upper and lower eyelid results in widening of the palpebral fissure with possible scleral show. Contracture of any of these lamellae or combination of lamellae can result in vertical shortening.

There are several indications for surgery. These include corneal exposure, lagophthalmos, chronic irritation, and cosmesis. It is crucial to determine which layers are shortened so that proper surgical repair can be achieved. In addition, patients with lower eyelid retraction must be assessed for horizontal eyelid laxity, as repair of the retraction alone might not be sufficient. Surgical repair of horizontal eyelid laxity and thyroid eyelid retraction is described in Chapters 24 and 20, respectively.

Preoperative Evaluation

A routine preoperative history and physical examination should be performed. Ophthalmologic examination should include measurements of the margin reflex distance, palpebral fissure width, levator function, eyelid crease height, Bell's phenomenon, amount of eyelid lag on downgaze, lagophthalmos with passive eyelid closure, and corneal evaluation for keratopathy secondary to exposure. Evaluation of vertical shortening is performed to determine if the anterior, middle, posterior, or any combination of lamellae is involved. For example, if there is pure anterior lamella shortage after transcutaneous lower eyelid blepharoplasty, this would typically result in a frank ectropion, whereas a middle lamellar problem would result in lower eyelid retraction without ectropion. A forced elevation test is necessary to establish where the disparity is occurring. This is performed by manually elevating the lower eyelid and determining the source of the tension (Figure 23-1). Most frequently, it is a result of involvement of both the anterior and middle lamellae.

Anesthesia

General, monitored, or local anesthesia may be used. The eyelid is locally infiltrated with 1% lidocaine with epinephrine (1:100,000) mixed with 0.5% Marcaine. Any donor site is locally infiltrated as well. The patient is then prepared and draped according to the surgeon's specifications.

Skin Incisions

Nidek surgical CO_2 laser, Ellman surgitron, or a scalpel can be used to make all skin incisions discussed in the procedures described next. Prior to the incisions, topical anesthetic is placed in the fornices, and appropriate eye shields with antibiotic ointment are placed to protect the eyes. In addition, any oxygen or other flammable gases must be turned off during the use of these devices unless confined to the patient's protected airway.

Levine MR.
Manual of Oculoplastic Surgery, Fourth Edition (pp 163-172).
© 2010 SLACK Incorporated

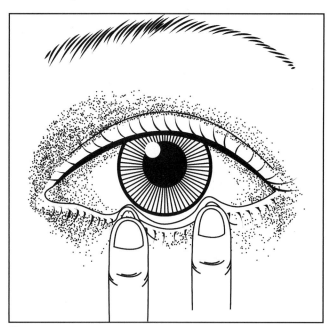

Figure 23-1.

Surgical Procedure

ANTERIOR LAMELLA SHORTAGE (LOWER EYELID)

The surgical treatment requires the use of a full-thickness skin graft. The donor site should be selected for thickness and color, depending on whether the upper or lower eyelid is involved. Because the eyelid skin is extremely thin, the best match is usually obtained from the ipsilateral or contralateral upper eyelid. Other donor sites are the supraclavicular regions, nonhair-bearing volar surface of the upper arm, and posterior or preauricular areas (Figure 23-2).

Step 1

A subciliary skin incision is made from the punctum, extending at the very least to the lateral canthus, or beyond as necessary, to release tension of the lower eyelid margin (Figure 23-3). The subcutaneous fascia is then opened using sharp Stevens scissors.

Step 2

Superior traction is then used while blunt and sharp dissection of the anterior and middle lamellar cicatrix is performed until the lower eyelid margin can be elevated easily to at least the center of the pupil in primary gaze (Figure 23-4).

Step 3

The eyelid is then checked for horizontal laxity. If present, surgical repair is performed (see Chapter 24).

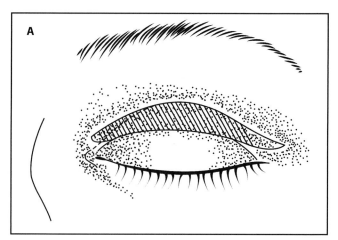

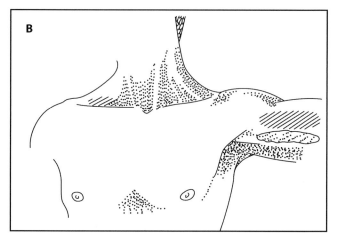

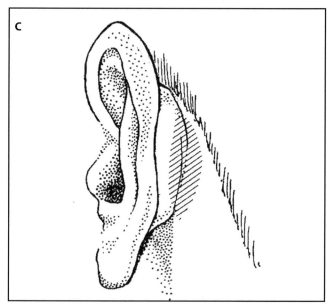

Figure 23-2.

Step 4

At this stage, the lower eyelid is placed on stretch, and the graft bed is measured (Figure 23-5). A full-thickness skin graft 20% larger in size is then obtained from the appropriate site for optimal color and texture match.

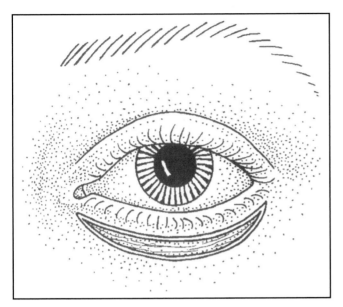

Figure 23-3.

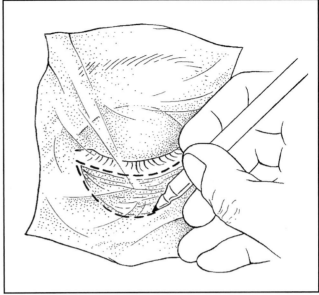

Figure 23-5.

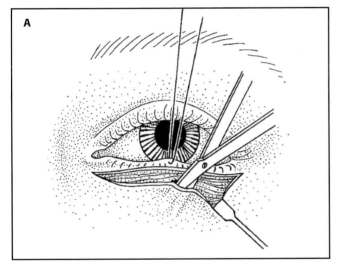

Figure 23-4.

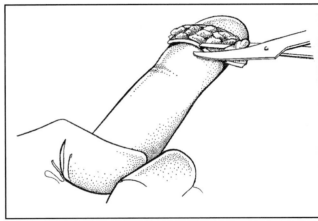

Figure 23-6.

Step 5
Once the graft is harvested, subcuticular tissue is debulked from the graft with Stevens scissors (Figure 23-6). The graft is then placed in the wound and conservatively trimmed to fit.

Step 6
Several interrupted 5-0 plain fast (fast-absorbing surgical gut suture) cardinal sutures are placed strategically to stabilize the graft.

Step 7
A running 5-0 plain fast suture is then used to approximate the skin edges (Figure 23-7). The graft may be fenestrated to avoid hematoma or if added coverage is necessary.

Step 8
A Telfa pad (or other bolster material) is then placed over the graft and secured with 4-0 prolene (polypropylene suture) horizontal mattress sutures (Figure 23-8). This maintains excellent approximation of the graft to the vascularized host site. It is important that the pad or bolster be larger than the

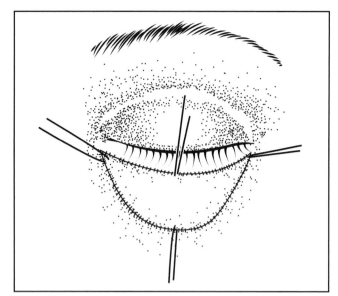

Figure 23-7.

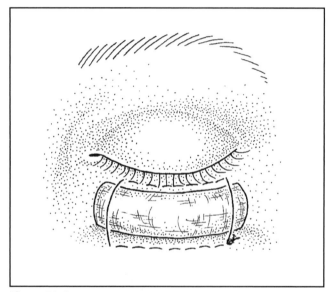

Figure 23-8.

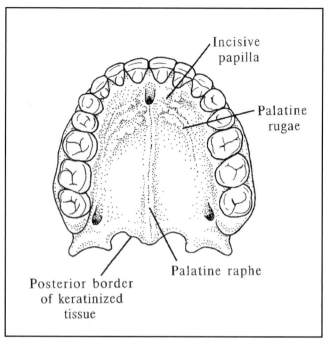

Figure 23-9.

graft so that a rim of adhesion between graft and host will not form.

Step 9
The bolster is left in place for 3 to 5 days.

Comments

The graft should be trimmed flush and left slightly larger than necessary, with shrinkage anticipated. If it is too large and a Telfa bolster is not used, the graft may corrugate and not be cosmetically acceptable.

Middle and Posterior Lamella Repair With Spacer (Lower Eyelid)

Many types of grafts can be used for posterior lamella repair, including acellular cadaveric dermal matrix (AlloDerm), porcine dermal collagen (Enduragen), and hard palate mucosa graft. We prefer the use of Enduragen. It is a relatively thin yet rigid graft that provides both functional eyelid support and excellent cosmetic results. Compared with the use of hard palate mucosa grafts, Enduragen decreases operating time for graft harvest, and patients have less discomfort postoperatively. Compared with AlloDerm, Enduragen has a more uniform and consistent thickness throughout the graft and appears to provide more long-term support to the eyelid with less loss of vertical height. Any of the 3 grafts can be used in the procedure described below.

In cases of severe eyelid retraction with associated malar ptosis or hypoplasia, a posterior spacer in conjunction with a supraperiosteal or subperiosteal midface lift can provide additional support and elevation of the lower eyelid. Silicone malar implants can also be used in patients with a "negative vector" (globe projecting anterior to face of maxilla) but are rarely necessary.

HARVESTING THE HARD PALATE GRAFT

A brief review of oral surgical anatomy is necessary (Figures 23-9 and 23-10). The anterior palatine nerve and artery exit the greater palatine foramen, which is one of the nerve block regions. This is anesthetized by identifying the third molar and injecting 1 mL of 1% lidocaine with epinephrine at the anterior edge approximately 3 mm in front of the border of the hard and soft palate. There should be minimal resistance in this region. If much resistance is met, then the area should be reidentified before continuing. The nasopalatine nerves are then blocked by injecting 0.5 mL of local anesthetic into the incisive papilla, which is exquisitely sensitive. The needle is then directed superiorly, medially, and posteriorly to reach the nasopalatine foramen, which lies immediately behind the central incisors. A small amount of local anesthesia is then infiltrated into the donor site mucosa for improved hemostasis and dissection.

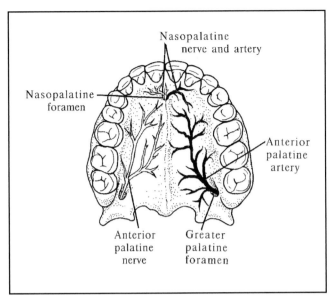

Figure 23-10.

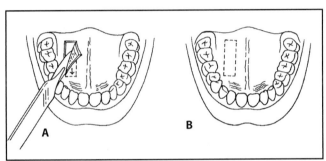

Figure 23-11.

Step 1
A self-retaining oral retractor can be used to improve exposure.

Step 2
The surgical site is identified, and local anesthesia is given as described previously.

Step 3
The graft size is then determined and marked with a methylene blue marking pen on the mucosa between the alveolar ridge and the median raphe.

Step 4
The preplaced marks are incised with a #15 Bard-Parker blade.

Step 5
The edge is then grasped with toothed forceps, and dissection is performed using the #64 Beaver blade (BD Beaver Mini Blade) (Figure 23-11).

Step 6
Pressure is applied with a dental roll for approximately 5 minutes, and then monopolar cautery is used sparingly for hemostasis, if necessary.

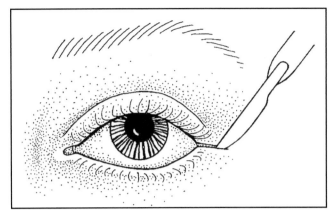

Figure 23-12.

PREPARATION OF ALLODERM AND ENDURAGEN

Both products are prepared according to protocol provided by each manufacturer. Keep in mind that AlloDerm must be rehydrated, and the process can take at least 20 minutes depending on the graft thickness. Enduragen does not require rehydration.

POSTERIOR LAMELLA REPAIR

Step 1
A lateral canthotomy skin incision is made (Figure 23-12).

Step 2
An inferior cantholysis is performed with monopolar cautery along with a transconjunctival incision 1 mm inferior to the tarsus extending medially toward the caruncle. This can also be performed sharply with a scissor or laser (Figure 23-13).

Step 3
The retractors and conjunctiva are dissected, allowing sufficient anterior lamella mobilization (Figure 23-14). If necessary, the dissection can be carried down to the orbital rim, releasing the orbitomalar ligament.

Step 4
The lower eyelid is placed on stretch superiorly, ensuring that it is freely mobilized and capable of being placed approximately 2 mm above the inferior limbus.

Step 5
The graft size is then determined.

Step 6
The graft is cut flush with the bed so that the eyelid margin covers approximately 2 mm of the inferior limbus.

Step 7
The graft is sutured into position with a running 5-0 plain suture (plain surgical gut suture) (Figure 23-15). If AlloDerm is being used, the basement membrane side should rest on the globe and the dermal side against the wound bed.

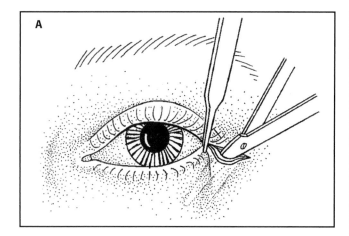

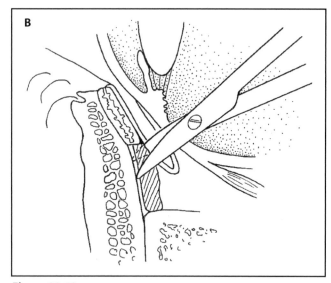

Figure 23-13.

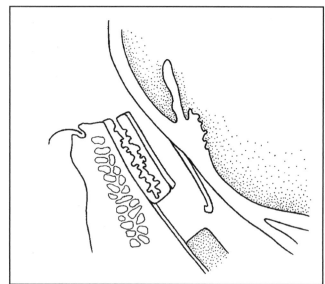

Figure 23-14.

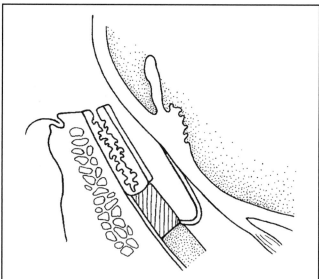

Figure 23-15.

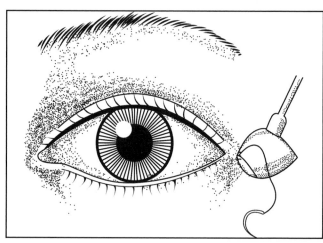

Figure 23-16.

Step 9

The lateral canthal angle is reformed with a deep 5-0 Vicryl suture (polyglactin 910). The needle is placed through the eyelid margin at the gray line of the upper and then lower eyelid and tied, and the distal end of the suture is kept long for use in the following suture tie. The same 5-0 Vicryl suture needle is then passed through the superior temporal orbital rim periosteum 1 to 2 mm above the medial canthal angle and then tied with appropriate tension using the distal suture end of the suture. This gives an excellent cosmetic reformation of the lateral canthal angle (Figure 23-16).

Step 10

The lateral canthotomy skin is then reapproximated with 5-0 plain fast-absorbing gut suture in a running fashion.

Step 11

Two Frost sutures with 4-0 prolene are then placed both laterally and medially through the lower eyelid and upper eyelid and then through the brow and tied

Step 8

The lower lid can be shortened as needed.

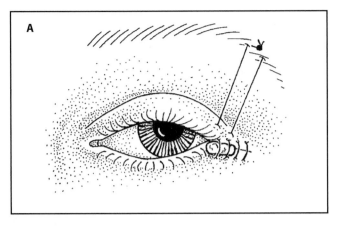

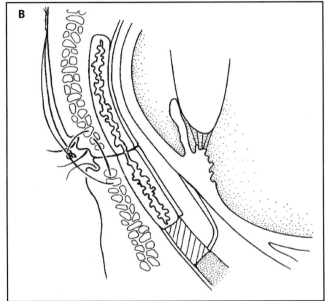

Figure 23-17.

securely over a bolster so that there is an upward traction during the initial healing phase (Figure 23-17). This is usually left in place for 7 days.

Comments

Although other grafts are available, hard palate grafts continue to be popular because they are an excellent substitute for reconstructing the posterior lamella and are thought to result in the least amount of graft contraction. They are of ideal stiffness, yet flexible enough to maintain the eyelid contour. Also, there is enough available for repair of essentially any size of posterior eyelid defect. Although the hard palate graft consists of a keratinized epithelium, it quickly undergoes metaplasia to a nonkeratinized epithelium secondary to vascularization. The quicker the metaplasia occurs, the less ocular irritation the patient has. The enhancement of vascularization of the graft occurs with proper graft thinning, meticulous surgical technique, and hemostasis. A small percentage of patients complain of postoperative oral pain and bleeding. If the patient uses a molded acrylic oral stent made before the procedure, it will keep the defect covered and decrease the discomfort. Also, if bleeding occurs, the patient can apply digital pressure to the stent, enhanc-

ing hemostasis. Postoperatively, the patient is placed on an oral antibiotic such as amoxicillin and clavulanate (Augmentin) or cephalosporin for 3 days. The patient should also use chlorhexidine gluconate (Peridex) as an oral rinse. Viscous lidocaine (Xylocaine) is helpful with pain management.

More recently, we have found that Enduragen provides excellent results without the second surgical site. Hard palate mucosal grafts are mainly used now in cases where Enduragen has failed, which is quite uncommon.

FULL-THICKNESS EYELID SHORTENING

The surgical procedures for repair of the external and internal lamellae can be used for full-thickness eyelid shortening; however, because a graft on top of a graft will not survive, the Brown-Beard split-level grafting technique may be used. This essentially places each graft at a different level so that they are not in direct apposition. Another method that is described in greater detail is Putterman's modification of the Hughes flap for lower eyelid vertical lengthening. This surgical treatment requires the use of a full-thickness skin graft.

ANESTHESIA

General, monitored, or local anesthesia may be used. The eyelid is locally infiltrated with 1% lidocaine with epinephrine (1:100,000) mixed with 0.5% Marcaine. The donor site is locally infiltrated as well. The patient is then prepared and draped in the usual sterile fashion.

FULL-THICKNESS LAMELLA SHORTAGE (LOWER EYELID)

Step 1

An external subciliary incision is performed approximately 1 mm below the lower eyelid margin. The lower eyelid is everted, and an incision is made 4-mm below the posterior eyelid margin through conjunctiva just below the tarsal border. The remaining tissue between the 2 bi-leveled incisions is then dissected with Westcott scissors around the tarsus, joining the 2 incisions (Figure 23-18).

Step 2

The upper eyelid is everted.

Step 3

An incision is made 4 mm above the upper eyelid margin through the conjunctiva and tarsus. The length of the incision corresponds to the retracted eyelid (Figure 23-19).

Step 4

Sharp Stevens scissors are used to make vertical cuts to the superior edge of the tarsus. The vertical cuts are then extended toward the superior fornix. The flap is separated from the underlying levator and Müller's muscle until it is freed up enough to advance it inferiorly under the bridged eyelid margin (Figure 23-20).

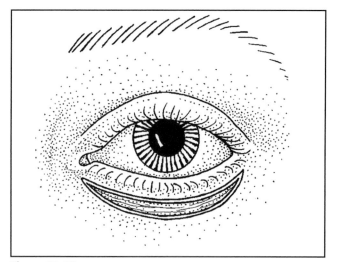

Figure 23-18.

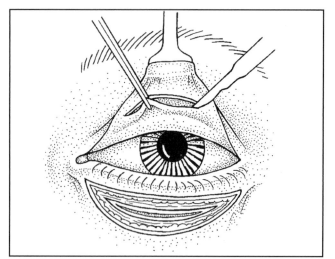

Figure 23-19.

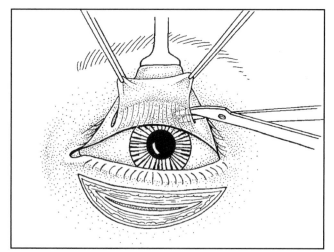

Figure 23-20.

Step 5

The tarsus from the inferior edge of the Hughes flap is then sutured to the inferior tarsus edge of the lower eyelid, or conjunctiva if tarsus is not present,

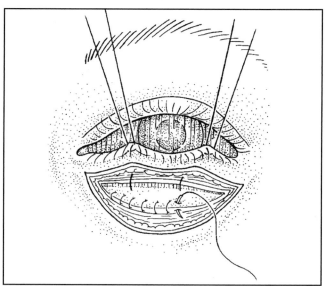

Figure 23-21.

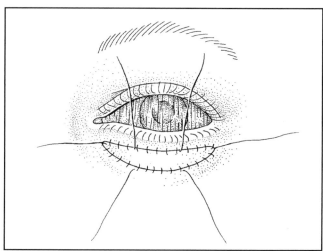

Figure 23-22.

with 6-0 Vicryl sutures anchoring it into position (Figure 23-21).

Step 6

The eyelid margin is elevated so that it lies approximately 2 mm above the limbus. The superior edge of the Hughes flap is sutured to the tarsus beneath the lid margin.

Step 7

The graft bed is measured, and a full-thickness skin graft that is slightly larger than this dimension is harvested.

Step 8

The graft is trimmed flush with the defect.

Step 9

The graft is initially secured with interrupted 5-0 plain fast cardinal sutures.

Step 10

The remaining edges are approximated with running 5-0 plain fast sutures (Figure 23-22).

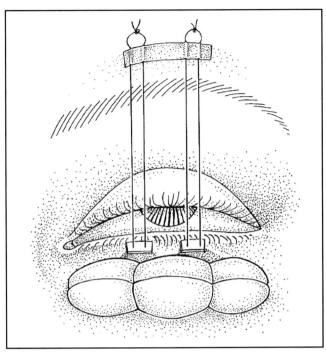

Figure 23-23.

Step 11

Two Frost sutures of 4-0 prolene are placed through the lower eyelid margin medially and laterally and brought out through the brow and tied securely over a bolster.

Step 12

Antibiotic ophthalmic ointment is placed on the graft and skin edges. A Telfa pad or dental roll is placed over the graft with the cardinal suture tied securely to bolster the graft (Figure 23-23).

Step 13

The bolster and silk sutures in the graft are removed after 7 days.

DIVIDING THE FLAP

The flap is divided after 6 weeks.

Step 1

Local infiltration of the upper and lower eyelid is performed.

Step 2

A grooved director can be placed under the flap or protection of the surgeon's choice.

Step 3

The flap overlying the protector is cut with scissors.

Step 4

The upper and lower eyelids are everted, and the remaining flap is cut flush at the base. Any scar tissue of the upper eyelid is released. Intralesional steroid can be placed in the upper lid to help avoid contraction.

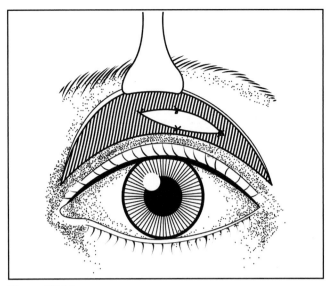

Figure 23-24.

Comments

This procedure is worthwhile because there is a predictable final eyelid level. Compared with free tarsoconjunctival grafts, a variable amount of resorption may occur. During dissection of the Hughes flap, care must be taken to avoid large buttonholes in the flap, which could compromise the vascular supply. Also, the upper eyelid height may be affected if Müller's muscle or levator aponeurosis is included in the Hughes flap. When dividing the flap, any upper eyelid scar tissue is excised to avoid upper eyelid retraction.

Posterior Lamella Repair With Spacer (Upper Eyelid)

A spacer for the upper eyelid differs from that of the lower eyelid due to its contact with the cornea. A hard palate mucosa graft can keratinize and Enduragen's rougher surface and increased firmness could potentially cause ocular surface irritation. We prefer the use of AlloDerm.

Step 1

A lid crease incision is made.

Step 2

Thermal cautery is then used to dissect through orbicularis and identify the septum. The septum is then incised in its entire length horizontally, exposing the preaponeurotic fat and levator aponeurosis.

Step 3

The levator is then recessed from the anterior superior edge of tarsus using Stevens scissors or thermal cautery. Depending on the degree of retraction, full-thickness blepharotomy may also need to be performed until the desired contour and eyelid height is reached.

Step 4

The graft size is then determined, and AlloDerm is trimmed to be the spacer between the tarsus and levator (Figure 23-24).

Step 5

The graft is then sutured into position with interrupted 5-0 plain fast suture, preserving the new eyelid height and contour.

Step 6

The upper eyelid skin is then closed with a running 7-0 nylon suture.

CHAPTER 24

INVOLUTIONAL ECTROPION REPAIR

David T. Tse, MD, FACS

Ectropion is a commonly encountered eyelid malposition characterized by eversion of the eyelid margin away from the globe. Although the upper or lower eyelid may be affected, this condition more commonly involves the lower eyelid. Chronic exposure of the globe and palpebral conjunctiva results in dry eye symptoms with reflex tearing. The exposed palpebral conjunctiva becomes inflamed and may develop metaplastic changes of epidermalization. An exposed punctum can become stenotic, contributing to tear outflow impairment. Additionally, corneal exposure may lead to epithelial breakdown, with increased risk of infectious keratitis. Upper eyelid ectropion often results from cicatricial changes of the anterior lamella related to previous injury, such as laceration or burn. Iatrogenic upper eyelid ectropion may occasionally occur after ptosis repair or blepharoplasty.

The pathogenesis of lower eyelid ectropion varies. Frueh and Schoengarth, in an excellent paper, succinctly summarized in a systematic fashion the evaluation and treatment of the 6 pathologic elements that may be present in an ectropic eyelid. These are (1) horizontal lid laxity, (2) medial canthal tendon laxity, (3) punctal malposition, (4) vertical tightness of the skin, (5) orbicularis paresis secondary to seventh nerve palsy, and (6) lower eyelid retractor disinsertion.

The presence of each factor is determined by clinical examination. One or more of these components may be present in an ectropic eyelid. Proper recognition of the underlying anatomic defect enables the surgeon to select the appropriate surgical procedure for correction. Many procedures have been described for the treatment of each of these pathologic elements. In this chapter, one practical technique is presented for each of the conditions.

Horizontal Lid Laxity

Horizontal lid laxity is most likely a result of stretching of the lateral and medial canthal tendons rather than actual elongation of the tarsal plate. This produces a redundancy in the lid tissues, causing the lid margin to fall away from the globe. Horizontal lid laxity can be corrected surgically by a number of procedures. One popular method is full-thickness excision of a wedge of eyelid tissue and primary closure of the defect. One disadvantage of this method of horizontal lid shortening is that it often leads to lateral canthal deformities such as blunting of the lateral canthal angle. Additionally, a block resection technique often exaggerates the laxity of the medial and lateral canthal tendon and may produce a horizontally narrowed palpebral fissure. More important, surgical correction is not aimed at the underlying pathologic condition, namely, stretching of the lateral canthal tendon.

In correcting this element of lid malposition, the "lateral tarsal strip" procedure advocated by Anderson and Gordy is preferred. In this technique, the eyelid is shortened at the lateral canthal end of the lid. The advantages of this technique are (1) surgery is directed at correcting the anatomic defect; (2) there are no marginal lid sutures; (3) the danger of lid notching or misdirected lashes irritating the cornea is avoided; (4) canthal malposition and lid shortening may be corrected simultaneously; (5) the procedure can be performed quickly; and (6) the almond-shaped canthal angle is preserved.

The procedure is also useful in correcting eyelid laxity and canthal malposition in an anophthalmic socket. This technique provides immediate lid strength, allowing it to support weight, as is needed when there is an ocular prosthesis.

Levine MR.
Manual of Oculoplastic Surgery, Fourth Edition (pp 173-182).
© 2010 SLACK Incorporated

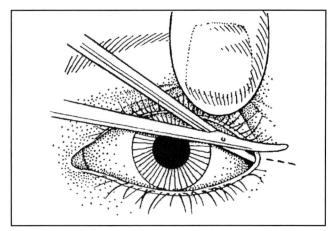

Figure 24-1.

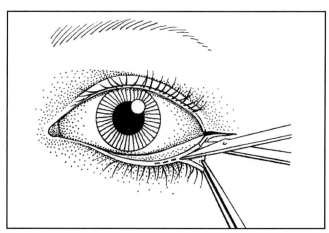

Figure 24-3.

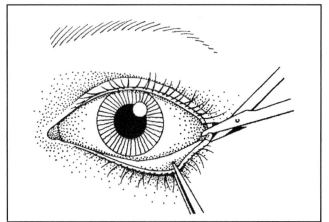

Figure 24-2.

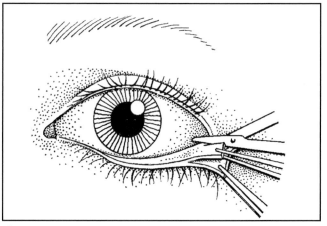

Figure 24-4.

PROCEDURE: LATERAL TARSAL STRIP

Step 1

Five minutes before anesthetic infiltration, a small cotton pledget moistened with 4% lidocaine is placed in the lateral inferior fornix to minimize the discomfort of needle prick. Lidocaine 2% with 1:100,000 dilution of epinephrine is injected into the lateral canthal region with a 30-gauge needle. A small amount of anesthetic is also delivered to the periosteum of the lateral orbital rim and the temporal inferior fornix. When injecting the inferior fornix, stand on the patient's opposite side while aiming the needle toward the ear, and inject slowly to prevent inadvertent globe penetration should the patient's head move reflexively in response to pain. Allow the anesthetic to hydraulically dissect ahead of the advancing needle tip. A lateral canthotomy is made with a Stevens scissors until the lateral orbital rim is exposed (Figure 24-1). Cutting into the periosteum should be avoided, as it will serve as an anchoring structure for the tarsal strip. All bleeding points are cauterized with a bipolar cautery. Hemostasis is imperative for visualization of anatomic landmarks and to minimize ecchymosis at the surgical site. An inferior cantholysis is performed by incising the attachment of the inferior

crus of the lateral canthal tendon from the lateral orbital rim (Figure 24-2). Once the inferior crus of the lateral canthal tendon is severed, the entire eyelid becomes mobile. Occasionally, the temporal pocket of the preaponeurotic fat pad may prolapse through this incision. The prolapsing fat pad can be cauterized with a bipolar cautery.

Step 2

With straight scissors, the eyelid is separated horizontally at the gray line into anterior and posterior lamellae (Figure 24-3). An incision should be made in the gray line, without cutting into the tarsal plate. At times, the gray line may be indistinct because of erythema from chronic irritation. One way to identify this landmark is to gently pinch on the lid margin with a nontoothed forceps to look for secretions from the meibomian gland openings. The gray line is located immediately anterior to the secretions. The length of incision along the gray line depends on the amount of lid shortening needed.

Step 3

A horizontal incision, equal in length to the amount of lid splitting, is made with a scissors at the inferior margin of the tarsal plate. This maneuver severs the conjunctiva and lower eyelid retractors from the tarsal plate, thus creating a 4.0- to 4.5-mm wide strip of tarsus (Figure 24-4).

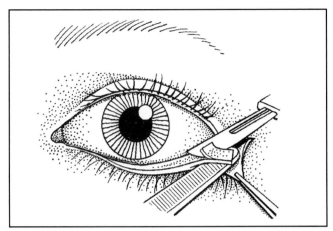

Figure 24-5.

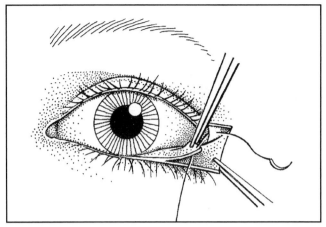

Figure 24-7.

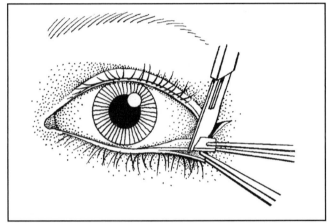

Figure 24-6.

Step 4

The mucosa along the superior border of the strip is excised, taking care to avoid excising any part of the tarsal plate. As the vertical height of the lower eyelid tarsal plate is only approximately 4.0 to 4.5 mm, inadvertent excision of tarsal substance narrows the strip, rendering it less effective as a fixation structure. While the tarsal plate is stabilized by a tissue forceps over a metal plate, a #15 Bard-Parker blade is used to scrape the palpebral conjunctiva off the tarsus (Figure 24-5). The tarsus must be denuded of conjunctiva to avoid formation of an epithelial inclusion cyst in the area of the new lateral canthus.

Step 5

The tarsal plate is grasped with a tissue forceps and pulled with sufficient tension in a lateral direction to place the lower punctum slightly lateral to the upper punctum. The amount of redundant lid tissue is determined by draping the tarsal plate over the lateral orbital rim. The excess tissue is excised with a scalpel blade (Figure 24-6). Usually, the redundant inferior cms of the lateral canthal tendon is excised. Rarely, the tarsal substance is excised. A strip of tarsus, free of any epithelial lining, is thus fashioned.

Step 6

The tarsal strip is sutured to the periosteum on the inner aspect of the lateral orbital wall with a 4-0 polyglactin (Vicryl) suture on a small half-circle spatula needle. The needle is first passed through the full thickness of the superior pole of the tarsal strip (Figure 24-7). A firm bite, at least 1.5 to 2.0 mm from the tarsal edge, should be taken; this avoids the potential problem of suture "cheese-wiring" through the tarsal substance. The needle then engages the periosteum immediately inside the lateral orbital wall and exits at the anterior surface of the rim to prevent anterior displacement of the canthus. Appropriate support for the tarsal strip is not provided if the tension-bearing periosteum is not engaged with the suture. To verify proper placement of the suture, gently pull the suture anteriorly. If the periosteum is properly engaged, there should be no movement of the tissue overlying the suture. Another suture is passed through the inferior pole of the tarsal strip and engages the periosteum in the same fashion. When correcting lid laxity and canthal malposition in an anophthalmic socket, an additional suture may be placed to augment lid support of the prosthesis. Larger needles are difficult to maneuver at the tight lateral orbital rim region, and needles with a lesser curvature may bend or break on attempted passage through the periosteum. A slight overcorrection in tautness and height is desired to allow for mild relaxation of the tissue in the early postoperative period.

Step 7

After the tarsal strip is secured to the orbital rim (Figure 24-8A), the lash-bearing portion of the anterior lamella overlying the tarsal strip is excised (Figure 24-8B).

Step 8

The skin edges are reapproximated with 6-0 or 7-0 nylon sutures placed in an interrupted fashion (Figure 24-9). Antibiotic ointment is applied 3 times daily. The sutures are removed in 7 days. It is imperative to recognize and treat concomitant medial canthal tendon laxity. The lateral tarsal

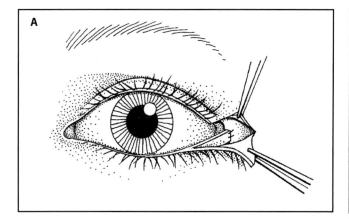

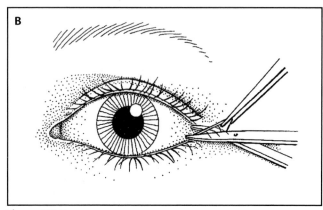

Figure 24-8.

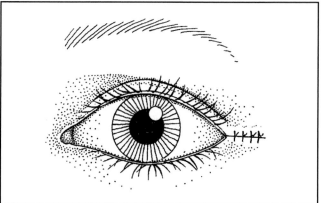

Figure 24-9.

strip procedure may be combined with medial canthal tendon plication in this setting. Tightening the eyelid laterally in the presence of unrecognized medial canthal tendon laxity displaces the inferior punctum away from the lacrimal recess, rendering the punctum ineffective for tear drainage.

Punctal Malposition

The inferior punctum is normally in apposition with the globe and in vertical alignment with the superior punctum. Occasionally, punctal eversion without horizontal eyelid laxity or anterior lamellae cicatrix can be seen. The exact cause of this condition is unclear, but segmental dehiscence or disinsertion of the lower eyelid retractors along the medial lid may be contributory. Punctal eversion can produce symptoms of exposure keratopathy due to disturbance of the tear meniscus and corneal wetting. Epiphora is another common symptom secondary to impaired tear drainage. The exposed medial palpebral conjunctiva is at risk for development of epidermalization, and stenosis of the punctum may result. Punctal eversion as a consequence of segmental retractor disinsertion must be differentiated from anterior lamella cicatrix. The skin is usually pliable in the former, but taut in the latter.

If punctal eversion is severe and the patient is symptomatic, surgical correction is necessary so that the punctum may return to its normal anatomic position and serve as a conduit for tears. A common approach is excision of tarsus, conjunctiva, and eyelid retractors as a horizontal fusiform wedge at the lower margin of the tarsal plate. The

conjunctiva is closed with 3 or 4 7-0 absorbable sutures. However, inadequate punctal inversion and recurrent punctal ectropion are frequent drawbacks of a simple ellipse closure. Failure to unite the lower eyelid retractors to the tarsal plate and lack of a cicatrix to maintain the punctum in an inverted position are factors contributing to the lack of precise and lasting correction of the condition. A modification of the simple closure technique is preferred. This technique emphasizes the union of the lower eyelid retractors, not just the conjunctiva, to the tarsal plate and the formation of a cicatrix to help keep the punctum in its normal anatomic alignment. This technique can be combined with a horizontal shortening procedure of the eyelid if laxity of the lower lid accompanies the punctal eversion; if not, it can be performed alone. If the punctum is stenotic secondary to chronic exposure, a 3-snip punctoplasty may also be done simultaneously.

PROCEDURE: MEDIAL SPINDLE

Step 1
A small amount of anesthetic is infiltrated under the skin approximately 10 mm below the punctum as well as along the medial forniceal conjunctiva.

Step 2
The medial eyelid is everted, and a diamond-shaped fusiform wedge of conjunctiva and lower lid retractors is excised inferior to the lower margin of the tarsal plate (Figure 24-10). The conjunctiva and underlying retractors are removed, with the vertical height measuring approximately 4 to 6 mm and the horizontal dimension approximately 6 to 8 mm. The vertical height of the fusiform excision depends on the amount of punctal ectropion. Its greatest vertical dimension should lie beneath the punctum. The inferior edge of this diamond-shaped incision points toward the inferior fornix and exposes the superior margin of the lower lid retractors. Cutting into the horizontal preseptal orbicularis muscle fibers should be avoided.

Step 3
The defect is closed with a double-armed 5-0 chromic suture in a horizontal mattress fashion. The suture is initially passed through the retractors at

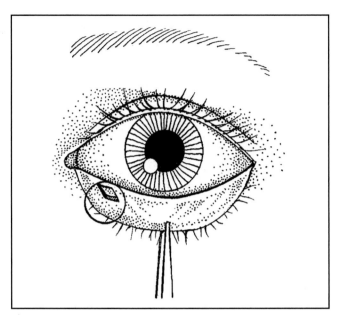

Figure 24-10.

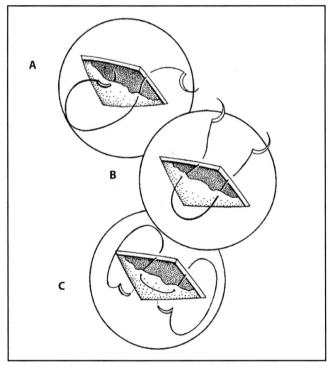

Figure 24-11.

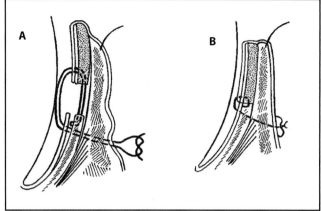

Figure 24-12.

needed to invert the punctum to the proper position. Care should be taken not to tie the suture too tightly as to overcorrect the medial eyelid margin and produce entropion. It may be helpful to have the patient sit up while the suture is being tied. The suture is left in place until it is absorbed.

The looping passage of the suture (Figure 24-12) induces a vector force that pulls the tarsal plate downward and rotates the punctum posteriorly. The passage of the suture through the full-thickness of the lower eyelid produces enough inflammatory reaction to create a cicatrix, augmenting the inversion effect and helping to keep the punctum in position after absorption of the suture. This procedure corrects mild and moderate degrees of punctal ectropion. In patients with concomitant horizontal lid laxity, a lateral tarsal strip procedure may also be required.

Medial Canthal Tendon Laxity

Medial canthal tendon laxity is detected by observing the lateral displacement of the lower punctum with lateral traction on the nasal eyelid. When the lower punctum is no longer aligned vertically with the upper punctum and can be displaced to the nasal limbus when the eye is in primary position, the medial canthal tendon should be repaired. It is unusual to find medial canthal tendon laxity alone without concomitant lateral canthal laxity. If both pathologic elements are present in the lid, the medial canthal laxity should be corrected first before proceeding with the horizontal shortening procedure.

Various surgical procedures have been described for correction of medial canthal tendon laxity. The medial tarsal strip may be used in the setting of a nonfunctioning inferior canaliculus, or when loss of function of the inferior canaliculus would be desirable. Otherwise, it is preferable to preserve the function of the canaliculus. The aim of medial canthal tendon plication is to restore the anatomic position of the inferior punctum so that it is in apposition with the globe and tear lake. The technique of medial canthal tendon plication involves exposing the tendon, anchoring the lid nasally and posteriorly while protecting the inferior canaliculus.

the lower edge of the incision in a backhanded pass, then uniting tarsal plate and conjunctiva on the upper edge (Figure 24-11A). After both arms of the suture have been passed, the suture is pulled superiorly, joining the edge of the retractors to the inferior tarsal border (Figure 24-11B). With forceps grasping the conjunctival edge of the lower border of the incision, the suture is passed full-thickness through the eyelid (Figure 24-11C). The needle should be brought through the skin 12 to 15 mm inferior to the lid margin. The other arm of the suture is passed in the same fashion. The sutures are tied on the skin surface. The suture tension should be adjusted as

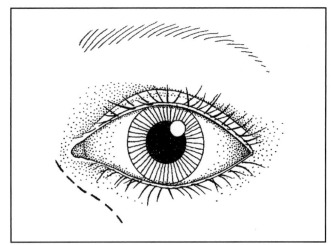

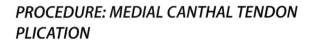

Figure 24-13.

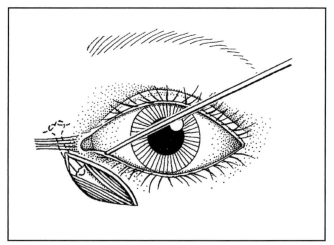

Figure 24-14.

PROCEDURE: MEDIAL CANTHAL TENDON PLICATION

Step 1

The medial canthus and medial lower eyelid are infiltrated with lidocaine 2% with 1:100,000 dilution of epinephrine. An incision is made over the medial canthal tendon, beginning in a vertical direction and curving inferolaterally along the medial lower eyelid margin, terminating approximately 3 mm below the punctum (Figure 24-13).

Step 2

A Bowman probe is placed in the lower canaliculus to identify and protect the structure throughout the operation. Blunt dissection is carried through the orbicularis muscle fibers with a Freer periosteal elevator to expose the medial canthal tendon and the nasal-most end of the tarsus beneath the punctum.

Step 3

A double-armed 5-0 Mersilene suture on a spatula needle is used. The suture passes through the nasal-most end of the tarsal plate, tunnels beneath the orbicularis muscle, and exits at the superior margin of the medial canthal tendon insertion (Figure 24-14). The other arm of the suture is passed parallel to the first in the same fashion. While the needle is being passed through the orbicularis, it is important to always keep the needle anterior to the Bowman probe. Passing the needle behind the Bowman probe incarcerates the canaliculus and compromises lacrimal drainage when the sutures are tied. Care should also be taken to avoid injuring the canaliculus. The 2 arms of the sutures are tied with sufficient tension to bring the lower punctum to a point just slightly lateral to the superior punctum. Over-tightening produces an accordion effect on the inferior canaliculus.

Step 4

The skin incision is closed with interrupted 7-0 nylon sutures. Horizontal laxity is then reassessed. If needed, a lateral tarsal strip procedure can be performed.

Vertical Tightness of the Skin

Cicatricial ectropion is caused by vertical tightness of the eyelid skin, which pulls the eyelid margin away from the globe. Actinic damage is a commonly encountered source of anterior lamella contracture with resultant lower eyelid ectropion. Other causes include thermal burn, chemical burn, trauma, laser resurfacing, chemical peel, or surgery. Inflammation due to dermatitis and infections such as herpes zoster may induce cicatricial alterations of the skin. Long-standing ectropion from other causes may predispose to secondary contracture of the anterior lamella, resulting in a complex ectropion.

Treatment of cicatricial ectropion must first be directed at releasing the scar bands to allow vertical lengthening of the anterior lamella. If a linear vertical scar is present, a Z-plasty may be performed. If more diffuse contracture is present, a full-thickness skin graft must be used to replace the deficit after releasing the scar bands. The skin may be harvested from the upper eyelid if dermatochalasis is present. Nonhair-bearing skin from the preauricular, retroauricular, or supraclavicular regions may be used. These techniques are illustrated in Chapter 25.

Horizontal eyelid tightening is often used to augment a skin-grafting procedure. Occasionally, a tarsal strip may not be long enough to reach the periosteum of the lateral orbital rim, or even if the strip reaches, there may be too much tension exerted against the strip. An effective method to augment the fixation is to reflect a piece of periosteum onto the anterior surface of the tarsal plate. A 5 mm x 7 mm periosteal flap, with the base at the anterior tip of the lateral orbital rim, is elevated off the temporal surface of the rim with a Freer periosteal elevator. The periosteal flap is reflected onto the tarsal plate and secured with 2 5-0 Vicryl sutures.

Orbicularis Paresis Secondary to Seventh Nerve Palsy

Permanent or temporary seventh nerve palsy commonly results in brow ptosis, lower eyelid ectropion, and reduced blink frequency. Exposure due to ectropion and the associated decreased blink and lagophthalmos from loss of orbicularis tone produce reflex tearing. Decreased tear pump function secondary to decreased orbicularis tone also contributes to tearing. Treatment is directed at minimizing exposure keratopathy and epiphora and preventing corneal ulceration.

For temporary loss of seventh nerve function, patients may only require frequent lubrication, taping of the lower eyelid, use of a nocturnal moisture chamber, or a combination of these. Patients with permanent seventh nerve palsy frequently require surgical intervention for treatment of exposure keratopathy. Horizontal eyelid tightening, such as the lateral tarsal strip procedure, provides immediate support to the lower eyelid. If secondary contracture of the anterior lamella has occurred, skin grafting may be required. Other procedures performed to promote eyelid closure include tarsorrhaphy and placement of a gold weight or palpebral spring in the upper eyelid.

Temporary paralytic ectropion may develop after botulinum toxin injection for treatment of essential blepharospasm. Because the effect of the toxin subsides within a few months, corneal protection can often be provided by lubrication while awaiting recovery of orbicularis tone. Occasionally, botulinum toxin injection unveils a subclinical case of involutional eyelid laxity, manifesting as profound ectropion. In this scenario, surgical intervention with a lateral tarsal strip or lateral tarsorrhaphy may become necessary.

Lower Eyelid Retractor Disinsertion

The lower eyelid retractors are referred to as the capsulopalpebral fascia and Müller's muscle. The capsulopalpebral fascia originates as the capsulopalpebral head with delicate attachments to the inferior rectus muscle and tendon. The capsulopalpebral head divides into 2 portions as it extends around and fuses with the sheath of the inferior oblique muscle. Anterior to the inferior oblique muscle, the 2 portions of the capsulopalpebral head rejoin to form Lockwood's ligament. The fascial tissue anterior to Lockwood's ligament is termed the *capsulopalpebral fascia*. A large portion of the capsulopalpebral fascia proceeds anteriorly to insert on the inferior fornix and to form Tenon's capsule on the globe. The rest of the capsulopalpebral fascia then proceeds upward to insert onto the inferior margin of the tarsal plate. Disinsertion of the retractors of the lower eyelid may manifest as ectropion or entropion. Differential vector forces between the anterior and posterior lamellae often determine whether ectropion or entropion will result. Lower eyelid retractor disinsertion in the absence of horizontal laxity or anterior lamella shortage is the most difficult element of an ectropic eyelid to recognize clinically. In patients with lower eyelid retractor disinsertion or dehiscence, there are 4 clinical clues that are similar to those found in an entropic eyelid:

1. Deeper inferior fornix (because the capsulopalpebral fascia sends attachments to the inferior fornix, the inferior fornix is pulled inward when the retractors are disinserted, thereby deepening the inferior fornix).

2. Higher resting lower lid position (because the retractors are no longer attached to the inferior margin of the tarsal plate, the involved eyelid often has a higher resting position of the lid margin when it is pulled out of its ectropic position).

3. Diminished lower eyelid excursion on downgaze (resulting from absence of attachment of the retractors to the tarsal plate).

4. A horizontal infratarsal red band and the edge of the disinserted retractor can be seen. (This red band is thought to be the orbicularis muscle fibers showing through the area of retractor disinsertion. However, this sign has not been too useful because the inferior fornix is often injected as the result of chronic lid eversion.) For correction of retractor disinsertion, a transconjunctival approach is used. This approach is similar to the technique described for the correction of punctal ectropion. The looping passage of the fornix sutures through the full-thickness of the eyelid and the formation of an inflammatory cicatrix produce a vector force that helps to effect and maintain an inward rotation of the lid margin. The key to success in this method is to unite the lower eyelid retractors, not just the conjunctiva, to the tarsal plate, because the retractors are responsible for the inversion effect.

PROCEDURE: SUTURE INVERSION TECHNIQUE

Step 1
The lower lid is anesthetized with lidocaine 2% with 1:100,000 dilution of epinephrine. Anesthetic is also injected under the conjunctiva along the infratarsal border. A 4-0 silk suture is placed through the central lid margin for traction.

Step 2
An infratarsal conjunctival snip incision is made with a Westcott scissors to enter the postorbicular fascial plane. The horizontal preseptal orbicularis muscle fibers can be seen through this opening. Medial and lateral infratarsal incisions are made across the length of the eyelid. Sharp dissection within this plane is carried toward the inferior orbital rim until the orbital fat pads are identified. The orbital fat pads are retracted anteriorly with a Desmarres retractor. Once the orbital fat is retracted, the disinserted anterior edge of the retractor can usually be seen several millimeters below the conjunctival incision.

Step 3
To identify the lower eyelid retractors with certainty, the disinserted edge of the retractor is grasped with a tissue forceps, and the patient is asked to look downward. A downward pull can be felt if the retractors are grasped by the forceps.

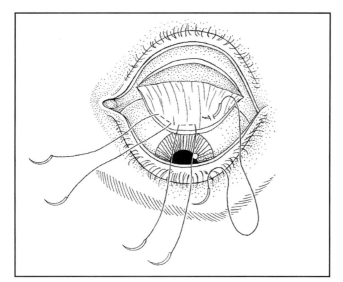

Figure 24-15.

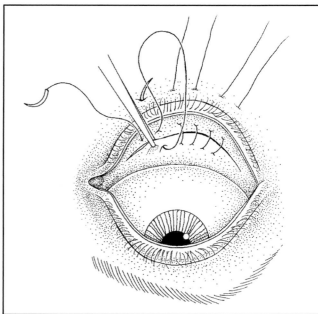

Figure 24-17.

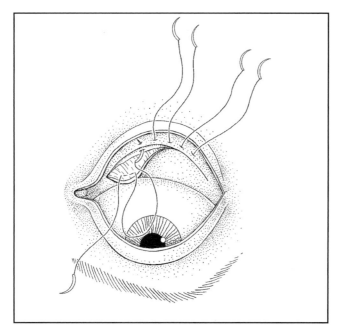

Figure 24-16.

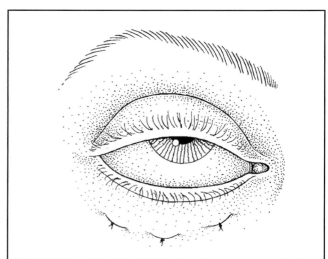

Figure 24-18.

Step 4

The disinserted edge of the lower eyelid retractor is then reattached onto the inferior border of the tarsal plate by using 3 sets of double-armed 5-0 chromic sutures. These sutures should be evenly spaced along the length of the lid. One arm of the suture is initially passed horizontally through the retractors at the lower edge of the incision (Figure 24-15). While the infratarsal edge is everted with a tissue forceps, the needle is passed through the tarsus in a backhanded fashion (Figure 24-16). The second arm is passed approximately 5 to 6 mm from the first in the same manner. After both arms of the suture have been passed, the suture is pulled superiorly, joining the edge of the retractor to the inferior tarsal border.

Step 5

With the forceps grasping the conjunctival edge of the incision, the needle is passed deep into the inferior fornix, through the full thickness of the eyelid, to emerge from the skin surface approximately 12 to 15 mm inferior to the lid margin (Figure 24-17). The other arm of the suture is passed in the same fashion.

Step 6

The other 2 sets of sutures are passed 4 to 5 mm apart in an identical manner. The 3 sets of sutures are then tied on the skin surface without the use of bolsters (Figure 24-18). When the sutures are tied, there is an immediate inversion of the lid margin. The sutures should not be tied too tightly as to overinvert the lid margin and produce entropion. To verify the proper reattachment of the retractors to the tarsal plate, the patient is asked to look downward; a smooth downward excursion of the lower lid should be seen. The looping passage of the sutures induces a vector force that pulls the tarsal plate downward and rotates the lid margin posteriorly. This inversion vector force counteracts any outward pulling effect imparted by the anterior lamella. The subsequent formation of an inflam-matory cicatrix induced by the absorbable sutures helps to maintain the eyelid in an upright posture. If concomitant horizontal lid laxity is present, a lateral tarsal strip procedure can be performed. Bacitracin ophthalmic ointment is applied on the suture knots and in the inferior fornix. The chromic sutures are usually absorbed within 10 to 14 days.

CHAPTER 25

CICATRICIAL ECTROPION

Michael J. Hawes, MD

The pathogenesis of cicatricial ectropion includes trauma, skin diseases, thermal and chemical injuries, and iatrogenic causes, such as excessive skin removal in lower blepharoplasty. Factors that may be present in cicatricial ectropion include vertical skin shortage or contracture and horizontal lid laxity. The surgeon should determine which of these factors needs correction and then select from the following surgical options.

Surgical Procedures

VERTICAL SKIN SHORTAGE OR CONTRACTURE

The anterior lamella of the lid is shortened in all cases of cicatricial ectropion. When the contracture is present in a single vertical line, a Z-plasty may correct it. If the shortening is generalized, a skin graft or skin-muscle flap should be performed. Another more recent concept is midface lift surgery, which can lessen or eliminate the need for adding tissue to the anterior lamella (see Chapter 11 on cheek-midface lift).

Z-PLASTY TECHNIQUE

The Z-plasty releases a line of tension by tissue transfer. The central line of the Z should be placed on the scar. The optimal angle for the triangular flaps is 60°.

Step 1

A marking pen is used to draw a line over the scar. Lines are drawn 60° from the superior and inferior ends of the vertical line, each measuring the same length as the vertical line (Figure 25-1A and 25-1B).

Step 2

Local anesthetic (2% lidocaine in a 50-50 mixture with 0.75% bupivacaine) is injected, and a 4-0 silk suture is placed through the eyelid margin at the termination of the scar. Traction on the eyelid is accomplished by gently pulling the suture.

Step 3

A #15 Bard-Parker blade is used to incise the skin. The skin flaps are undermined with a tenotomy or Westcott scissors and are transposed with skin hooks (Figure 25-1C).

Step 4

Interrupted 7-0 polypropylene sutures join the skin edges of the transposed flaps (Figure 25-1D). The previously placed traction suture is taped to the forehead or cheek for 3 to 7 days (Figure 25-1E). Skin sutures are removed in 5 to 7 days.

SKIN GRAFT TECHNIQUE

Full-thickness skin grafts are preferable to split-thickness grafts because the former are less likely to contract postoperatively. Potential donor sites include the retroauricular region, the upper eyelid, the supraclavicular region, and the inner aspect of the upper arm (Figure 25-2).

Step 1

A marking pen is used to outline the incision, which should be made at the desired upper lid crease location, or 2 to 3 mm beneath the cilia in the lower eyelid.

Step 2

Local anesthetic is injected in the involved eyelid and at the donor site. A 4-0 silk suture is placed in the eyelid margin at the center of the traction. A hemostat is used to exert tension on the suture.

Levine MR.
Manual of Oculoplastic Surgery, Fourth Edition (pp 183-188).
© 2010 SLACK Incorporated

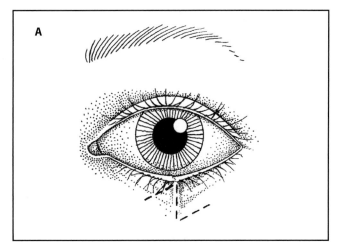

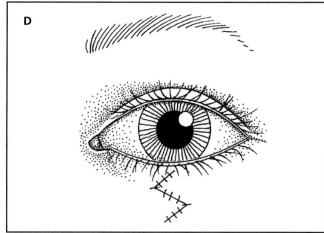

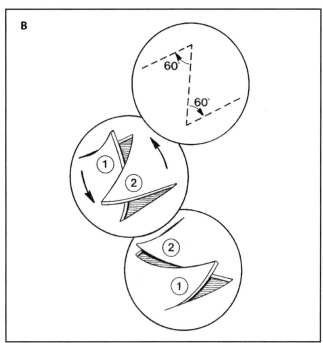

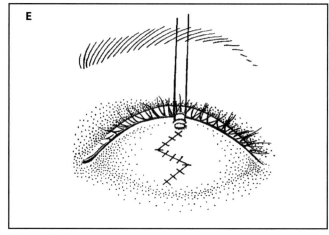

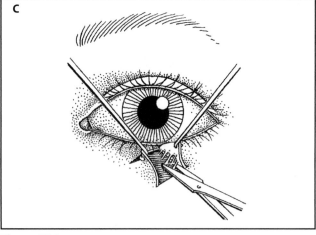

Figure 25-1.

Figure 25-1.

ally deeper until all bands of vertical scar tissue are incised. Although it is not essential to excise the scar tissue, release of all vertical scar tissue by incision is necessary (Figures 25-3B and 25-3C). Bleeding should be stopped completely before graft placement. The use of topical thrombin and Gelfoam is less traumatic than cautery.

Step 4

A template of the defect is made by tracing the defect with a translucent drape. The tracing should be done with the eyelid slightly on stretch and with an effort to make the template 25% larger than the defect, thus allowing for graft shrinkage (Figure 25-3D).

Step 5

The template is placed over the donor site and traced with a marking pen. When harvesting a graft from the retroauricular area, skin should be removed in equal amounts from both sides of the retroauricular crease to make closure easier. A #15 Bard-Parker blade at a 45° angle can be used to separate the skin from the underlying tissue (Figure 25-4). Closure of the donor site is accomplished with 4-0 polyglycolic acid suture subcutaneously and 4-0 silk or nylon in the skin. Skin sutures are removed in 7 days.

Step 3

A #15 Bard-Parker blade is used to incise the eyelid (Figure 25-3A). The incision is carried gradu-

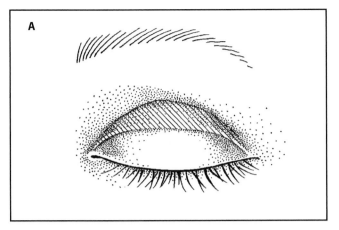

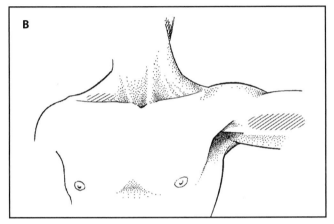

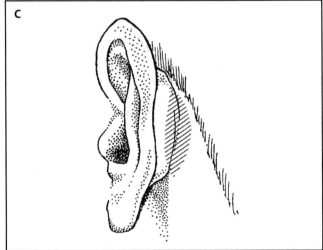

Figure 25-2.

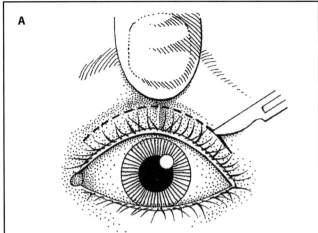

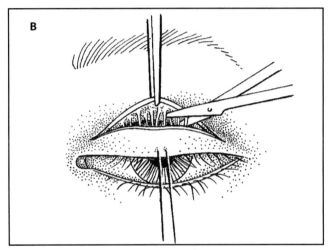

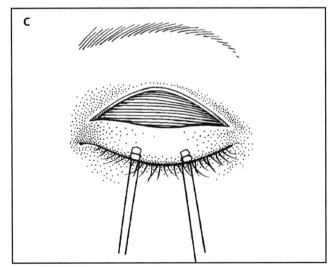

Figure 25-3.

Step 6

The skin graft is draped over the surgeon's finger; subcutaneous tissue is trimmed with scissors. This approach thins the graft, increases graft viability, and gives a nicer cosmetic result (Figure 25-5).

Step 7

The graft is now sewn to the recipient site with 6-0 plain, polypropylene, silk, or nylon sutures (Figure 25-6A). If the upper lid is being grafted, consideration should be given to placing deeper 6-0 polygly-colic acid sutures from the underside of the graft to the tarsus in an effort to define the upper lid crease in the desired location, usually near the top of the tarsus in the Western lid.

Step 8

Cardinal sutures are placed in each quadrant, followed by interrupted or running sutures. Any

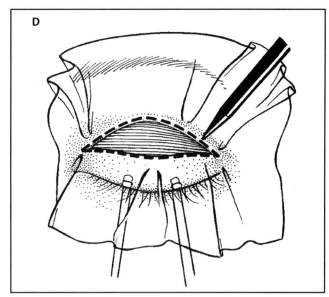

Figure 25-3.

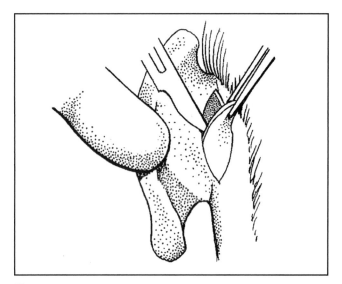

Figure 25-4.

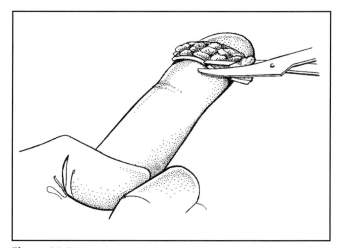

Figure 25-5.

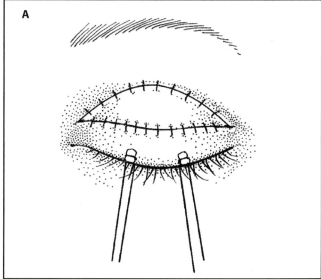

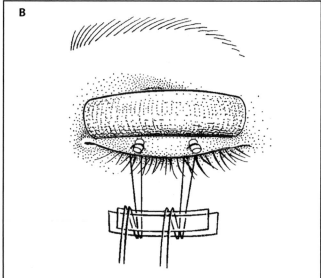

Figure 25-6.

excess graft should be trimmed, but it is wise to delay trimming until the suturing is nearly complete. Stab incisions should be made in the graft to allow blood and fluid to emerge. A hematoma under the graft often leads to graft necrosis.

Step 9

A bolster should be placed over the graft to push the skin gently against the recipient bed. Many surgeons leave the silk sutures long and tie them over the bolster. My preference is to use antibiotic-soaked dental rolls, which are not sewn to the graft. Ointment is used to coat the bolster, and 2 eye pads are placed over it after the previously placed traction suture(s) have been taped to the cheek (Figure 25-6B).

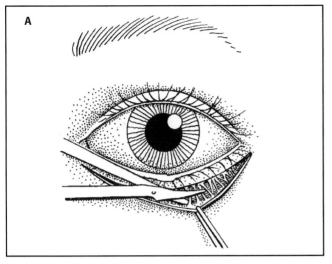

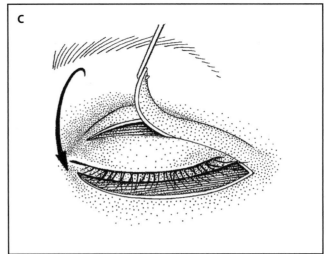

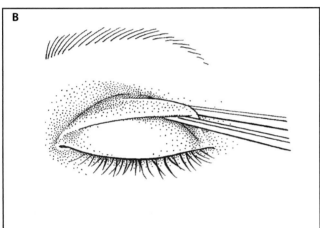

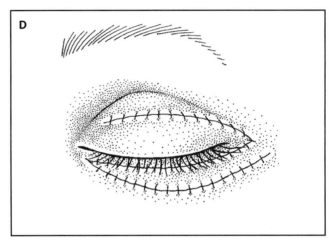

Figure 25-7.

Step 10
The dressing, bolster, and traction suture are removed in 1 to 5 days. The skin sutures are removed in 5 to 7 days.

SKIN-MUSCLE FLAP TECHNIQUE

In repairing a lower cicatricial ectropion, an alternative approach is to use redundant upper lid tissue as a flap to the lower eyelid. Advantages include better cosmesis and upward pull exerted on the lower lid. Disadvantages include the potential for creation of cicatricial lagophthalmos or asymmetry between the upper lids. Steps 1 to 3 are the same as for the skin graft technique (Figure 25-7A).

Step 4
The upper lid crease is traced with a marking pencil. A forceps is placed at the lid crease and is used to pinch the skin above the crease. The location of the forceps when slight lagophthalmos appears shows the maximum amount of tissue that can be safely spared (Figure 25-7B). This is outlined with a marking pencil and is infiltrated with anesthetic. The incision is made, leaving a hinge laterally in most cases, although it can also be placed medially when there is a medial ectropion. Scissors are used

to raise a flap in a plane between the orbicularis muscle and the orbital septum (Figure 25-7C).

Step 5
The lower lid incision is extended laterally to accommodate transposition of the skin-muscle flap. The flap is sewn to the recipient site with 6-0 plain, polypropylene, or silk sutures (Figure 25-7D). If inadequate tissue is obtained from the upper lid, it is necessary to add a skin graft to the recipient site. The opposite upper lid is a suitable source. The upper lid is closed with 6-0 plain, polypropylene, or silk sutures. Stab incisions are not necessary in the skin-muscle flap. Dressings and a bolster are applied as described in Steps 9 and 10 in "Skin Graft Technique."

HORIZONTAL EYELID LAXITY

The cicatricial forces may cause stretching of the medial and lateral canthal tendons. This problem is most significant in the lower lids and rarely needs to be addressed in the upper lids. When the vertical contracture is released by scar incisions, the horizontal laxity is more apparent. Observation of the lid is inadequate to judge horizontal laxity when the patient is supine. A good technique is to use a tenotomy muscle hook to compare the horizontal tension of the lower lids.

Repair can best be accomplished by a tarsal strip procedure, as described in Chapter 24. This repair should be performed after scar incision and before the donor tissue is harvested.

Complications

The most common complications after repair of a cicatricial ectropion are undercorrection and misdirected lashes. Undercorrection or recurrence of ectropion should prompt the surgeon to reconsider the various factors contributing to the ectropion. The surgeon should then decide whether each causal factor has been corrected. For example, was the skin graft or flap of adequate size and location to correct the vertical skin shortage? Could a disinsertion of the lower eyelid retractors be present and has it been corrected with the surgery performed? Has the horizontal eyelid laxity been adequately corrected at both the medial and lateral canthus?

Misdirection of eyelashes is frequently noted after ectropion repair. Inflammation and contraction of the palpebral conjunctiva often rotate the lash follicles inward and result in a more vertical orientation of the lashes. When the ectropion is initially repaired, the vertical position of the lashes may persist. The result may be good position of the eyelid margin but contact of the lashes with the globe. This problem tends to resolve in a few weeks or months as the inflamed palpebral conjunctiva returns to normal. Persistent trichiasis may require treatment with marginal rotation, cryosurgery, electrolysis, or excision of the misdirected follicles.

TRICHIASIS AND DISTICHIASIS

James R. Boynton, MD and Thomas C. Naugle, Jr, MD

Trichiasis

Trichiasis (Greek for hair) refers to a condition of abnormal eyelash growth. Normal eyelashes emerge from their follicles and bend outward, curving away from the eye (Figure 26-1A). In trichiasis, the eyelashes can be directed posteriorly toward the eye, often rubbing on the surface of the globe (Figure 26-1B). The difference between entropion and trichiasis is in the position of the lid margin. In entropion, the lid margin is turned inward. In trichiasis, the lid margin is in a normal position, but the eyelashes can be turned inward. The unfortunate results of trichiasis can be pain and corneal scarring, with decreased vision.

The pathogenesis of trichiasis involves the creation of microcicatrices in the area of the eyelash follicles. The follicles are distorted, and the lashes become misdirected because of scarring of the lid margin. The underlying pathologic process may also cause keratinization of the lid margin mucosa, which further aggravates the ocular surface problems. In addition, abnormalities of tear production often result from conjunctival changes, which cause further difficulties. The more common diseases that cause trichiasis include trachoma, ocular pemphigoid, erythema multiforme (Stevens-Johnson syndrome), blepharitis of any sort, and chemical burns.

Distichiasis

Distichiasis refers to an abnormality characterized by a second row of eyelashes located behind the normal lash line. The abnormal or accessory eyelashes grow from, or adjacent to, the sebaceous gland orifices and usually rub against the cornea (Figure 26-1C). There are 2 types of distichiasis: congenital and acquired. Congenital distichiasis may be inherited as a dominant trait with variable penetrance, or it may be sporadic. The eyelashes may be heavy, dark, and sharp or thin and pale. Depending on the type of eyelash and the relationship to the cornea, the patient may be miserable or almost without symptoms.

Congenital distichiasis may result from arrested differentiation. Multipotential primary epithelial germ cells migrate from the primitive epidermis into the dermis. They then differentiate into hair follicles, sebaceous glands, and sweat glands. These elements are found combined in pilosebaceous units throughout the skin. The eyelid glands (meibomian and Zeis) are specialized sebaceous glands. Incomplete differentiation might well result in hair production within these glands.

Acquired distichiasis may appear clinically similar to the congenital form. The acquired type probably is a reaction to a noxious stimulus. The normal non-hair-producing sebaceous glands are transformed into hair follicles by mechanical or chemical stimuli. Evidence of this metaplasia may be seen in cases of Stevens-Johnson syndrome, ocular pemphigoid, and other inflammatory conditions. In such cases, distichiasis may coexist with trichiasis and other eyelid abnormalities.

Treatment

Because many lash problems are the manifestations of an underlying disease, prevention or cure of the primary disorder is the first line of defense. Reducing the incidence of injuries and treating injuries and cicatrizing disease early (eg, herpes zoster) may improve the acute course in many patients. Likewise, improved treatment of blepharitis, conjunctival shrinkage conditions, and similar problems reduces the incidence and severity of morbidity secondary to aberrant lashes.

The 2 approaches to treatment of aberrant eyelashes are destruction of the eyelash follicles or repositioning of the lash-bearing areas so that the lashes no longer rub against the globe. The eyelashes can be removed by simple epila-

Levine MR.
Manual of Oculoplastic Surgery, Fourth Edition (pp 189-194).
© 2010 SLACK Incorporated

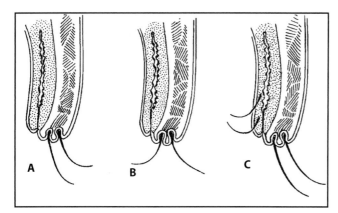

Figure 26-1.

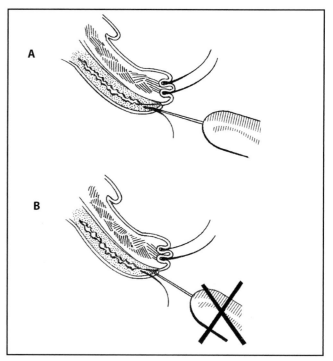

Figure 26-2.

tion, electrolysis, cryotreatment, argon laser, or surgical excision.

Frequent epilation of multiple eyelashes may result in exuberant regrowth and a magnification of the problem. If the eyelashes break off rather than emanate from the follicle, the lash stub may be extremely sharp and may injure the cornea more than the original lash. Very fine, thin, pale eyelashes may be difficult to see and almost impossible to grasp.

ELECTROLYSIS

Electrolysis may be effective as a means of removing a few isolated lashes.

Step 1

Local anesthesia is injected, and the needle tip of the instrument is placed in the depth of the follicle (Figure 26-2A).

Step 2

Current is applied until a frothing or bubbling is seen at the base of the eyelash (usually 15 seconds).

Step 3

The procedure must be done under magnification if the eyelashes are small.

COMMENTS

Electrolysis may eradicate eyelashes, but it is not without problems. The needle tip may not follow the follicle to its base (Figure 26-2B) but bypass it. It is often hard to place the tip into a small follicle, and short, fine lanugo lashes are difficult to treat. The destructive electric current produces scarring of the lid, which can aggravate a tendency toward entropion. This is particularly worrisome if multiple eyelashes are treated close together. Eyelashes do recur after electrolysis. The procedure can be time consuming and tedious when more than one or two eyelashes are being treated.

CRYOSURGERY

The use of cryosurgery to treat eyelid tumors afforded an opportunity to observe the effects of freezing on lid lashes. The permanent loss of eyelashes that occurred in treated areas provided an example for the procedure to be used as therapy for trichiasis. The results of cryotreatment of eye lids in experimental animals originally suggested that freezing to -30°C is a safe and effective method of eradicating eyelashes. Clinical experience has subsequently shown that cryosurgery (at temperatures of -20°C) can be used with good success to ablate unwanted eyelashes.

The differential sensitivity of various cells to cold injury provides the basis for the practicality of cryotreatment. Thus, the cells within the eyelash follicle are more sensitive to freezing and undergo necrosis, whereas the rest of the eyelid recovers from the cold insult. Achieving the proper temperature at the level of the lash follicle is therefore important. If the temperature does not get low enough, the eyelashes will regrow. By contrast, excessive freezing can result in permanent alteration and loss of normal eyelid tissue.

The biophysical mechanisms of cold injury are complex: (1) when intracellular ice crystals form, they expand, which can cause a mechanical rupture of cell membranes; (2) the pH value of intracellular fluids is altered and may result in protein denaturation; (3) cold injury to blood vessels may cause thrombosis with secondary ischemia and infarction; and (4) it is possible that cryotreatment may release antigens, triggering an immune response that adds to tissue insult and destruction. Optimum cellular injury is achieved by a rapid freeze and slow thaw, which is then repeated.

Step 1

Local infiltrative anesthesia with epinephrine is used. Vasoconstriction speeds freezing and slows thawing.

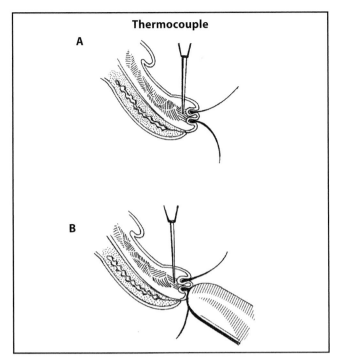

Thermocouple

A

B

Figure 26-3.

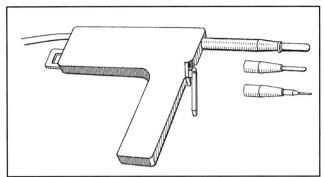

Figure 26-4.

Step 2

A plastic corneoscleral shell is used to protect the globe. Use of a lid clamp such as those designed for chalazion excisions or other stabilizing lid clamps may make the procedure technically easier and reduce blood flow, facilitating a fast freeze and slow thaw.

Step 3

A thermocouple is used to monitor the temperature of the tissue at the base of the eyelashes. The needle tip of the thermocouple is placed under the skin 3 to 4 mm below the lid margin in the area to be treated (Figure 26-3A). It is usually easiest to place the needle parallel to the lid margin. Proper placement is essential, or the information gained from the thermocouple is useless. If the probe is placed too superficially, the follicles are undertreated, but if the needle tip is too remote from the eyelash bases, overtreatment can occur. It usually takes 30 to 60 seconds to reach -20°C. Originally, the eyelids were frozen to -30°C, but the side effects are greater with this temperature, and good results can be attained with -20°C. The tissue is allowed to thaw slowly and the procedure is repeated. The second freeze usually takes a shorter time. Overlapping applications are made along the involved area of the eyelid.

Step 4

After secure placement of the thermocouple needle, the cryoprobe is applied to the lid margin and the eyelid is frozen (Figure 26-3B). Moisture between the tissue and the probe helps attain a rapid spread of the freeze. However, the probe must be in firm contact with the lid tissue before freezing to ensure optimum ice ball formation.

Step 5

The probe may be placed against the posterior aspect of the lid margin or on the skin surface of the lid. Advantages of posterior placement include the ability to push the eyelid away from the globe with the probe. There may be less damage to the anterior lid margin using this technique. This includes less loss of skin pigment, less intense alterations of the tissue at the lash line, and possible sparing of normal eyelashes in some cases. The conjunctiva and tarsus recover well from freeze injury. By contrast, the eyelash follicles in some cases may lie closer to the anterior lid surface, and it may be easier in these cases to obtain a rapid freeze with anterior placement of the probe. Only the tip of the thermocouple needle is temperature sensitive, so placement of the cold probe near the shaft of the needle is not a problem.

The maximum inflammatory reaction usually occurs within 48 to 72 hours. There is edema, erythema, and surface exudation, but little pain. The reaction subsides in 1 to 2 weeks, and the eyelashes shed spontaneously or may be easily removed without resistance. Antibiotic ointment is given after treatment for 7 to 10 days.

COMMENTS

The use of the proper freezing equipment is most helpful. The cryoprobes for retinal cryopexy do not produce temperatures that are cold enough in general, and a higher incidence of eyelash recurrence follows their use. Liquid nitrogen is more cumbersome to use and store and can easily overfreeze the eyelid margin. A nitrous oxide-cooled probe made by Cryomedics (Kry-Med model MT 650, Cryomedics, Bridgeport, CT) is the tool of choice (Figure 26-4). Interchangeable tips are available with which to tailor the freezing procedure to each individual problem.

Experimental treatment of rabbit eyelids has provided specimens for histologic study. The general architecture of the eyelid is preserved, but scar formation occurs in the deeper structures and hyperplastic changes of the epithelial surfaces. Sebaceous glands may be reduced in number.

The results of cryosurgery treatment for trichiasis are gratifying. Up to 85% of treated patients may have permanent loss of eyelashes. Recurrences can easily be retreated, with equally good expectations in most cases.

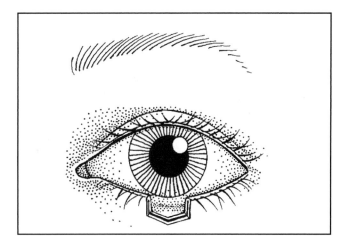

Figure 26-5.

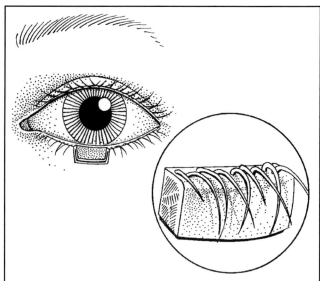

Figure 26-6.

No procedure is without complications, and it is important to be aware of the potential adverse effects of the application of cryosurgery to the eyelids. Complications have been reported in up to 25% of treated eyelids, although many are minor. Complications have included loss of vision, corneal ulcers, lid notching, symblepharon, xerosis, cellulitis, activation of herpes zoster, tissue necrosis, loss of pigment, and, possibly, induced trichiasis adjacent to the treatment site. Extreme edema is occasionally seen but is transitory. In general, patients with conjunctival shrinkage diseases are more likely to experience complications. If the underlying disease process is activated by the cryosurgery procedure, loss of vision can occur. Therefore, caution is in order when considering the use of cryosurgery in the management of patients with cicatricial pemphigoid, Stevens-Johnson syndrome, and other shrinkage disorders.

ARGON LASER

Ablation of aberrant lashes with argon laser has recently been investigated. Lashes are individually treated. The lid usually heals rapidly with minimal discomfort. Recurrent lashes are treated as easily as the primary ones. Loss of pigment and dimpling of the lid margin may occur.

Step 1
Local infiltrative anesthesia is used.

Step 2
The patient is positioned at the slit lamp, and a protective corneoscleral shell is used.

Step 3
Laser settings of 1.0 to 2.5 W, 0.2- to 0.5-second duration, and 50-μm spot size are selected.

Step 4
The lid margin is everted so that laser burns can be applied coaxially with the lash follicle.

Step 5
Burns are applied to a depth of approximately 2 mm to destroy the lash follicle.

SURGICAL PROCEDURES

The problem of in-turned eyelashes may be treated with a number of surgical procedures. Many of these procedures are aimed at correcting cicatricial entropion. Basically, they reposition the lid margin. Surgical procedures directed at removing in-turned lashes are presented in the following discussion. Some procedures are applicable to trichiasis and distichiasis, whereas others are specific for one entity.

Problem I: Localized Trichiasis

If the area of trichiasis is localized and fairly small and adequate laxity is present, a full-thickness excision of the involved lid margin cures the problem. The lid edges must be rejoined carefully under magnification for optimum results (Figure 26-5).

Problem II: Moderate Trichiasis

In lower lids, where the trichiasis is slightly more extensive, the involved area of abnormal eyelashes can be excised as a strip of anterior lamella, including the lashes (Figure 26-6). The inferior skin edge is freed so that there is no downward traction on the lower lid margin. The raw area is allowed to epithelialize. In similar situations involving the upper lid, the anterior lamella including the aberrant lashes can be recessed (Figure 26-7A). The recessed lash line is tacked down to the tarsus 3 mm above the lid margin, and the lashes are everted with the help of sutures and excision of skin (Figure 26-7B). With the passage of time, the aberrant lashes may migrate inferiorly and have to be excised.

An additional technique involves raising a skin-muscle flap to expose the bulbs at the lash roots (Figure 26-7C). Each bulb is destroyed with bipolar cautery. The aberrant lashes are epilated easily to confirm bulb destruction and the flap is sutured back into place. This procedure has the advantage of minimal lid margin scarring and avoidance of trauma to the conjunctival surface.

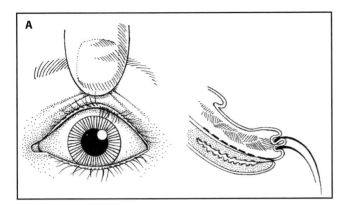

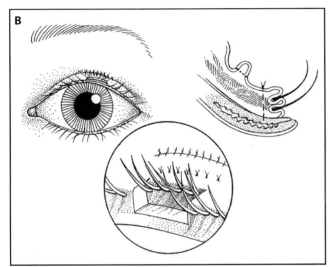

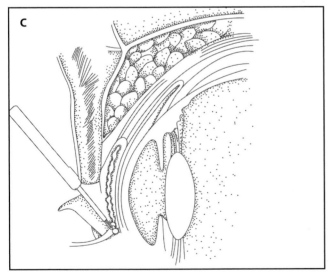

Figure 26-7.

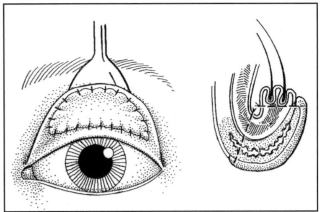

Figure 26-8.

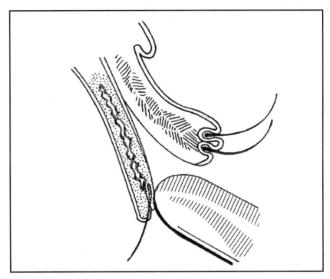

Figure 26-9.

Problem III: Extensive Trichiasis

More extensive disease of the lid margins may best be treated by recession or excision of the lash line and placement of a buccal mucosal graft (Figure 26-8). Mucous membrane from the hard palate may also be used as a free graft. Hard palate mucosa, however, is keratinized and can damage the cornea, especially in the upper eyelid. It is more useful in the lower eyelid.

Problem IV: Distichiasis

Distichiasis may be managed by simple cryotreatment. Alternatively, splitting the eyelid into anterior and posterior lamellar layers before freezing has been suggested as a means of preserving normal lashes and avoiding damage to the anterior lid margin (Figure 26-9). This technique can result in cicatricial ectropion in some cases. Excision of individual eyelash follicles under high magnification has been suggested as a means of treating distichiasis. Although this approach may be effective and may minimize trauma to the eyelid, it is tedious and time consuming. Abnormal lashes cannot always be followed from the lid margin to their origin. Excision of eyelashes in distichiasis may be easier to perform if a flap of tarsus is elevated to expose the follicles (trap door technique) (Figure 26-10). An effective but more traumatic surgical procedure is excision of the posterior lash line including the involved posterior lid margin. The raw area can be left to heal spontaneously if the excision is not extensive. It may be best to place a mucous membrane graft in cases of larger excisions (Figure 26-11).

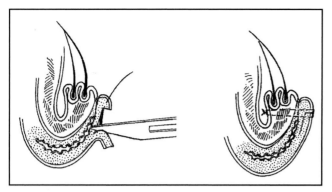 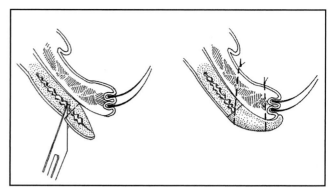

Figure 26-10.   **Figure 26-11.**

All cases of trichiasis and distichiasis are best managed on an individual basis. The nature, severity, and extent of the problem, along with the presence of other lid or ocular disease, should be considered when choosing therapy. Appropriate treatment can most often be selected if each patient's situation is carefully evaluated. In spite of numerous good therapeutic options, the management of trichiasis and distichiasis can be a difficult and frustrating experience for both patient and surgeon. There is good evidence that the stem cells for lash growth are located in the upper portion of the follicle rather than deep in the bulb as previously thought. Further studies of hair cell growth may allow selective manipulation of the process at key control points such as ascension of the dermal papilla. Knowledge of biochemical details of the growth process may allow enzymatic control of follicular cells.

Little is now known about factors responsible for the direction of hair growth or curvature of the hair itself. Control of these 2 variables would be of enormous help in managing trichiasis.

CHAPTER 27

TARSORRHAPHY AND EYELID TRACTION SUTURES

Steven Fagien, MD, FACS

Tarsorrhaphy is the surgical fusion of the upper and lower eyelid margins. It is most commonly performed to protect the cornea from exposure resulting from proptosis, seventh nerve (facial) paralysis, neuroparalytic keratitis, indolent corneal ulcers, tear film deficiencies, and a variety of other ocular and eyelid disorders.

Tarsorrhaphies can be temporary or permanent, in which case raw tarsal edges are created to form a lasting adhesion with the option of eventual reversal in the long or short term (fusion). They may be total or partial, depending on whether all or a portion of the palpebral fissure is occluded. In addition, they may be classified as lateral, medial, or central, according to the position in the palpebral fissure affected.

The procedure to be described is based on an anatomic approach. It is usual to consider the eyelid margin as being composed of an anterior lamella, consisting of skin (with cilia) and orbicularis muscle, and a posterior lamella, consisting of tarsus and conjunctiva. In most cases where tarsorrhaphy is performed with the anticipation of long-term or even permanent effects, tissue excision can still be confined exclusively to the posterior lamella, whereas the anterior lamella and lash line are preserved. This approach results in an excellent cosmetic result if the tarsorrhaphy is opened at a later date. It may also prevent the complications of an irregular eyelid margin (after release), entropion, and trichiasis, which may prove to be at least as detrimental to the cornea as the initial exposure.

Surgical Procedure

Step 1

Local anesthesia with 2% lidocaine with epinephrine is administered by local infiltration. The length of the eyelid adhesion necessary to produce the desired effect is determined by gently pinching the upper and lower eyelids together with either forceps or fingers. The proposed area for tarsorrhaphy is then marked onto the upper and lower eyelid medially and laterally with a marking pen. It is recommended that 2 to 3 mm be added to the desired horizontal width, as there is a natural tendency for the resultant eyelid fusion to be slightly less (long term) than the anticipated total horizontal width of the tarsorrhaphy initially performed.

Step 2

The anterior and posterior lamellae of the upper eyelid are split with a stab incision at the posterior gray line using a #11 Bard-Parker blade (Figure 27-1). Separation of the anterior and posterior lid lamellae is carried to a depth of approximately 3 to 4 mm using Stevens or Westcott scissors. This allows a large surface area for adhesion and spares the cilia within the anterior eyelid lamella. After the incision in the gray line has been carried along the predetermined length, an identical incision is performed in the opposing eyelid to the desired length.

Step 3

The surface epidermis (epithelium) of the posterior lamella at the eyelid margin of the upper and lower eyelid is then excised using the #11 Bard-Parker blade or iris or Westcott scissors (Figure 27-2). There should be minimal excision of the tarsal plate, and the de-epithelialized edges should be even to ensure good apposition.

Step 4

Tarsal sutures of 5-0 or 6-0 polyglactin (Vicryl) or polyglycolic acid (Dexon) on a spatulated needle are passed through the half-thickness of the tarsus beginning 2 to 3 mm superior to the upper eyelid margin and brought out through the meibomian

Levine MR.
Manual of Oculoplastic Surgery, Fourth Edition (pp 195-198).
© 2010 SLACK Incorporated

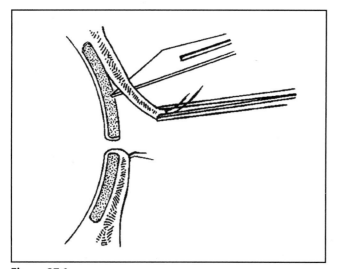

Figure 27-1.

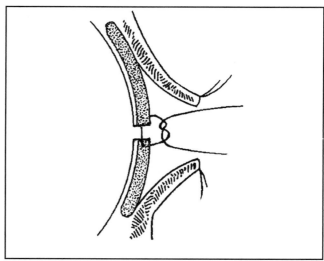

Figure 27-3.

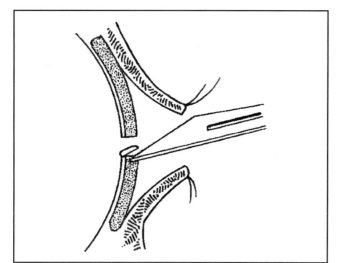

Figure 27-2.

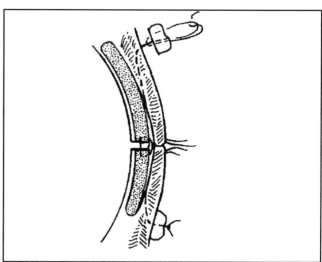

Figure 27-4.

gland orifices (middle of the tarsus). They are then passed into the lower eyelid through the meibomian gland orifices and exit anteriorly at a point 2 to 3 mm inferior to the lower eyelid margin (Figure 27-3). It is important not to pass these sutures through the full thickness of the tarsus because they will likely rub against the cornea in the immediate postoperative period. In addition, it is important for these lamellar sutures to exit and enter within the plane of the meibomian gland orifices at the eyelid margin because sutures placed more anteriorly are likely to erode. Three or 4 sutures are required for tarsorrhaphy of the lateral one third of the eyelid. When the sutures are tied, the bared edges of the tarsus will then be brought together. Vicryl and Dexon sutures usually dissolve within approximately 40 days, by which time a firm adhesion should be present. This tarsal adhesion should be permanent.

Step 5

The anterior lamella may be left untouched in most cases. However, when the anterior lamella appears to be under tension after the tarsus has been sutured, or when a previous tarsorrhaphy has broken down, the tarsal bite should be reinforced with anterior eyelid lamella sutures. This procedure can also be performed in all cases to unequivocally ensure a reduction in the tension of the posterior lid lamella closure. These are usually double-armed 4-0 polypropylene (Prolene) or silk sutures passed through a rubber or silicone sponge. The sutures enter the anterior lid lamella of the upper eyelid approximately 4 mm above the lash line and exit through the "split" at the eyelid margin. They are passed into this "split" between anterior and posterior lid lamellae on the lower eyelid margin and exit through skin 4 mm below the lower eyelid margin. The suture needles are passed again through a lower eyelid silicone or rubber sponge and are tied securely (Figure 27-4). If significant cicatricial forces are present that might actively pull the eyelids apart (eg, third-degree burns of the eyelids), a "tongue-in-groove" tarsorrhaphy may be performed. In this procedure, the eyelid is again

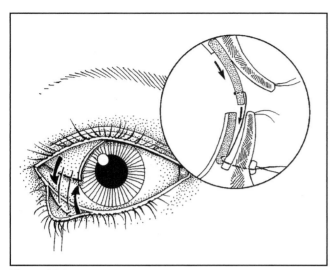

Figure 27-5.

split at the gray line, and the epithelium is denuded at the margin of the posterior lamella. However, rather than suturing the tarsal plates edge-to-edge, the posterior conjunctival surface of the upper eyelid tarsal plate is de-epithelialized and sandwiched between the lower tarsal plate posteriorly and lower eyelid anterior lamella anteriorly. It is sutured in place with a horizontal mattress suture of double-armed 5-0 Vicryl. Again, care is taken to make the tarsal "bites" in the inferior tarsal plate partial thickness. The sutures are brought out through the superior tarsal plate and tied over a silicone or rubber sponge (Figure 27-5).

Temporary Suture Tarsorrhaphy

At times, patients may have exposure symptoms, and it is not certain that their symptoms and signs would be relieved by tarsorrhaphy. They may also be somewhat apprehensive regarding even a minor surgical procedure and would like to be convinced that their symptoms will be resolved by such a procedure. In these situations, a temporary suture tarsorrhaphy is an ideal procedure. Also, in patients who have exposure keratopathy, eyelid retraction secondary to blepharoplasty, or other signs of exposure, including chemosis (especially in patients with thyroid disease), a temporary tarsorrhaphy would be quite useful to resolve their symptoms expeditiously. Other patients who would benefit from a temporary suture tarsorrhaphy are those with acute Bell's palsy and symptoms of lagophthalmos and exposure keratopathy and patients who are comatose or who have sustained severe facial trauma (especially those intubated in intensive care settings), in whom a quick temporary solution is ideal. More recently, temporary suture tarsorrhaphy has been routinely incorporated in primary blepharoplasty and midface/cheek lift procedures to promote optimum long-term lower eyelid position as well as to reduce short-term exposure/dryness symptoms and chemosis. The theory and mechanism for improvement of ocular signs and symptoms is the same as for a permanent suture tarsorrhaphy, but such instances

may require only several days or weeks of treatment and are less likely to need a "permanent" surgical procedure.

Step 1

Local anesthesia is the same as for a permanent tarsorrhaphy (2% lidocaine with epinephrine). In cases where tarsorrhaphy is used in cosmetic lower blepharoplasty, the eyelid is infiltrated with local anesthetic in the usual fashion, and the tarsorrhaphy suture is placed as the last component of the surgery. The procedure is usually performed laterally; however, it can be performed medially and laterally for more complete eyelid closure. In cases where it is anticipated that the suture will remain in place for weeks (such as in facial paresis), 5 mm x 3 mm (approximate) rectangular bolsters are cut from the synthetic sponge-like material contained within the double-armed 4-0 silk suture supplied by Ethicon Inc. Each arm of the double-armed 4-0 silk suture (needle) is passed through one end of the sponge to exit in the posterior aspect of each sponge. Each arm of the suture is then passed approximately 4 mm below the lower eyelid margin through skin and orbicularis muscle to enter into the middle of the tarsus and exit through the eyelid margin at the meibomian gland orifices. In cases where it is expected that the suture will be removed within 2 weeks (such as in cosmetic blepharoplasty), bolsters are usually not necessary, and the suture material can be varied from whatever suture material is used for skin closure or an alternate suture of choice.

Step 2

Each suture is then passed through the meibomian gland orifices at the upper eyelid margin and exits the tarsus, orbicularis, and skin approximately 4 mm above the eyelid margin. The double-armed suture is then passed through a similar-sized synthetic sponge and tied securely. The suture should tie fairly snugly; otherwise, an incomplete lid opposition may result when the initial intraoperative and postoperative edema resolves.

The advantage of such a procedure, especially in blepharoplasty patients, is that, when combined with the use of a topical antibiotic/corticosteroid, chemosis secondary to exposure is rapidly resolved. Lid retraction is also somewhat relieved by eye and eyelid movement (particularly upgaze) because this acts as a continuous massage to release cicatricial adhesions in the lower eyelid that may be contributing to the lower eyelid retraction. The sutures can remain for several weeks or be removed at any time with a simple snip of the suture. When the tarsorrhaphy is needed for longer periods of time, suture reaction is minimized by using antibiotic-corticosteroid ointment on the sutures at bedtime.

This procedure leaves no (lasting) eyelid margin deformity after release. In cases in which there is uncertainty about the need for tarsorrhaphy, such a trial can prove whether this will resolve exposure symptoms. Permanent surgical tarsorrhaphy can then be performed—even in the same area—immediately after removal of the suture or if signs and symptoms of exposure recur at a later date.

Eyelid Traction Sutures

Eyelid traction sutures are used for a variety of oculo-plastic surgical procedures. They are particularly useful when repairing congenital ptosis or myogenic ptosis with reduced motility (especially frontalis sling procedures), when multiple lower eyelid traction sutures can be released sequentially to ensure corneal protection in the immediate postoperative period. They are also commonly used in the lower eyelid with the repair of cicatricial ectropion with skin grafts, tarsal strip procedures for a variety of eyelid malpositions, correction of the lower eyelid retraction (especially in patients with thyroid disease), lower eyelid blepharoplasty, and after removal of eyelid margin malignancies to prevent postoperative lid retraction and ectropion. They are also occasionally used in the upper eyelid for patients who have undergone upper eyelid levator recessions (and Müller's muscle extirpation) for upper eyelid retraction associated with thyroid ophthalmopathy.

Eyelid traction sutures promote an elevated position of the lower eyelid margin and a depressed position of the upper eyelid (ie, as in upper eyelid retraction surgery for patients with thyroid disease) when there is the possibility of migration of the eyelid toward the opposite (unwanted) direction. For example, horizontal shortening tarsal strip procedures or cicatricial ectropion repairs with skin grafts are aided by elevating the lower eyelid with a traction suture in the immediate postoperative period. It has also been helpful in patients undergoing either standard transcutaneous blepharoplasty with skin removal as well as when surgery is performed (even in part) via a trans-conjunctival approach to ensure an elevated lower eyelid position for the first day or two after surgery.

In patients undergoing cosmetic lower eyelid surgery (without skin grafting, which is typically bolstered to provide support to the skin graft), ice packs are commonly applied for the first few days after surgery. The usual tendency, however, is for the patient to apply the ice packs in a manner that may force the lower eyelid into a retracted state unless there is an attempt to massage the eyelid superiorly. Additionally, elevating the lower eyelid margin in those individuals who have had surgical incision/release of the lower eyelid retractors via a transconjunctival approach may benefit from traction. In these cases, traction sutures aid in maintaining a good lower eyelid position, while enabling the patient to apply ice to the lower eyelids in a more carefree manner.

Anesthesia

Local anesthesia with 2% lidocaine (Xylocaine) with epinephrine, 0.75% bupivacaine, or both is administered by local infiltration. At times, however, this is not needed, because the eyelid has already been anesthetized for the primary procedure.

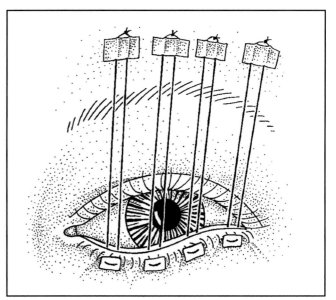

Figure 27-6.

Surgical Procedure

Step 1

The position of the lower eyelid to be elevated (or the upper eyelid to be depressed) is determined. A double-armed 4-0 silk suture is passed through a pre-tarsal segment of the eyelid margin, usually approximately 1 to 3 mm from the lashes (a preconstructed synthetic bolster/sponge can be fashioned if necessary).

Step 2

Each arm of the double-armed 4-0 silk suture is passed through the eyelid margin (or sponge first) and then enters through the skin and orbicularis muscle 1 to 3 mm below (or above in the upper lid) the lower eyelid margin. Each needle of the double-armed suture exits through the meibomian gland orifices, and the sutures are tied to each other (Figure 27-6).

Step 3

The eyelid is elevated (or lowered in the upper eyelid) to the desired position. Tincture of Benzoin (or Mastisol) solution, or a similar liquid adhesive, is applied to the skin area where the suture will be fixated. When the suture and eyelid are in good position, the suture is fixed to the skin area using 0.5-inch Steri-Strip adhesive bandages.

Step 4

The traction sutures may be left in for 1 to 7 (or more) days. The antibiotic or antibiotic/steroid ointment applied to the surgical area can also be applied to the traction suture area.

CHAPTER 28

FLOPPY EYELID SYNDROME REPAIR

Julian D. Perry, MD and Thu Pham, MD

Floppy eyelid syndrome produces easily everted upper eyelids and conjunctivitis. Symptoms are nonspecific and overlap with other causes of ocular irritation. Patients often present with chronic complaints of ocular irritation, redness, and mucous discharge. Some patients or their family members may report spontaneous eversion of one or both eyelids during sleep. Often, the affected side corresponds to the side on which the patient sleeps. In patients with no sleeping preference or those who sleep face down, bilateral eyelid involvement often exists.

Preoperative Evaluation

The hallmark of floppy eyelid syndrome remains the easily everted upper eyelid. The tarsus is soft and foldable, in contrast to the normal tarsus, which has a rigid structure that functions to maintain the integrity of the eyelid. On examination, gentle lifting of the upper eyelid demonstrates the ease of eyelid eversion. In addition to significant horizontal eyelid laxity, the eyelid may also demonstrate abnormal thickness and a rubbery consistency. Other eyelid findings include dermatochalasis, blepharochalasis, blepharoptosis, eyelash ptosis, blepharitis, tear dysfunction, and lower eyelid laxity and ectropion.

Although overweight middle-aged men represent the majority of patients with floppy eyelid syndrome, not all patients with floppy eyelid syndrome are overweight, and the disease occurs in women as well. Floppy eyelid syndrome has been reported to occur in conjunction with multiple systemic conditions, most commonly obstructive sleep apnea and obesity. The disease causes loss of elastin within the tarsal plate; however, the fibers remain mostly preserved around meibomian glands, and collagen fibers appear to be unaffected. Sleeping position may cause mechanical upper eyelid eversion from contact with the pillow or bed sheets to produce keratoconjunctivitis. Pressure-induced ischemia along with oxidative reperfusion injury may represent the causative mechanism. Hormonal factors may also play a role.

Conservative treatment options include lubricating drops and ointments, patching, and nightly placement of an eyeshield or eyelid taping. Many patients with floppy eyelid syndrome and sleep apnea use continuous positive airway pressure machines, which may further aggravate symptoms by increasing airflow around the exposed eye. Refitting of the continuous positive airway pressure mask may improve signs and symptoms.

Surgical Techniques

Surgical treatments typically address the horizontal eyelid laxity and/or the lash ptosis. Many surgical techniques have been described to address the horizontal eyelid laxity, including full-thickness eyelid excision and the lateral tarsal strip procedure. The tarsal strip procedure is addressed in Chapter 24.

Standard full-thickness pentagonal block resection typically improves the laxity; however, it results in incisions perpendicular to the relaxed intention lines, which may lead to visible scarring. Anterior curvilinear incisions with squared posterior incisions through tarsus may lead to a more desirable external scar. A second modification of standard full-thickness excision involves medial eyelid excision in conjunction with blepharoplasty-type skin excision. This procedure addresses horizontal eyelid laxity as well as the cutaneous redundancy that often coexists in this syndrome.

WEDGE RESECTION WITH ANTERIOR CURVILINEAR INCISION

Step 1

The lateral aspect of the upper eyelid is infiltrated with lidocaine 1% with 1:100,000 dilution of epinephrine through a 30-gauge needle. When injecting the upper eyelid, care is taken to inject directly into the eyelid margin to achieve

Levine MR.
Manual of Oculoplastic Surgery, Fourth Edition (pp 199-202).
© 2010 SLACK Incorporated

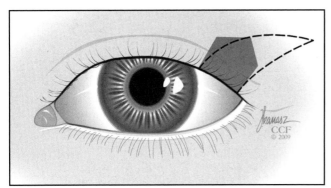

Figure 28-1. (Reprinted with permission, Cleveland Clinic Center for Medical Art & Photography © 2009. All Rights Reserved.)

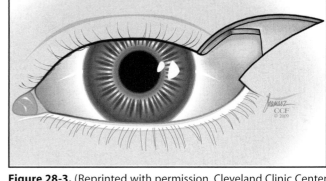

Figure 28-3. (Reprinted with permission, Cleveland Clinic Center for Medical Art & Photography © 2009. All Rights Reserved.)

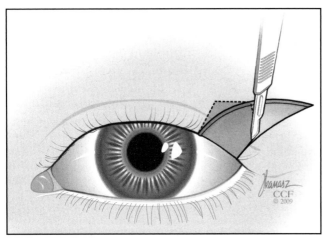

Figure 28-2. (Reprinted with permission, Cleveland Clinic Center for Medical Art & Photography © 2009. All Rights Reserved.)

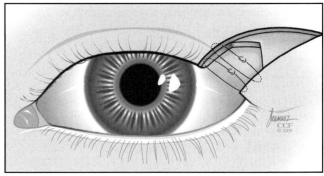

Figure 28-4. (Reprinted with permission, Cleveland Clinic Center for Medical Art & Photography © 2009. All Rights Reserved.)

anesthesia in this area. Castroviejo forceps are used to determine the amount of tissue to be resected by advancing the lax upper eyelid toward the lateral canthus at the proposed medial incision line until the eyelid is under surgical tension. A curvilinear anterior marking is created with a marking pen (Figure 28-1).

Step 2

The central aspect of the eyelid to be removed is grasped at the eyelid margin with forceps, and a #15 blade is used to make vertical incisions through full-thickness eyelid margin and then vertically along the tarsus (Figure 28-2). After the posterior pentagonal incision has been created, the blade is then used to incise the skin along the curvilinear markings. Remaining orbicularis attachments between the pentagonal posterior incision and the curvilinear anterior incision can be lysed with Stevens scissors to remove the full-thickness eyelid tissue (Figure 28-3).

Step 3

The full-thickness defect closure begins with re-alignment of the tarsus with a mattress suture of 5-0 polyglycolic acid. A spatulated needle is passed through the tarsus approximately 3 mm inferior to the lid margin, exiting immediately inferior to the

lid margin. It is then passed through the opposite aspect of the wound in a similar fashion and tied.

Step 4

Two or 3 polyglycolic acid sutures are then used to close the remainder of the tarsus, with care to avoid penetration through conjunctiva, which may result in corneal breakdown (Figure 28-4). The needle enters the orbicularis and exits through the tarsus, anterior to the conjunctiva. The needle is then passed in a similar fashion through the opposite aspect of the wound and tied. In this way, the knot resides superficially, away from the conjunctiva, to decrease the risk of erosion through the palpebral conjunctiva.

Step 5

A vertical mattress suture of 6-0 mild chromic is used to align the meibomian gland orifices and avert the eyelid margin wound edge. The needle is passed parallel to the plane of meibomian glands approximately 1 mm from the cut edge and exits from the cut edge tarsus about 1 mm inferior to the margin. The needle passes through the opposing wound edge in a similar fashion, exiting about 1 mm from the wound edge. The needle is then reintroduced about 3 mm from the cut edge, emerging in the plane of the meibomian gland orifices 3 mm from the opposing cut edge (Figure 28-5). This "near-near, far-far" suture allows for excellent eversion of the lid margin to avoid notching. The following pearl allows for easier placement of the "far-far" needle pass: after the "near-near" pass, the surgeon grasps both ends of

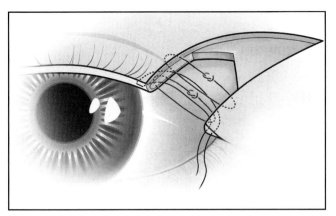

Figure 28-5. (Reprinted with permission, Cleveland Clinic Center for Medical Art & Photography © 2009. All Rights Reserved.)

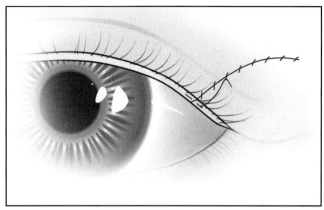

Figure 28-6. (Reprinted with permission, Cleveland Clinic Center for Medical Art & Photography © 2009. All Rights Reserved.)

the suture and gently lifts superiorly. This aligns and stabilizes the lid margin for the "far-far" pass. The "far-far" pass is made with the dominant hand while the nondominant hand lifts both ends of the suture.

Step 6

This suture is tied, leaving the tail end about 3 to 4 cm long so that it can be incorporated into the inferior knot of the cutaneous running suture in order to keep the suture tails away from the eye (Figure 28-6). Prior to running this cutaneous suture, the orbicularis is closed with a deep polyglycolic acid suture. The previously placed vertical mattress suture is then used to close the cutaneous aspect of the wound in running fashion. The tail of this suture is then incorporated into the knot for cutaneous closure in order to keep the tail away from the eye.

The patient is instructed to use ice compresses for 2 days and antibiotic ointment for 2 weeks postoperatively. All sutures that have not absorbed are removed under the slit lamp 2 to 3 weeks postoperatively. The mild chromic gut suture elicits a mild inflammatory reaction, causing some erythema and induration along the wound that resolves several weeks after surgery.

Complications include eyelid notching and mechanical keratopathy due to the lamellar sutures through the tarsus or the suture knot along the eyelid margin. Careful surgical technique minimizes the risk of suture-related injury. If the patient develops keratopathy due to erosion of a tarsal suture, it can be removed under the slit lamp. If the vertical mattress knot along the eyelid margin produces symptoms, a bandage contact lens can be placed until the suture dissolves or until it is removed 2 to 3 weeks postoperatively. Occasionally, redundant cutaneous tissue along the superior aspect of the wound produces a dog-ear deformity. Small redundancies often improve spontaneously, but larger ones can be addressed by removing a small Burrow's triangle superior to the wound after healing.

WEDGE RESECTION WITH CONCOMITANT BLEPHAROPLASTY-STYLE SKIN REMOVAL

This technique involves full-thickness excision of the upper eyelid medial to the laterally displaced tarsus in conjunction with blepharoplasty-type skin excision. The superior aspect of the cutaneous pentagonal incision is curved within the relaxed skin tension lines, and a blepharoplasty-type skin incision is performed as well. This technique results in an incision that runs mainly within the relaxed skin tension lines. The technique addresses not only the horizontal laxity, but also the redundant cutaneous tissues found in many patients with floppy eyelid syndrome. This procedure also avoids significant removal of tarsus; while the tarsus exhibits more elasticity in floppy eyelid syndrome, it still likely acts as a significant eyelid scaffold and support structure.

Step 1

The entire upper eyelid is infiltrated with lidocaine 1% with 1:100,000 dilution of epinephrine through a 30-gauge needle with care to infiltrate directly within the eyelid margin medially where the full-thickness eyelid excision will take place and anteriorly along the entire upper eyelid where skin removal will occur.

Step 2

A pentagonal area is marked medially. The medial aspect of the full-thickness eyelid removal will be 2 mm lateral to the upper punctum, and the lateral aspect will be in the area to produce the desired amount of surgical tension on the wound for appropriate eyelid shortening. A blepharoplasty-type incision is then marked as well. This incision is marked similar to standard upper blepharoplasty, using the eyelid crease as the inferior border, and the superior border running parallel, with care to avoid lagophthalmos (Figure 28-7). Pinching the skin to be removed with forceps until just before lagophthalmos is produced will aid in determining the superior marking for incision.

Step 3

The pentagonal area is removed in a similar fashion as described in the previous technique. The blepharoplasty skin-muscle flap is incised with a #15 blade and excised with electrocautery, radiofrequency, laser, or a sharp instrument such as scissors or a #15 blade.

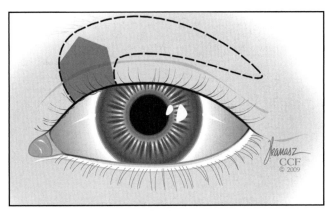

Figure 28-7. (Reprinted with permission, Cleveland Clinic Center for Medical Art & Photography © 2009. All Rights Reserved.)

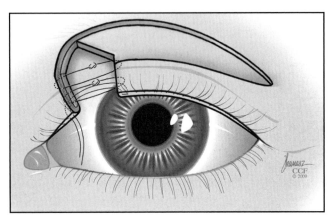

Figure 28-8. (Reprinted with permission, Cleveland Clinic Center for Medical Art & Photography © 2009. All Rights Reserved.)

Step 4

The pentagonal area is closed in a similar fashion as described in the previous technique with 6-0 mild chromic gut suture (Figure 28-8). The tail of the

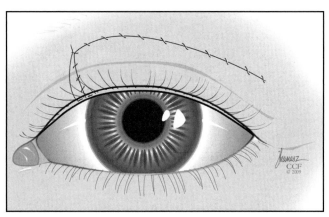

Figure 28-9. (Reprinted with permission, Cleveland Clinic Center for Medical Art & Photography © 2009. All Rights Reserved.)

suture is trapped beneath the running suture at the superior extent of the cutaneous incision, and the blepharoplasty-type horizontal incision is closed with the same running 6-0 mild chromic gut suture (Figure 28-9).

Similar to the technique of full-thickness eyelid excision, complications include eyelid notching and mechanical keratopathy due to the lamellar sutures through the tarsus or the suture knot along the eyelid margin. Persistent redundant cutaneous tissue can be excised. Lagophthalmos due to excessive skin removal can be minimized by performing the pinching maneuver to determine the amount of skin resection. Importantly, neither technique addresses the lash ptosis and upper eyelid entropion commonly encountered in floppy eyelid syndrome. Techniques to address upper eyelid entropion are addressed elsewhere in the text. Full-thickness eyelid removal does result in some elevation of the eyelid in floppy eyelid syndrome, but severe ptosis may require staged surgical repair.

SECTION VII

FACIAL NERVE DYSFUNCTION

CHAPTER 29

FACIAL NERVE PALSY

Rodger P. Davies, MBBS, FRANZCO, FRACS, FANZSOPS

The facial nerve has 4 major functions, which are supplied by 4 brain stem nuclei. The facial motor nucleus innervates the facial muscles, the superior salivatory nucleus supplies secretomotor innervation to the lacrimal and palatine glands via the greater palatine nerve, the nucleus solitarius receives sensation from the anterior two thirds of the tongue via the chorda tympani, and the trigeminal nucleus receives fibers of sensation from part of the external ear.

The nerve leaves the brain stem at the cerebellopontine angle inferior to the trigeminal nerve (Figure 29-1A). It enters the temporal bone via the internal auditory canal; within the temporal bone, the greater and lesser superficial petrosal nerves, the nerve to the stapedius muscle, and the chorda tympani arise. The nerve leaves the temporal bone via the stylomastoid foramen and passes through the parotid gland, where it divides into 5 branches that supply the facial muscles (Figure 29-1B).

Etiology of Facial Palsy

Bell's palsy is the most common cause of facial nerve palsy, with an incidence of 20 per 100,000 people per year. By definition, it is an idiopathic lower motor neuron facial palsy. The typical course is sudden onset of varying degrees of facial palsy, with gradual recovery over weeks to months. Complete resolution occurs in 80% of cases. Prognosis for recovery is worse with more severe palsy and increasing age. Atypical presentations suggest specific causes of the palsy. Tumors such as acoustic neuroma, meningioma, primary facial nerve tumors, or parotid carcinoma cause progressive facial palsy that does not improve. Other causes include parotid surgery and severe head injury, cerebrovascular accident, infections such as herpes zoster (Ramsay Hunt syndrome), acute or chronic otitis media, and cholesteatoma. Infants with congenital facial palsy caused by complicated forceps

delivery usually recover fully. Mobius' syndrome, which results from hypoplasia of the facial motor nucleus and abducens nucleus, is congenital bilateral facial and lateral rectus palsies.

Clinical Features

Facial palsy causes poor lid closure, lower lid ectropion, and upper lid retraction because of unopposed levator action. Exposure keratopathy occurs as a result of a combination of lagophthalmos, decreased blinking, and decreased tear production and can progress to ulceration, perforation, scarring, and decreased vision. Epiphora may result from reflex tearing, punctal eversion, and decreased lacrimal pump function. Associated cranial nerve abnormalities may occur with intracranial lesions such as acoustic neuroma. Fifth nerve involvement with corneal anesthesia decreases corneal protection and may cause neurotrophic corneal ulceration. Cosmetic abnormalities include eyebrow ptosis and dermatochalasis.

Evaluation

Clinical evaluation should include assessment of visual acuity, ocular motility, corneal sensation, lid closure (forced and blinking), lower lid and punctal position, Bell's phenomenon, basal tear production, corneal epithelial condition, and the optic nerves for papilledema caused by intracranial tumor. Involvement of other cranial nerves and other seventh nerve functions, such as decreased lacrimation, hyperacusis, and diminished taste sensation, may help identify the site of the lesion.

A computed tomographic or magnetic resonance imaging scan can demonstrate the facial nerve from the brain stem to the facial muscles. Other investigations that may be useful include electrodiagnostic studies of the facial

Levine MR.
Manual of Oculoplastic Surgery, Fourth Edition (pp 205-210).
© 2010 SLACK Incorporated

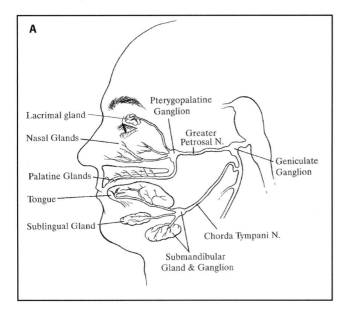

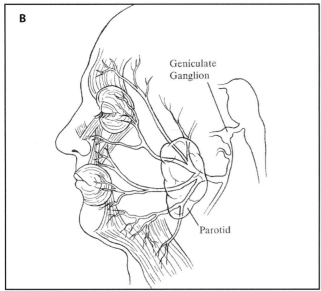

Figure 29-1.

nerve, salivary flow testing, taste testing, and audiology testing for changes caused by stapedius muscle dysfunction.

Management

The oculoplastic surgeon is concerned with maintenance of lid position, lid closure, protection of the cornea from exposure, and control of symptoms such as epiphora and ocular discomfort. A stepwise regimen of management can be followed with good results.

OCULAR LUBRICANTS

Ocular lubricants are the mainstay of treatment. Drops are given by day as frequently as required to keep the eye comfortable, with the more viscous drops providing better corneal epithelial protection. Ointment is used at night in combination with an eye cover such as cellophane, an adhesive bubble, or a pad. Care needs to be taken when a pad is used because the lids may open under the pad with subsequent trauma to the cornea.

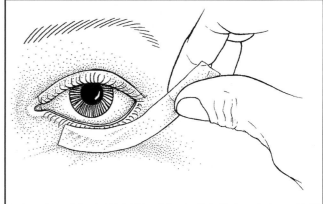

Figure 29-2.

BOTULINUM TOXIN-INDUCED PTOSIS

Botulinum toxin-A (Botox) can be injected into the levator muscle to induce ptosis to protect the cornea if lubricants are inadequate. This is an alternate to padding or taping the eye closed and can be repeated as needed. An injection of 0.1 mL (5 U) of botulinum toxin-A is given subconjunctivally with the lid everted and just above the tarsus. Maximum effect is seen in 2 to 7 days, and the ptosis may last for 6 to 8 weeks. Diplopia may occur if the superior rectus is involved.

TARSORRHAPHY

Tarsorrhaphy gives suboptimal cosmesis, limitation of the visual field, and may obscure the visual axis, but can be useful in protecting the cornea if the patient is unable or unwilling to have other surgery. A 5-mm lateral tarsorrhaphy reduces lagophthalmos by 70% to 80%. Temporary tarsorrhaphy is indicated if the cornea is decompensating, recovery of function is expected, and the patient is unable to have other procedures performed. Permanent tarsorrhaphy is indicated if the cornea is decompensating, there is no prospect for recovery of function, and the patient is unwilling to have other procedures performed.

Lower Eyelid Ectropion Correction

Lower lid ectropion causes discomfort because of conjunctival exposure, contributes to lagophthalmos, causes epiphora by punctual eversion, and is not cosmetically appealing. Taping of the lid to pull it up and laterally can provide temporary correction (Figure 29-2). Surgical correction is best attained by a lateral tarsal strip procedure to horizontally tighten the lower lid.

Gold Weight Insertion

Gold is used because it is inert, has a high weight-to-volume ratio, and is a good color match for the skin. Gold implants come in 0.6, 0.8, 1.0, 1.2, 1.4, 1.6, 1.8, 2.0, and 2.2 gram weights, and the gold is 99.9% pure 24K. The weight is contoured to match the tarsus and has fixation holes (Figure 29-3).

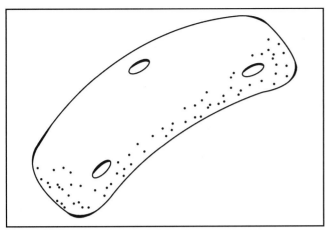

Figure 29-3.

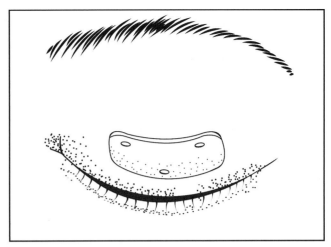

Figure 29-5.

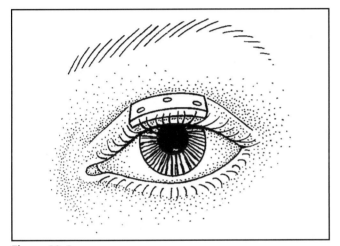

Figure 29-4.

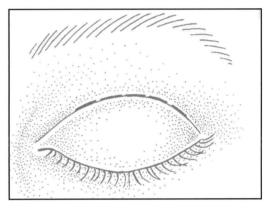

Figure 29-6.

The gold weight can be used as early as several days after the onset of facial palsy because it is easily reversible if orbicularis function returns and can greatly reduce the need for supportive care.

INDICATIONS

The indications for gold weight insertion are exposure keratopathy or marked irritation despite intensive medical therapy in short- or long-term facial palsy. It is more likely to be required if tear production is poor, if there is loss of corneal sensation, and with poor Bell's phenomenon.

SURGICAL TECHNIQUE

Step 1

Preoperatively, the appropriate weight is selected by taping, or sticking with tincture of benzoin, different weights to the eyelid over the center of the tarsus (Figure 29-4). The correct weight places the lid 2-mm below the limbus with the eye open and causes complete closure in the erect position (Figure 29-5). The patient may need to sleep with his or her head slightly elevated to get the required effect of gravity at night.

Step 2

The upper eyelid crease is marked, and the upper lid is injected with lidocaine 2% with 1:100,000 epinephrine (Figure 29-6).

Step 3

An incision is made in the eyelid crease through skin, orbicularis, and levator aponeurosis down to the tarsal plate.

Step 4

The dissection is continued inferiorly in the pretarsal space so that anterior tarsus is bared at the site for implantation (Figure 29-7).

Step 5

The gold weight is placed into this space with the top edge of the weight level with the top edge of the tarsus and fixed to the tarsus with 7-0 nylon sutures (Figure 29-8).

Step 6

To prevent ptosis, the levator aponeurosis can be closed; however, it is often desirable to leave a small recession and to decrease exposure. The orbicularis is carefully closed with 7-0 polyglactin to prevent exposure of the gold weight (Figure 29-9). Then, the skin is closed with 7-0 polyglactin (Figures 29-10 and 29-11).

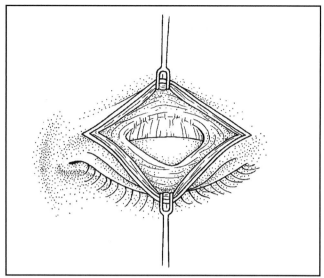

Figure 29-7.

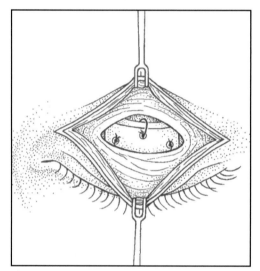

Figure 29-8.

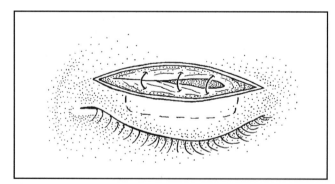

Figure 29-9.

COMPLICATIONS

Migration is prevented by good fixation to the tarsus and closure of levator aponeurosis over the weight. Persistent inflammation in response to the gold weight or fixation sutures may necessitate removal. Extrusion may occur if the gold weight is placed anterior to the orbicularis or if poor wound closure and delayed heal-

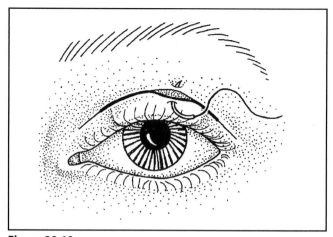

Figure 29-10.

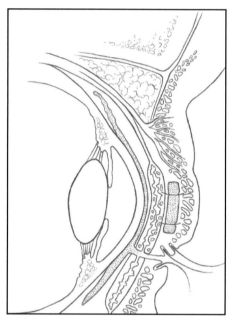

Figure 29-11.

ing occur. Infection is uncommon with sterile technique. Astigmatism has been described in 2 cases.

Facial Reinnervation, Reanimation, and Suspension

Reinnervation of the facial nerve by reanastomosis of cut ends of the nerve may be performed at the time of surgical transection. Autogenous nerve grafting, using the sural nerve, for instance, can bridge a gap between the cut ends. Crossover nerve grafts by either facial nerve to facial nerve (7 to 7) or hypoglossal nerve to facial nerve (12 to 7) anastomosis provide innervation when the proximal facial nerve is not accessible. Muscle grafting techniques use temporalis muscle to reanimate the orbicularis oculi or the orbicularis oris. Facial suspension or face-lift procedures can be performed to raise the brow, cheek, corner of mouth, and jowl. These techniques are beyond the scope of this book.

Brow Ptosis and Dermatochalasis Correction

Brow ptosis and dermatochalasis are corrected after all other procedures are done, after maximal recovery is complete, and only if there is no corneal decompensation. Brow ptosis is best corrected by direct brow lift and should be performed before blepharoplasty, as it corrects some of the skin overhang. Alternatively, endoscopic brow lift can be done to hide scars behind the hairline. Blepharoplasty is then done to correct any remaining dermatochalasis.

Direct Brow Lift

Direct brow lift has been described in Chapter 9. An ellipse of skin of height equivalent to the amount of lift is required. A scar is often visible unless the brow is very bushy.

Blepharoplasty

Upper eyelid blepharoplasty, for dermatochalasis, should be conservative to minimize danger of corneal exposure.

Management of Aberrant Regeneration of the Facial Nerve

Patients with aberrant regeneration of the facial nerve have mild ptosis and blinking with oral movements and lower facial spasms with eyelid closure. It is important to explain the anatomy and pathology of this condition and have the patient observe him- or herself in the mirror to demonstrate eyelid closure with movements of the mouth. Dilute botulinum toxin injections (2.5 to 5.0 U/mL) can be used to inhibit these unwanted movements by injecting the toxin in the temporal upper and lower eyelids and lateral canthal area. Caution should be used when injecting the corner of the mouth to prevent mouth droop, slurring, and buccal mucosal biting.

CHAPTER 30

HEMIFACIAL SPASM

Essam A. El-Toukhy, MD, FRCOph

Hemifacial spasm is a progressive disorder of intermittent, irregular contraction of one side of the face. It usually begins with unilateral fasciculation of the periocular orbicularis oculi and surrounding muscles and gradually spreads to involve the muscles of facial expression including the platysma.

Hemifacial spasm is typically unilateral, involves the whole side of the face, and may continue during sleep. Mild facial weakness is usually present. Hemifacial spasm is usually caused by irritation of the facial nerve near its origin in the brain stem, usually by a kink in the anterior inferior or posterior inferior cerebellar artery, although other vessels may be involved. Magnetic resonance imaging is usually recommended in the work-up of these patients to rule out posterior fossa lesions that should be treated surgically.

Hemifacial spasm must be differentiated from myokymia and facial tics. Myokymia is a continuous unilateral localized fasciculation within the orbicularis muscle of the eyelid that occurs in normal individuals under conditions of stress and fatigue. It is usually transient and nonprogressive. Facial tics are habitual and usually begin in childhood and can be suppressed voluntarily.

In cases in which vascular compression of the facial nerve is confirmed by magnetic resonance imaging and magnetic resonance arteriography, microvascular decompression of the facial nerve (Janetta procedure) can be used with a success rate of more than 80%. However, serious complications such as hearing loss, otitis media, permanent facial palsy, epilepsy, and even death can occur.

Botulinum toxin (Oculinum) has become the first line of treatment for hemifacial spasm. It interferes with acetylcholine release at the presynaptic nerve terminal and causes a temporary muscle paralysis and denervation atrophy that abolishes abnormal movements. It is simple and effective and has a success rate of more than 90%. The toxin is supplied as a freeze-dried residue in 100 U per vial. This is diluted with 2 to 4 cc of nonpreserved saline to yield a concentration of 2.5 to 5.0 U per 0.1 mL.

Injection Technique

Step 1

The patient is carefully examined, and the sites of spasms are carefully recorded.

Step 2

A 30-gauge needle is used to inject 2.5 to 5.0 U of the toxin in the preselected sites. Injections are given first in the orbicularis oculi muscle, the procerus and corrugator muscles, and the frontalis muscle (Figure 30-1). The injections within the orbicularis muscle are quite superficial, whereas those into the corrugator superciliaris and procerus are deeper. Injections are avoided in the medial aspect of the lower lid to avoid tearing from lacrimal pump dysfunction. Similarly, postinjection ptosis can be reduced by avoiding injections in the central upper lid.

Step 3

Injections are then given into the nasal fold, upper lip, chin, and other musculature of the face. However, the retractor muscles at the corner of the mouth should be avoided to prevent drooping of the mouth.

Step 4

Sensitivity to botulinum toxin varies among patients, so the sites and doses of injections can be modified according to the patient's response. Due to the associated facial palsy, a dose lower than that needed for blepharospasm is usually sufficient. Approximately 25 to 30 U are usually needed for one side of the face.

Levine MR.
Manual of Oculoplastic Surgery, Fourth Edition (pp 211-212).
© 2010 SLACK Incorporated

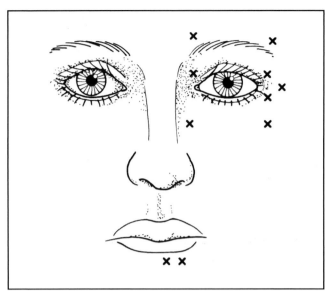

Figure 30-1.

Step 5

After injection, profound paralysis of the injected muscles usually starts in 24 to 48 hours and lasts for approximately 4 to 6 months. Patients are given artificial tears to guard against dry eyes, which is a common side effect. Most patients report a satisfactory improvement in their condition with a sustained benefit from repeated injections.

Complications

Complications are usually a result of paralysis of the facial musculature. Ptosis can be prevented by avoiding injections in the central part of the upper lid. Drooping of the angle of the mouth can be prevented by avoiding injections in the area. Lagophthalmos, mild ectropion, and tearing can occur because of orbicularis paralysis. The use of artificial tears is a safeguard against exposure keratitis. No major systemic side effects have been reported with the use of botulinum toxin.

CHAPTER 31

BLEPHAROSPASM

Essam A. El-Toukhy, MD, FRCOph

Essential blepharospasm consists of bilateral involuntary spasmodic contractions of the orbicularis oculi. In addition, the corrugator superciliaris and procerus muscles are commonly affected. The condition usually starts with periods of increased blinking that gradually increase in duration. The eyelids are relaxed between spasms, but the condition is invariably progressive, with the periods of spasms becoming more frequent and the periods of relaxation becoming shorter. In some patients, there is difficulty or failure to open the eyelids between the spasms (apraxia of lid opening). It is worsened by stress, fatigue, and bright light and is improved by rest and sleep. Involvement of the lower face and mouth is usually referred to as Meige's syndrome.

Essential blepharospasm occurs in middle age and old age, and women are more commonly affected. The condition is believed to be a result of an organic neurologic disorder, probably in the basal ganglia or thalamus, although the exact anatomic lesion has not been determined. However, it usually leads to significant vision impairment, ocular irritation, and social embarrassment.

The forceful contractions of the orbicularis oculi and the forced attempts to open the eyelid often lead to brow ptosis, levator aponeurosis disinsertion and blepharoptosis, dermatochalasis, and laxity of the canthal tendons and ectropion. Dry eyes are frequently present. Conditions that should be considered in the differential diagnosis include psychic blepharospasm, habitual spasms, tardive dyskinesia, Parkinson's disease, and the use of antipsychotic drugs. A complete ophthalmologic and neurologic examination is required to establish the diagnosis.

Botulinum toxin (Oculinum) has become the first line of treatment for blepharospasm. It interferes with acetylcholine release at the presynaptic nerve terminal and causes a temporary muscle paralysis and denervation atrophy that abolishes abnormal movements. It is simple, effective, and has a success rate of more than 90%. The toxin is supplied as a freeze-dried residue in a 100-U vial. This is diluted with 2 to 4 cc of nonpreserved saline to yield a concentration of 5.0 U/0.1 mL or 2.5 U/0.1 mL, as needed.

Injection Technique

Step 1

The patient is carefully examined, and the sites of spasms are carefully recorded.

Step 2

A 30-gauge needle is used to inject the toxin in the preselected sites in the periocular region (Figure 31-1). The injections within the orbicularis muscle are quite superficial, whereas those into the corrugator superciliaris and procerus are deeper. Some people advise the use of a topical anesthetic cream before injections to reduce pain; however, I have not found this necessary. Injections are avoided in the medial aspect of the lower lid to prevent tearing and to keep the lacrimal pump going. Similarly, postinjection ptosis can be reduced by avoiding injections in the central upper lid.

Step 3

Sensitivity to botulinum toxin varies among patients, so the sites and doses of injections can be modified according to the patient's response. Usually, 20 to 25 U are needed on each side.

Step 4

After injection, profound paralysis of the injected muscles usually starts in 24 hours and lasts for approximately 3 to 4 months. Patients are given artificial tears to guard against dry eyes, which is a common side effect. The average duration between injections is approximately 4 months. Most patients

Levine MR.
Manual of Oculoplastic Surgery, Fourth Edition (pp 213-214).
© 2010 SLACK Incorporated

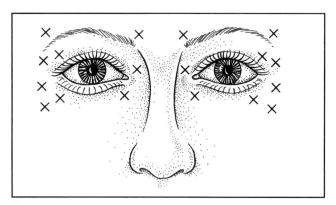

Figure 31-1.

report a satisfactory improvement in their condition with a sustained benefit from repeated injections.

Complications

Complications are usually a result of paralysis of the periocular musculature. Mild ptosis occurs in less than 10% of patients and is usually transient. It can be avoided to a great extent by making sure the injections are superficial and avoiding injections in the central part of the upper lid. Similarly, lagophthalmos, mild ectropion, and tearing can occur because of orbicularis paralysis. The use of artificial tears is a safeguard against exposure keratitis. No major systemic side effects have been reported with the use of botulinum toxin, although some abnormalities of neuromuscular transmission have been reported at remote sites as muscle weakness.

In a few patients, the toxin may become less effective over time, possibly due to the development of an antitoxin. These patients may require larger doses, up to 70 U.

Surgical Management

Surgical management of blepharospasm by orbital myectomy is usually reserved for cases in which botulinum toxin is ineffective, injections are required too frequently, or in which it is part of another procedure (eg, blepharoptosis repair). The procedure involves complete removal of the orbicularis oculi, corrugator superciliaris, and procerus muscles. Not infrequently, botulinum toxin injections are still used after the procedure. Selective facial nerve avulsion is no longer recommended due to a higher rate of complications.

SECTION VIII

EYELID FLAPS

CHAPTER 32

PERIOCULAR FLAPS

Eugene O. Wiggs, MD

A flap is tissue with its own blood supply that is transferred to another bodily area. Most flaps used in periocular reconstruction are random pattern flaps (ie, flaps that are not based on an axial arterial blood supply). In the periorbital area, the flap length-to-width ratio can exceed the 3:1 or 5:1 ratios needed for survival in nonfacial areas. This happy circumstance is due to an abundant blood supply.

In oculoplastic surgery, flaps are usually classified as (1) sliding, (2) advancement, (3) rotation, or (4) transposition. A sliding flap is one in which more skin relaxation is obtained by undermining. Undermining is also used in an advancement flap, but relaxing incisions are used on either side of the flap to obtain greater tissue mobilization. A rotation flap involves rotation of the flap around an axis, with closure of the remaining defect directly, with another flap or with a skin graft. A transposition flap consists of tissue that is transposed over intervening normal tissue into an adjacent area. An interpolation flap is one that is transferred into a defect that is not immediately adjacent; interpolation flaps are infrequently used in oculoplastic surgery.

Maintenance of blood supply to the flap is obviously essential for its survival. Therefore, a surgeon must exercise great caution in using a flap from an irradiated area because of the compromised blood supply. In general, flaps from irradiated areas are contraindicated. Patients should avoid tobacco use of any kind for 2 to 3 weeks after a flap procedure. Tobacco produces arteriolar constriction that can endanger flap survival.

Flaps have numerous advantages over skin grafts, which include the following:

❋ A flap brings its own blood supply.

❋ A flap avoids sacrifice of normal tissue and unsightly linear scars.

❋ There is minimal contracture in a flap compared with a skin graft.

❋ There is generally a better color and texture match.

❋ There is increased bulk; however, in some instances, this is not always advantageous because a thicker flap can mask the recurrence of a tumor.

❋ Flaps resist infection better than skin grafts.

❋ Flaps generally produce fewer ocular adnexal deformities than skin grafts.

General Principles of Periocular Flap Surgery

❋ In any flap design, it is important to avoid distorting landmarks such as the eyebrows or hairline.

❋ Do not excise a dog ear on the flap because this can compromise the blood supply. Any cosmetic blemish resulting from a dog ear can be treated at a later date. Resection of a small dog ear(s) on a larger thicker advancement flap is an exception to this admonition.

❋ Close any existing dead space.

❋ Any blanching or cyanosis of the flap indicates a need to delay the flap. Delay techniques can be found in standard texts. Delay of a flap augments its survival, probably by improving the vascularity of the flap.

ANESTHESIA

The procedure can be performed with the patient under general or attended local anesthesia. The areas to be incised are infiltrated with a long-acting local anesthesia

Levine MR.
Manual of Oculoplastic Surgery, Fourth Edition (pp 217-220).
© 2010 SLACK Incorporated

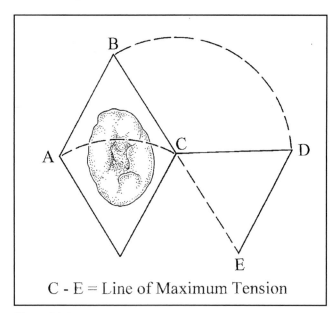

C - E = Line of Maximum Tension

Figure 32-1.

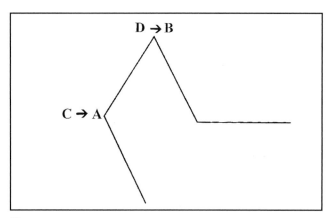

Figure 32-2.

with epinephrine, which provides hemostasis and blunts acute postoperative pain. A frontal nerve block may be used as needed.

RHOMBIC ROTATION FLAP

The rhombic rotation flap has erroneously been called a rhomboid flap when, in fact, it is a rhombic flap as elegantly described by Borges.[1] A rhomboid is a parallelogram that does not have equal sides. The rhombic flap is designed so that the sides are equal. If the surgeon anticipates that the area to be resected will be covered by a flap, an attempt is made to resect the tumor in the shape of a rhombus. In Figure 32-1, note that the rhombic defect will be covered by the flap outlined by the points C, D, and E. C-D and D-E are equal in length to the sides of the rhombus. The flap is designed so the line C-E, which is the line of maximum tension, is generally parallel to a line of maximum elasticity in the face. The "donor" area is closed first, thus minimizing tension on the flap. The flap is then easily rotated into position with point C rotating to point A, and point D rotating to point B (Figure 32-2). The exception to this rule is when such a flap is used in the lower eyelid. The line of maximum elasticity in the lower eyelid

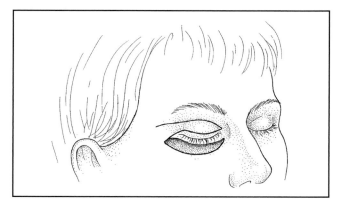

Figure 32-3.

and malar area is vertical. However, by placing the line of maximum tension parallel to the line of maximum elasticity, the result often is ectropion of the lower eyelid, even if the eyelid is shortened horizontally. The obvious way to avoid this problem is to design the flap so that the line of maximum tension is essentially horizontal. The ability to close the donor area of the flap can be tested by what has been termed the pinch test—that is, bringing the 2 points along the line of maximum tension together to ensure that closure can be accomplished.

Even if this exception to the general rule regarding the line of maximum tension of the flap and the line of maximum elasticity of the face is used, ectropion can result in the lower eyelid because of the weight of the flap and poor lower eyelid tone. If this is anticipated, a horizontal shortening procedure should be performed on the lower eyelid to avoid ectropion. An excellent procedure for shortening the lower eyelid is the lateral tarsal strip procedure. Frequently, it is necessary to splint the lower eyelid upward using a monofilament suture for 3 to 5 days postoperatively in an effort to avoid postoperative ectropion. If the surgeon thinks that the weight of the flap will still produce lower eyelid ectropion in spite of horizontal eyelid shortening and intermarginal suture, an additional "antiectropion" method must be used. A reliable method uses a nonabsorbable monofilament suture that secures the dermis of the flap (or the tissue inferior to it) to the infraorbital rim via a periosteal bite; alternatively, a hole can be drilled in the infraorbital rim. Another method to avoid ectropion induction is to use fascia lata to suspend the lower eyelid.

TRANSPOSITION FLAPS

Three types of transposition flaps are discussed here: (1) the skin-muscle flap from upper eyelid to lower eyelid, (2) the forehead to lower eyelid flap, and (3) the nasolabial flap.

Skin-Muscle Flap From Upper Eyelid to Lower Eyelid

The skin-muscle flap from the upper eyelid to the lower eyelid is useful with small to moderate degrees of lower eyelid cicatricial ectropion and in lower eyelid reconstruction. A blepharoplasty ellipse is marked out on the upper eyelid with the ellipse left open laterally (Figure 32-3). Via a lower eyelid subciliary incision, a

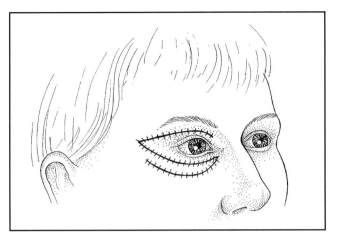

Figure 32-4.

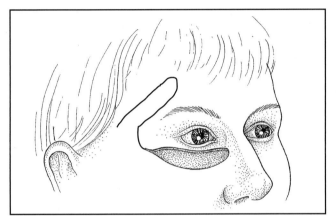

Figure 32-5.

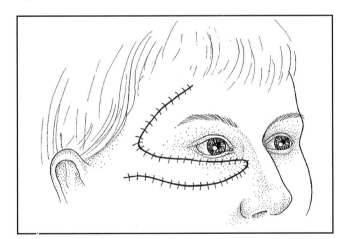

Figure 32-6.

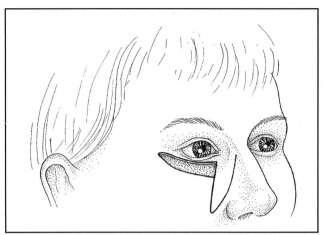

Figure 32-7.

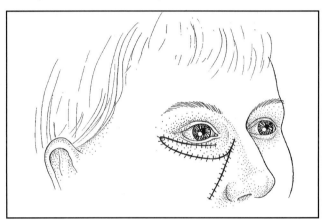

Figure 32-8.

skin muscle flap is elevated to the infraorbital rim and allowed to retract. The lower eyelid is horizontally shortened as needed. The upper eyelid flap is transposed into the lower eyelid and the wounds closed. Intervening tissue at the lateral canthus is resected as needed, allowing transposition of the upper eyelid skin muscle flap into the lower eyelid defect (Figure 32-4).

Forehead to Lower Eyelid Flap

The forehead to lower eyelid flap is useful only for serious, significant structural defects. The flap is best

mobilized from the temporal area just in front of the hairline (Figure 32-5). If there is a significant eyebrow ptosis, the flap is mobilized from above the eyebrow to neutralize the brow ptosis. The donor area is closed with deep interrupted 4-0 monofilament sutures, and the skin of the donor area is closed with a running 5-0 polypropylene suture that is also used to sew the flap in place. This flap is most useful when there is a need for support and bulk in the lower eyelid (Figure 32-6).

Nasolabial Flap

The nasolabial flap is most useful in patients in whom there is a medial cicatricial ectropion and lower eyelid retraction or in eyelid reconstruction in which the major component of the defect is medial. A significant disadvantage of the flap is that it is somewhat thicker and heavier than what is usually used in oculoplastic surgery. As in the forehead to lower eyelid flap, the thickness can be an advantage, however, in providing needed bulk and support in some patients. Closure is the same as for the forehead to lower eyelid flap (Figures 32-7 and 32-8).

RHOMBUS-TO-W FLAPS

The rhombus-to-W flap has been advocated by Becker[2] and is useful when the defect to be closed is situated between 2 landmarks, thus obviating the use of other types of flaps. This particular flap also has a better

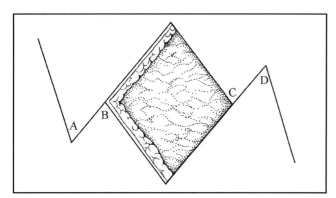

Figure 32-9.

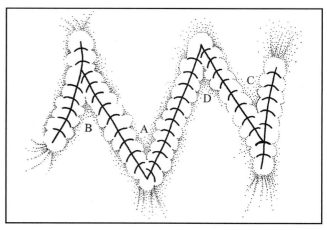

Figure 32-11.

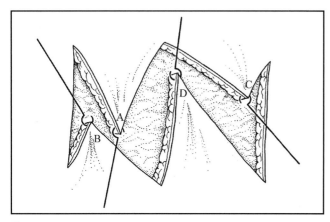

Figure 32-10.

postoperative scar pattern than a rhombic flap. The flaps are first incised, the skin is undermined, and the flaps transposed (Figures 32-9 to 32-11). Then, 6-0 silk or polypropylene sutures are used to secure the flaps in place.

Conclusion

The ability to conceptualize and use flaps in periocular surgery enormously extends the surgeon's capabilities to produce optimal results for the patient and avoids the problems inherent in skin grafts, including not having to incise another body area.

PRIMARY REPAIR OF A LID DEFECT WITH OR WITHOUT CANTHOLYSIS

Daniel E. Buerger, MD; David G. Buerger, MD; and George F. Buerger, Jr, MD

The excision of a lid lesion must be done with total removal of the lesion as the first priority. You cannot excise a lesion less than completely based on a type of repair you might like to perform. The type of repair chosen is based on the size of the defect so created, in conjunction with the degree of laxity of that eyelid.

Reparative techniques must be approached as a continuum of repair, using the simplest, least complicated technique possible and progressing to larger and more complicated procedures as the situation dictates. Although the exact extent of the repair technique is not known preoperatively, it is wise to at least have a game plan in mind. Although we are primarily concerned here with surgically created defects, the same principles and techniques apply also to traumatic defects.

Preoperative Management

Before the patient arrives in the operating suite, the surgeon should provide the patient with a thorough explanation of the nature of the problem, possible extent of the surgical procedure, postoperative course, possible complications, and expected results. Once this discussion is completed, the patient can sign the permission for surgery.

If the lid to be operated on is on the same side as the patient's only seeing eye, then the surgeon must discuss these implications with the patient and the family. This can obviously change the postoperative plans, such that the patient will wear no eye patch at all or will wear one for only 1 or 2 hours before discharge. The procedures discussed here can be carried out on an outpatient/same day surgery basis or even performed in the office if the necessary facilities and equipment are available.

The patient is brought to the operating room and prepared for surgery. The surgical preparation should include the area of both eyes and one postauricular area if

the need for a skin graft is a possibility, although we prefer a full-face preparation.

Anesthesia

Although general anesthesia may be used, particularly in an anxious, apprehensive patient, this is seldom necessary. For an anxious patient, intravenous sedation usually produces the desired calming effect and allows regional block or local infiltration anesthesia to be used. We usually use a combination of regional block and infiltration anesthesia to take advantage of the hemostasis of the epinephrine contained in the local anesthetic agent. Either 1% or 2% lidocaine with 1:100,000 epinephrine may be used. To give the patient a longer pain-free postoperative period, a mixture of equal parts of lidocaine with epinephrine and 0.75% bupivacaine may be used.

A properly placed nerve block requires only 0.5 mL of the anesthetic agent. The extent of the defect and the proposed reconstructive technique determine the extent of anesthesia required (ie, infraorbital nerve block, lacrimal nerve block, frontal nerve block, superior or inferior trochlear nerve block, or zygomaticofacial nerve block).

Surgical Procedure

Step 1

The involved lid is inspected, and the proposed medial and lateral incision sites are marked with a marking pen. Approximately 1.5 to 2.0 mm of normal-appearing tissue is included beyond the lesion borders. In certain types of lesions, even this amount may be inadequate. The frozen section report from the pathologist will indicate whether the lesion resection is complete. If there is residual tumor present on a border, additional resection of

Levine MR.
Manual of Oculoplastic Surgery, Fourth Edition (pp 221-224).
© 2010 SLACK Incorporated

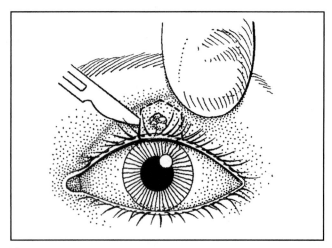

Figure 33-1.

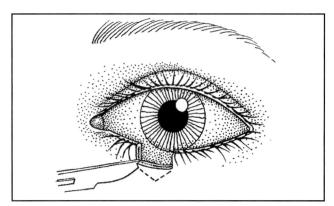

Figure 33-2.

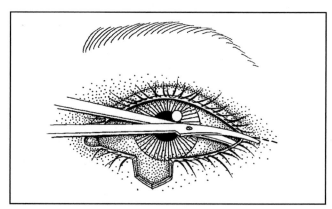

Figure 33-3.

tissue must be performed until a tumor-free border is obtained. If the patient had a Mohs' histologically controlled excision performed, it is at this point that the surgeon enters the picture.

Step 2

A colored protective corneal-scleral lens is placed on the globe before the surgical excision. We prefer colored lenses to clear lenses to reduce the chance that the lens will be left in place at the conclusion of the procedure.

Step 3

The important point in excising a lesion is to make the vertical cuts on the lid perpendicular to the lid margin through the total height of the tarsus. This applies to both upper and lower lids. A V-cut must not be used to resect the lesion unless the creation of a lid notch or margin defect is desired.

Step 4

Once the distal end of the tarsus has been reached, the incision lines are angled together, forming the pentagon-shaped resection (Figures 33-1 and 33-2). The cut through the lid margin can be performed with a sharp blade through the tarsus moving toward the lid margin or with a heavy scissors. We have found that the scissors is the easier way to perform this cut. It is easy to stabilize the lid adjacent to the cut site with a Graefe forceps.

Step 5

Bleeding will be occurring by now. Pressure on the lid for several minutes decreases or abolishes the bleeding. Electrocautery can be used to accomplish this faster. If cautery is used, the lightest setting possible that allows cauterization should be used.

Step 6

This is the point at which the surgeon determines how to perform the closure of the defect, depending on the size of the defect created and the degree of laxity of the lid. By picking up each cut edge with forceps or a pair of skin hooks and pulling them together, the surgeon can directly see whether the edges will approximate each other. If the 2 edges approximate each other, then a direct closure is possible. If the 2 edges leave a gap of only several millimeters, then a lateral canthotomy with a cantholysis should provide enough relaxation to allow a direct closure. If a gap of more than several millimeters exists, then the semicircular flap technique is used.

Step 7

If it has been determined that a lateral canthotomy with cantholysis is necessary, attention is turned to the lateral canthus. Using a small blade or scissors, the skin is carefully cut starting at the lateral canthus; the cut is extended for 5 to 7 mm lateral to the lateral canthal angle (Figure 33-3).

Step 8

The cut as started in Step 7 is continued through the underlying orbicularis muscle and then through the appropriate branch of the lateral canthal tendon (ie, the inferior branch for the lower lid, and the superior branch for the upper lid). By putting some medial traction on the lid, the surgeon can tell when an adequate lysis of the branch of the lateral canthal tendon has been accomplished. The lid then has the several additional millimeters of medial movement and thus allows approximation of the cut edges. By using a careful dissection through the skin, orbicularis muscle, and then the branch of the tendon, cutting through the conjunctiva is avoided. If such a thing should occur, there is usually no real harm done (Figure 33-4).

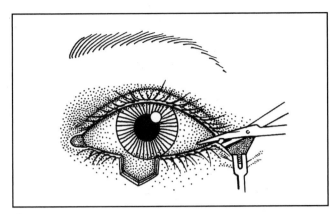

Figure 33-4.

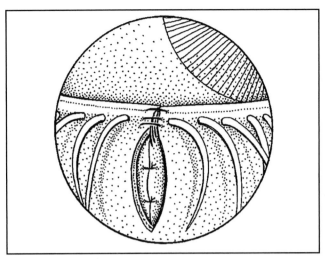

Figure 33-6.

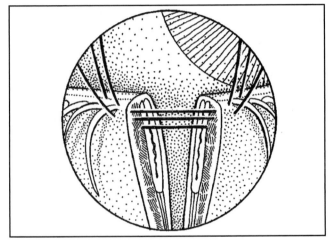

Figure 33-5.

Step 9

By leaving the conjunctiva intact, the cut edge of skin can be readily sutured back to the conjunctiva with a fine absorbable suture. We use several interrupted 7-0 polyglactin (Vicryl) sutures for this. These sutures need not be removed, but if they do remain after several weeks, the knots can be easily cut.

Step 10

With or without the lateral cantholysis having been performed, attention is now directed to the closure of the lid defect. Whether the lid margin or tarsus is closed first is a personal preference. We usually close the tarsus first, being sure, however, that the lid margin will be in perfect alignment and there is no degree of step defect. If such a defect is created, then the sutures must be removed and replaced correctly. No such step defect should exist at this point or it will persist forever (Figure 33-5).

Step 11

The tarsus is closed with a 6-0 polyglycolic acid synthetic absorbable (Dexon) suture and a PR-1 needle. This small half-curve needle allows for an easy bite into the tarsus; it is easy to go through only tarsus and not exit through the conjunctiva during the placement of this suture. If the suture is placed through the conjunctiva, it could produce some

corneal irritation, more particularly on the upper lid. It is for that reason better not to go through conjunctiva. The knot of this suture is placed on the anterior surface of the tarsus. The knot should never be allowed to sit at the posterior tarsus or conjunctival area, or both, as this could easily erode and irritate the cornea (Figure 33-6). On the lower lid, 2 or 3 such sutures are sufficient. On the upper lid, 4 or 5 sutures suffice. Some surgeons include some posterior orbicularis tissue in this bite; others close the orbicularis muscle separately.

Step 12

Attention is directed to the lid margin. The traditional margin closure uses 3 sutures: posterior lid margin, gray line, and lash line. Some oculoplastic surgeons have eliminated the posterior margin suture and use only 2 sutures for the margin closure. With a good high tarsal closure, this is possible. We usually use 3 sutures on the lid margin, but in a slightly different format (see Figure 33-5). Using a 6-0 black silk suture, one suture is placed through the gray line, starting back approximately 3 to 4 mm from the cut edge and carried in a slightly posterior direction so as to include some tarsus in this bite. A similar bite is secured through the other cut edge of the lid. The suture is knotted, but the ends are left long for later use. Next, a suture is placed approximately 1.5 mm back and deep from the cut edge in the posterior area of the lashes and exiting through the corresponding area of the other side of the lid margin; this suture is knotted, and the ends are also left long. The third suture is placed in the area of the most anterior lashes on the lid margin, again, approximately 1.5 mm back and deep. After this suture is knotted, the ends of the other 2 sutures are carried forward, and 2 additional throws are placed on the anterior-most suture. This carries the lid margin knots forward from the cornea and prevents possible corneal irritation.

Step 13

If there is any significant gap in the area of the orbicularis muscle, especially if one did not pick up a bite of it in the tarsal suture, then a 6-0 Vicryl or Dexon suture can pick up a small bite of muscle; the suture is placed so the knot is on the deep side of the muscle and not immediately underneath the skin. Several such sutures may be used.

Step 14

The skin is then closed either with a continuous or interrupted suture closure technique mild gut suture. The 6-0 fast-absorbing suture is only for skin closure. When using this suture, there cannot be any tension on the skin, and approximately 5 throws should be placed on the knot because it has a tendency to untie fairly easily. This suture remains in place for 4 to 6 days. At that time, much of the suture has dissolved. The choice for skin closure is ultimately up to the surgeon.

Step 15

The protective corneal-scleral lens is removed.

Step 16

Antibiotic drops are instilled on the eye, and antibiotic ointment is placed on the skin incision areas. A small Telfa pad and an eye pad are placed on the eye and taped for a light pressure dressing. If the eye that has been operated on is the patient's only seeing eye, the patch is removed approximately 1 hour after surgery, before the patient's departure for home.

Postoperative Care

By using the mild gut suture for the skin closure, the only sutures that need to be removed are the 6-0 silk sutures on the lid margin. The patient is seen initially between 12 and 14 days after surgery for such suture removal. The patient is instructed to leave the patch intact until the following morning, then to remove it, keep the lids clean (gently), and instill antibiotic drops 4 times a day for 1 week, then twice a day until the margin sutures have been removed. The patient is instructed to use a small amount of antibiotic ointment (0.25 to 0.50 inch on a cotton swab) and apply it to the incision area 3 times a day for 1 week, then once a day until the margin sutures are removed. The use of prophylactic postoperative medications is a personal choice. Some oculoplastic surgeons never use drops or ointments postoperatively.

Most patients require very little pain medication after this surgery. We usually give the patient a prescription for acetaminophen (Tylenol) with 30 mg codeine to be taken every 3 to 4 hours for moderate pain in case regular Tylenol is not sufficient for pain relief. We strongly recommend to the patient that if the excised lesion was malignant, follow-up examinations should occur at 6 and 12 months after surgery, then yearly for 4 additional years.

Complications

Preventing problems is easier than curing problems. To a great degree, most of the potential problems or complications can be prevented by meticulous surgery in the preparation and closure of such lid defects. Attention to details as just described, along with some specific comments made in this section and previously, should help you avoid most problems.

If the lid margin or skin closure does not look perfect—that is, if you note a step defect or notch of the lid margin—then remove all sutures and start over. This is why some surgeons advocate placing the 6-0 silk sutures on the lid margin first, to give good anatomic alignment there, followed by closure of the tarsus. Meticulous hemostasis avoids the possibility of continued oozing or bleeding and the development of a hematoma. Complete and understandable communications with the patient and his or her family about postoperative home care is an absolute necessity. Exact and specific instructions must be given so the patient knows what is expected because his or her actions can adversely affect postoperative outcome. We always tell patients that good surgery must be followed by good postoperative care.

Cleansing of the surgical incision area must be explained, as well as the use and application of antibiotic drops and antibiotic ointment. Advise the patient whether face washing, hair washing, bathing, or showering is permitted. Advise the patient to refrain from heavy or dirty work for several weeks to help prevent the chances of postoperative bleeding or infection. In discussing when the patient can resume normal work activities, it is important to note whether the patient has a desk-type job or works in a dirty environment. Obviously, the latter might require additional time off compared with the patient who performs desk work.

If the patient reports that the incision area is becoming more painful or erythematous, then suspect an infection. Perhaps systemic antibiotics should be instituted, if such symptoms or findings begin or worsen. The only way the surgeon would know that such is the case is by instructing the patient and the family to call if any problems arise or such symptoms are occurring. Obviously, the earlier that corrective actions are taken, the faster the problem disappears and the better the recovery will be.

REPAIR OF LID DEFECTS
USING A SEMICIRCULAR FLAP

Daniel E. Buerger, MD; David G. Buerger, MD; and George F. Buerger, Jr, MD

We will follow the concept of the continuum of repair necessary for increasingly larger eyelid defects as discussed in Chapter 33. After the lesion is excised, if the gap is greater than approximately 3 mm when the 2 edges of the lid are grasped with forceps or skin hooks and pulled together, a repair technique that permits closure of this larger defect must be used. The Tenzel rotational flap, or semicircular flap, proves to be an ideal technique.

The semicircular flap can be used for either upper or lower lid reconstruction. It is useful for defects affecting up to 40% to 50% of the medial or central portion of the eyelid. Because the necessity for this technique is determined in Step 6 of Chapter 33, we will start at that point.

Upper Lid Defects

Steps 1 to 6

See Steps 1 to 6 in Chapter 33.

Step 7

An inferiorly directed semicircle is drawn on the skin with a marking pen, starting at the lateral canthus. It is the size of one half of a quarter (ie, imagine the coin positioned at the lateral canthus and trace around it). The skin and underlying muscle are cut with a #15 Bard-Parker blade. Electrocautery is used to achieve hemostasis while this musculocutaneous flap is dissected from the underlying tissue (Figure 34-1).

Step 8

A small lateral canthotomy is made with scissors, and dissection is continued to cut through the upper branch of the lateral canthal tendon, detaching it from the remainder of the lateral canthal tendon (Figure 34-2). With additional undermining, the flap along with the lateral portion of the

upper lid can now be mobilized medially to allow approximation of the 2 cut edges of the lid defect. Sometimes, additional mobilization requires cutting the lateral part of the orbital septum.

Step 9

The closure of the lesion defect area is as described in Steps 10 to 14 of Chapter 33. After the lesion defect area is closed, attention is redirected to the rotational flap laterally (Figure 34-3).

Step 10

The lateral canthal area is reformed by suturing the deep edge of the flap to the periosteum at the inner aspect of the lateral orbital rim/lateral canthal tendon area using a 4-0 polyglycolic acid (Dexon) suture with the PR-1 needle (see Figure 34-3).

Step 11

Several deep sutures of 4-0 Dexon or polyglactin (Vicryl) are used to close the area of the orbicularis muscle laterally.

Step 12

With all tension off the skin, the skin incision can then be closed with the 6-0 mild gut suture. If a dog ear is encountered in the skin closure, a small triangle can be excised laterally.

Step 13

Conjunctiva can be undermined and advanced to the edge of the flap/new lid margin laterally and sutured to it with several interrupted 7-0 Vicryl sutures. The knots can be clipped off several weeks later if the suture has not dissolved (Figure 34-4).

Step 14

The protective corneal-scleral lens is removed. If difficulty is encountered in undermining the conjunctiva, the inner aspect of the flap can be left as

Levine MR.
Manual of Oculoplastic Surgery, Fourth Edition (pp 225-228).
© 2010 SLACK Incorporated

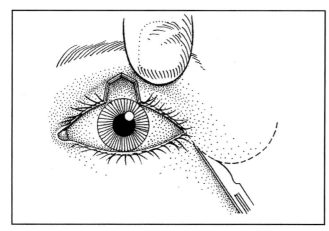

Figure 34-1.

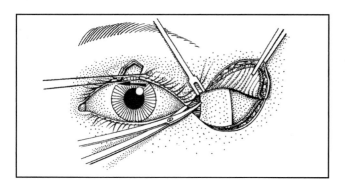

Figure 34-2.

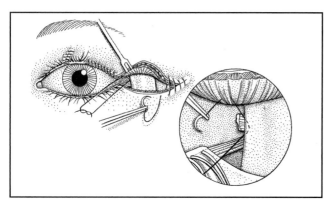

Figure 34-3.

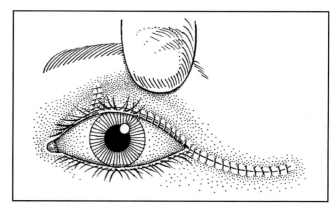

Figure 34-4.

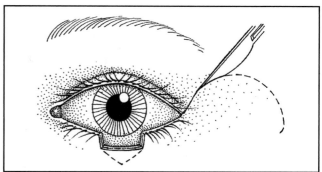

Figure 34-5.

is, and conjunctival epithelium can be allowed to epithelialize this area. Because bulbar conjunctiva is intact opposite this defect area, re-epithelialization should proceed without symblepharon formation.

Lower Lid Defects

Steps 1 to 6
See Steps 1 to 6 in Chapter 33.

Step 7
A superiorly directed semicircle is drawn on the skin with a marking pen, starting at the lateral canthus. It is the size of one half of a quarter, but, as opposed to an upper lid procedure, it is now directed above the lateral canthus. The skin and underlying muscle are cut with a #15 Bard-Parker blade. Electrocautery is used to achieve hemostasis while this musculocutaneous flap is dissected from the underlying tissue (Figure 34-5).

Step 8
A small lateral canthotomy is made with scissors, and dissection is continued to cut through the lower branch of the lateral canthal tendon, detaching it from the remainder of the lateral canthal tendon (Figure 34-6). With additional undermining, the flap, along with the lateral portion of the lower lid, can now be mobilized medially to allow approximation of the 2 cut edges of the lid defect. If the lower eyelid cannot be sufficiently mobilized medially, a Stevens scissors is used to cut the retractors and orbital septum of the lower eyelid beneath the inferior tarsal border, starting laterally with a scissors blade placed behind the conjunctiva and the other blade anterior to the septum and posterior to the orbicularis muscle. This maneuver frees the restricting orbital septum and the inferior retractors.

Step 9
The closure of the lesion defect area is as described in Steps 10 to 14 of Chapter 33. After the lesion defect area is closed, attention is redirected to the rotational flap laterally (Figure 34-7).

Step 10
The lateral canthal area is reformed by suturing the deep edge of the flap to the periosteum at the inner

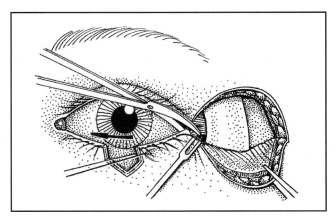

Figure 34-6.

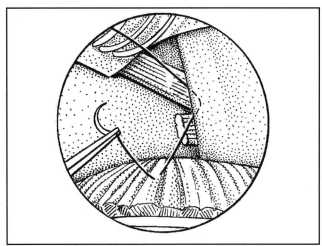

Figure 34-8.

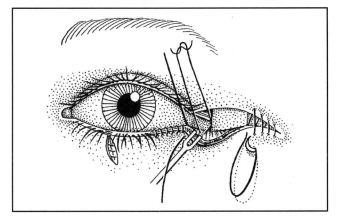

Figure 34-7.

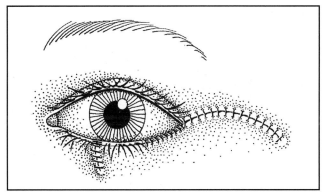

Figure 34-9.

aspect of the lateral orbital rim/lateral canthal tendon area, using a 4-0 Dexon suture with the PR-1 needle (Figure 34-8). It is of utmost importance in re-forming the lower lid aspect of the lateral canthus to have this suture well secured because lower lid droopiness or a frank ectropion could develop. If the retractors and orbital septum have been cut, the conjunctiva may be sutured to the inferior tarsal border with 7-0 Vicryl sutures, providing there is no eyelid malposition (entropion) as a result.

Steps 11 to 13

Closure is essentially identical to closure for the upper lid (see Upper Lid Defects) (Figure 34-9).

Step 14

The protective corneal-scleral lens is removed.

Step 15

Antibiotic drops are instilled on the eye, and antibiotic ointment is placed on the skin incision areas. A small Telfa pad is placed over the eye and adnexal area, along with a light pressure dressing. If the eye that has been operated on is the patient's only seeing eye, the patch is removed approximately 1 hour after surgery, before the patient's departure for home.

Postoperative Care

The patient is instructed to leave the patch intact until the second postoperative day, then to remove it, keep the lids clean (gently), and instill the antibiotic drops 4 times a day for 1 week, then twice a day until the margin sutures have been removed. The patient is told to apply a small amount of antibiotic ointment to the incision areas 3 times a day for 1 week, then once a day until the sutures are removed. The patient is advised to use acetaminophen (Tylenol) with 30 mg codeine for the first 24 hours, then switch to regular Tylenol.

By using the mild gut suture for the skin closure, the only sutures that need to be removed are the 6-0 silk sutures on the lid margin. The patient is seen initially between 12 and 14 days after surgery for such suture removal. We strongly recommend to the patient that if the excised lesion was malignant, follow-up examinations should occur at 6 and 12 months after surgery, then yearly for 4 additional years.

Complications

As stated in Chapter 33, preventing problems is easier than curing problems, and potential problems or complications can be prevented by meticulous surgery, as just described. To re-emphasize a couple of points made, but perhaps overlooked, the incision for the Tenzel semicircular flap is started immediately at the lateral canthal angle. As stated in Chapter 33, the concept of a continuum of repair necessary for a lid defect is essential. You cannot perform a lateral cantholysis using a straight, laterally placed horizontal incision only to discover that there is not enough mobilization of the lid and then try to convert to the Tenzel flap. You must know that the lateral cantholysis will only give several millimeters, and if the potential defect to be closed is more than approximately 3 mm, you must immediately plan for a Tenzel semicircular flap. The major complication that occurs if this is not done is a depression of the lower lid in the very lateral aspect just medial to the lateral canthus. This is totally preventable if the flap incision is started upward at the lateral canthus for a lower lid defect and downward for an upper lid defect.

The second pearl in preventing lateral displacement of the lid is meticulous closure of the deep orbicularis muscle to the lateral canthal tendon/angle area using the half-curved needle to secure a small bite of periosteum. This gives a good, secure reconstruction of the lateral canthal angle and prevents future problems, particularly when the reconstruction involves the lower lid.

We frequently insert a suture tarsorrhaphy using a 5-0 or 6-0 polypropylene (Surgilene or Prolene) suture in and out of the gray line of the lower lid and upper lid in the lateral half of the lid, keeping the knot lateral. This gives good stabilization, particularly for a reconstructed lower lid, during the first 10 to 12 days. We usually remove that suture at the same time that the marginal sutures are removed. If the lid that is operated on is the only seeing eye for the patient, then either a smaller intermarginal suture tarsorrhaphy or none at all is used, depending on the need for such support.

Because diabetics are more susceptible to infection, if surgery is performed on a diabetic patient, be all the more firm with the patient regarding the use of antibiotic drops or ointment and regarding the reporting of any adverse problem to you so that systemic antibiotics can be instituted immediately. We do not advocate the routine use of oral antibiotics on a prophylactic basis.

TARSAL-CONJUNCTIVAL ADVANCEMENT FLAP IN LOWER EYELID RECONSTRUCTION

Eugene O. Wiggs, MD

Wendell Hughes described an upper eyelid tarsal-conjunctival advancement flap for posterior lamellar reconstruction of full-thickness defects of the lower eyelid.[1] In this procedure, the anterior lamina of the eyelid is covered with a skin-muscle flap or a full-thickness skin graft. A modification of this technique avoids splitting the upper eyelid margin, thereby obviating secondary upper eyelid margin deformities.

Large full-thickness lower eyelid defects can be reconstructed by (1) a tarsal-conjunctival graft and skin-muscle advancement flap from below or a skin-muscle transposition flap from the ipsilateral upper eyelid; (2) the Tenzel semicircular lateral canthal rotation flap, which is useful for full-thickness defects of moderate size in the central or lateral portion of the upper or lower eyelid; (3) a tarsal-conjunctival transposition flap from the ipsilateral upper eyelid combined with a skin-muscle flap or full-thickness skin graft; or (4) the Hughes procedure, which is described here.

The Hughes procedure is useful when one of the other techniques noted previously cannot be used. One indication might be resection of lesions that extend far enough inferiorly to make application of one of the previous techniques (1, 2, or 3, noted in the previous paragraph) unsuitable. The procedure can also be useful in selected trauma situations. The major disadvantage of the procedure is that the patient is monocular during the interval between stage I and stage II of the operation if the flap covers the pupil. Leibsohn and colleagues suggested a buttonhole in the flap to overcome this disadvantage.[2] The Hughes procedure for lower eyelid reconstruction has, in my view, limited applications. However, it is reliable and has withstood the test of time. The other techniques noted previously do not render the patient monocular for a central defect of the lower eyelid. The Hughes procedure is most useful for full-thickness lower eyelid defects medial or lateral to the pupillary axis.

Anesthesia

The procedure can be performed with the patient under attended local or general anesthesia. The use of long-acting local anesthesia with epinephrine provides hemostasis and blunts acute postoperative pain. Frontal nerve block is a useful adjunct for upper eyelid anesthesia in selected cases.

Surgical Technique

Step 1

After frozen section clearance has been obtained, or if the patient has previously undergone Mohs' surgery, the apposing upper eyelid is everted.

Step 2

A scalpel incision is made 3 to 4 mm above and parallel to the upper eyelid margin, through the tarsus and conjunctiva so as to enter the pretarsal space.

Step 3

The length of this incision is the width of the tarsal-conjunctival advancement flap. This determination is made by bringing the 2 ends of the remaining lower eyelid snugly toward each other while keeping the eyelids in contact with the globe. In other words, the flap is not quite as wide as the original lower eyelid defect.

Step 4

The initial scalpel incision is extended to the appropriate length with fine-pointed scissors.

Step 5

Vertical cuts are made to the top of the tarsus on both sides of the potential flap (Figure 35-1).

Levine MR.
Manual of Oculoplastic Surgery, Fourth Edition (pp 229-232).
© 2010 SLACK Incorporated

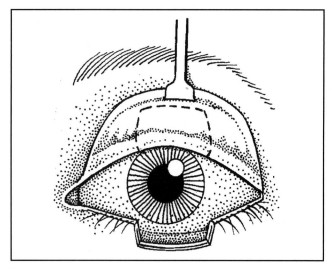

Figure 35-1.

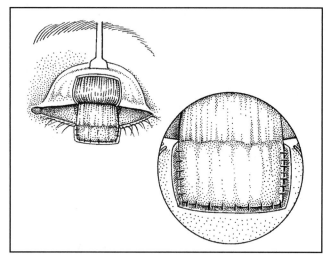

Figure 35-2.

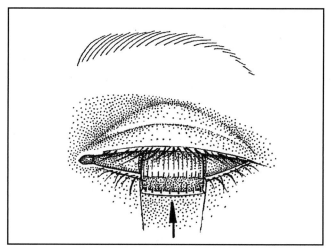

Figure 35-3.

Step 6

The tarsal conjunctival flap is then elevated and separated from its anterior attachments; vertical cuts are made with scissors through conjunctiva on both sides of the flap, extending the incisions to the upper fornix.

Step 7

The conjunctiva is then separated from the underlying Müller's muscle and levator aponeurosis, carrying the dissection to the upper fornix. Frequently, in elderly patients, Müller's muscle laminates between the flap and the levator aponeurosis. Müller's muscle also tends to be atrophic in elderly patients. In younger patients, Müller's muscle tends to hug the levator aponeurosis, and in these patients, a plane is usually easily developed between the Müller's muscle and conjunctiva. Müller's muscle can also be left attached to the flap, if one wishes; this increases the vascularity of the flap but is unnecessary in my experience.

Step 8

The flap is then advanced into the lower eyelid defect so that the top of the tarsus of the tarsal-conjunctival advancement flap is flush with the remaining lower eyelid margin.

Step 9

The flap is anastomosed to the tarsus and conjunctiva of the lower lid with 5-0 or 6-0 chromic gut sutures (Figure 35-2). If the eyelid is not snug against the globe, the flap is too wide and should be shortened.

Step 10

The anterior lamina of the defect is then covered with an advancement skin flap from below. This technique is often feasible in elderly patients because of excess skin; in younger patients, however, it has the potential to induce ectropion because of a lack of stretch, and in this situation, a full-thickness skin graft is useful.

Step 11

Scissors are used to make 2 parallel vertical cuts through skin inferiorly (Figure 35-3).

Step 12

The skin flap is mobilized inferiorly and advanced to 1 mm below the top of the remaining eyelid margin. To avoid retraction, the skin advancement flap should not be under any tension.

Step 13

The redundant skin at the base of the advancement flap is removed by excising a triangle of skin on each side (Figure 35-4).

Step 14

The skin advancement flap is closed with 6-0 silk.

Step 15

A skin-muscle transposition flap from the upper eyelid can also be used for the anterior lamina of the reconstructed lower eyelid. If a small amount of lower eyelid skin remains laterally, skin and muscle are removed over the lateral portion of the eyelid.

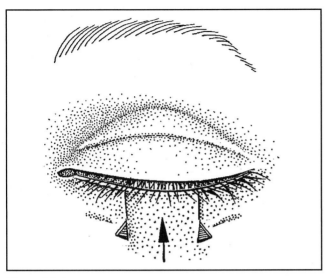

Figure 35-4.

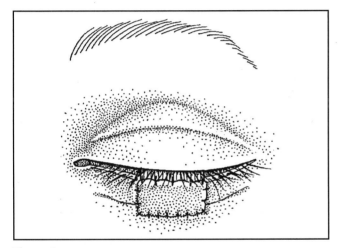

Figure 35-5.

Usually, the skin-muscle transposition flap has less tendency to induce ectropion than an advancement flap from below and has a better appearance than a skin graft. In general, I prefer flaps to skin grafts because they generally have a better color and texture match, and the flap has its own blood supply. The transposition flap is sutured in place using 6-0 black silk; a 6-0 monofilament suture is used to close the defect from the transposition flap in the upper eyelid.

Step 16

If a skin graft is needed, a postauricular graft, supraclavicular graft, or skin from the apposing upper eyelid may be used (Figure 35-5).

Step 17

The skin graft is sutured with 5-0 or 6-0 black silk and stented with a sponge. The upper eyelid donor area is closed with a 6-0 polypropylene suture. The postauricular wound is closed with interrupted 4-0 absorbable dermal sutures and a running 4-0 polypropylene suture. The supraclavicular wound

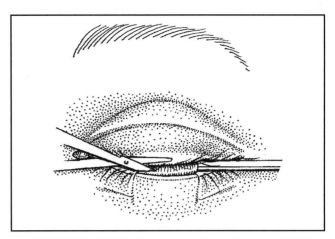

Figure 35-6.

is closed with 4-0 polypropylene sutures and deep sutures as needed.

Dividing the Flap

The eyelids are opened as a secondary procedure 6 to 12 weeks after the primary reconstruction. Stage II reconstruction is done after the flap has stretched sufficiently so that upper or lower eyelid retraction does not occur. However, in a monocular patient, the flap may be divided if necessary after 2 weeks without compromising the blood supply to the new lower eyelid. For obvious reasons, this flap is generally unsuitable for the monocular patient.

Step 1

Topical anesthetic drops are placed on the eye. A frontal nerve block and local infiltration anesthesia of the upper and lower eyelids are performed.

Step 2

A grooved director is placed beneath the flap, inserting it from a lateral to medial direction, and the director is moved approximately 2 mm higher than where the site of the reconstructed lower eyelid margin will be (Figure 35-6). This maneuver neutralizes the effects of lower eyelid retraction, which occurs postoperatively.

Step 3

A straight cut is then made in the grooved director with the straight scissors or scalpel beveled so that the posterior lamina of the reconstructed lower eyelid is higher than the remaining normal eyelid margin, about 2 mm.

Step 4

The remaining flap attached to the upper eyelid is cut off at its base, making sure to remove all keratinized epithelium, which has frequently advanced up the flap. No repair is done on the small epithelial defect remaining on the upper eyelid.

Step 5

Horizontal mattress sutures of 6-0 mild chromic are then used to ensure that the conjunctiva is

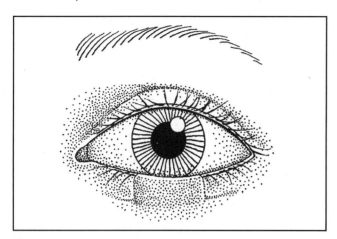

Figure 35-7.

2 mm higher than the skin on the reconstructed lower eyelid. In general, the conjunctiva tends to retract more than skin; suturing minimizes this potential. Conjunctiva is preferred to skin for the reconstructed eyelid margin to prevent keratinized epithelium and lanugo hairs from irritating the eye (Figure 35-7).

Remarks

Several important facts need to be emphasized in performing the modified Hughes tarsal-conjunctival advancement flap technique for lower eyelid reconstruction. The tarsal-conjunctival advancement flap should be narrower in width than the lower eyelid defect so that the reconstructed eyelid hugs the globe. It is important to remember that the reconstructed eyelid is a tonic lid over most of its length. The flap should not be started at the eyelid margin, but 3 to 4 mm above the margin; undermining should be extended to the upper fornix to prevent postoperative upper eyelid retraction. If damage to the levator aponeurosis occurs, ptosis can ensue postoperatively; however, this problem is extremely rare in my experience. If damage to the aponeurosis does occur intraoperatively, it should be repaired. There should be no hesitation in sacrificing small or moderate amounts of lower eyelid tissue laterally if a transposition flap of skin muscle from the upper lid can be used in place of a skin graft.

CHAPTER 36

Tarsal-Conjunctival Graft or Flap and Skin-Muscle Transposition Flap in Lower Eyelid Reconstruction

Eugene O. Wiggs, MD

Lateral and total lower eyelid defects can be nicely reconstructed in a one-stage procedure using a tarsal-conjunctival graft and skin-muscle transposition flap from the ipsilateral upper eyelid.

Anesthesia

The procedure can be performed under general or attended local anesthesia. The upper eyelid, lower eyelid, and lateral canthus are infiltrated with a 1:1 mixture of 2% lidocaine with epinephrine and bupivacaine 0.5%. The use of long-acting local anesthesia with epinephrine provides hemostasis and blunts the acute postoperative pain. Frontal nerve block is a useful adjunct for upper eyelid anesthesia in selected cases.

Surgical Technique

Step 1

The tumor is excised using frozen section control or Mohs' surgery. If a remnant of lower eyelid remains laterally, it is sacrificed for structural purposes.

Step 2

A skin-muscle flap is mobilized from the ipsilateral upper eyelid, leaving the flap based and widened at the lateral canthus (Figure 36-1). The lower border of the flap corresponds to the upper eyelid crease. The flap is wrapped in a saline sponge and reflected laterally. Some patients may request/require upper blepharoplasty on the other side for cosmetic or functional purposes.

Step 3

The upper eyelid is everted; 3- to 4-mm above and parallel to the eyelid margin, a scalpel incision is made through tarsal-conjunctiva, and the pretarsal space is entered. Scissors lengthen the incision for the full extent of the tarsus.

Step 4

A horizontal conjunctival incision is made at the top of the tarsus for the full length of the tarsus. Vertical cuts are made in the tarsus medially and laterally; the tarsus is freed up anteriorly and the resultant tarsal-conjunctival graft is placed in a saline sponge (Figure 36-2).

Step 5

The conjunctiva is undermined to the superior fornix as a precaution against upper eyelid retraction postoperatively. The conjunctiva is then sewn to the remaining upper eyelid tarsus-conjunctiva with a running 6-0 or 5-0 plain gut suture. The ends of the gut sutures are tied anteriorly. By not tying the knot posteriorly, a suture keratopathy is avoided.

Step 6

The tarsal-conjunctival graft is sewn into the lower eyelid defect under slight tension using 6-0 or 5-0 chromic gut. The tarsal-conjunctival graft should be 1 to 2 mm higher than the remaining lower eyelid margin as the graft contracts slightly postoperatively. Laterally, a 5-0 absorbable monofilament suture is placed through the lateral aspect of the tarsal-conjunctival graft and sewn to the periosteum at the lateral canthal angle just posterior to the rim. This suture should make the eyelid rest snugly against the eye.

Step 7

Tissue is excised laterally between the lateral aspect of the surgical defect and the lower aspect of the skin-muscle transposition flap to allow the skin-muscle flap to be transposed into the lower eyelid defect (Figure 36-3).

Levine MR.
Manual of Oculoplastic Surgery, Fourth Edition (pp 233-236).
© 2010 SLACK Incorporated

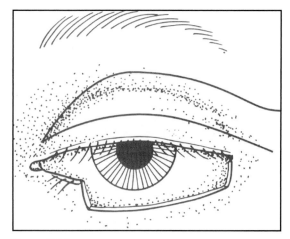

Figure 36-1.

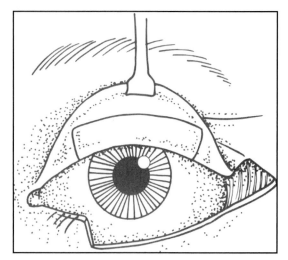

Figure 36-2.

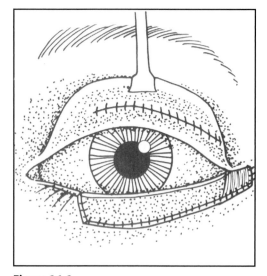

Figure 36-3.

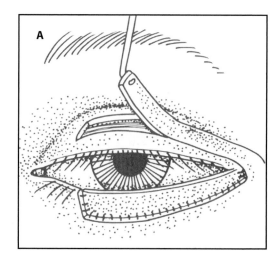

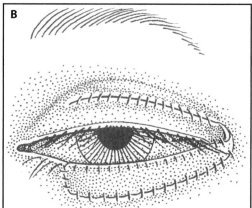

Figure 36-4.

Step 8

The upper eyelid skin-muscle flap is elevated, transposed into the lower eyelid defect, and excess flap is trimmed medially, placing the flap under slight tension (Figure 36-4A). Horizontal mattress sutures of 6-0 mild chromic are used to recess the top of the skin-muscle flap from the top of the tarsal-conjunctival graft to prevent keratinized epithelium from irritating the eye. The flap is sewn in place with 6-0 black silk or 6-0 polypropylene. The upper eyelid wound is closed with 6-0 polypropylene (Figure 36-4B). Upper blepharoplasty may be performed on the other upper eyelid as necessary.

Step 9

One or 2 intermarginal sutures tied over Weck cell pegs are placed to splint the lower eyelid upward and decrease the eyelid's movement. In the elderly, a skin-muscle advancement flap from inferiorly can sometimes be used instead of a skin-muscle upper eyelid transposition flap (Figure 36-5). Ectropion, however, is more likely to occur than with the upper eyelid transposition flap.

In 1976, Hewes, Sullivan, and Beard[1] described a one-stage method for reconstruction of a full-thickness lower eyelid defect using a transposition flap of tarsus-conjunctiva from the apposing upper eyelid. The flap is rotated so that the conjunctiva is posterior (Figure 36-6). The

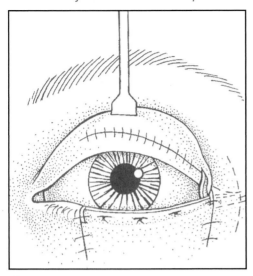

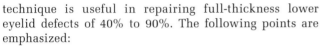

Figure 36-5.

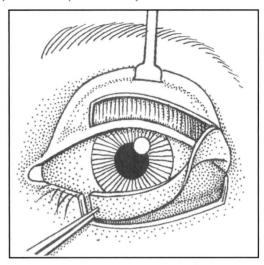

Figure 36-6.

technique is useful in repairing full-thickness lower eyelid defects of 40% to 90%. The following points are emphasized:

* The flap requires special attention to 2-point fixation—good medial closure of the medial tarsus to the inferior crus of the medial canthal tendon, and laterally to the periosteum of the orbital rim.

* Any remaining lateral lower eyelid must be removed to complete the procedure.

* Because of a precarious blood supply to the inner lamella, a skin-muscle advancement flap from the lower eyelid and premalar area is used to complete the reconstruction, although a thin skin graft from the apposing eyelid can be successful. In my hands, a tarsal-conjunctival graft with upper eyelid skin-muscle transposition flap produces a superior cosmetic result to use of a tarsal-conjunctival transposition flap. The tarsal-conjunctival transposition flap procedure is also more technically difficult.

Complications and Their Management

Complications related specifically to these procedures are infrequent. Generally, I have found these operations reliable and predictable. Therefore, the thrust of these observations relate to prevention of complications via proper intraoperative technique. Some intraoperative maneuvers have been described in the section Surgical Technique but are included in this discussion for the sake of completeness. Improved blood supply of the skin-muscle upper eyelid flap is accomplished by using a thicker flap, especially laterally. A thin flap means less blood supply. The flap should also be widened laterally. In removing the tarsal conjunctival graft from the upper eyelid, avoid making the tarsal incision closer than 3- to 4-mm from the eyelid margin to avoid postoperative entropion.

Conjunctival undermining to the superior fornix is essential to avoid postoperative upper eyelid retraction. Closure of the posterior eyelid defect with a 6-0 or 5-0 plain gut suture is accomplished by running the suture in a subepithelial fashion. This technique, combined with tying the knots anteriorly, prevents suture-induced keratopathy. If suture keratopathy does occur, it can be managed by the use of ointment. A soft contact lens would also be beneficial but would be difficult to insert.

Postoperative lower eyelid ectropion is avoided by sewing the tarsal-conjunctival graft into the surgical defect under slight tension. This means decreasing the length of the graft or flap as needed and anchoring the graft securely to the periosteum of the lateral orbital rim just anterior to the lateral orbital tubercle in total eyelid reconstruction or with lateral defects. The graft should also be approximately 2 mm higher than the upper edge of the skin muscle transposition flap. The purpose of the skin muscle recession on the graft is to reduce lanugo hair contact, keratinized epithelium, or both from irritating the cornea. Sewing the tarsal graft into the surgical bed approximately 2-mm higher than the adjacent eyelid margin minimizes eyelid notching.

To avoid kinking of the skin-muscle transposition flap laterally, it is essential that the upper eyelid flap be extended onto the lateral canthus. The lateral extension allows a less acute angle where the flap crosses the lateral canthus. Kinking of the flap can impair its blood supply. Compromised circulation to the distal flap results, however, if the flap is too long.

A suture tarsorrhaphy (intermarginal suture) is performed with a monofilament suture tied over Weck cell sponges. This maneuver immobilizes the reconstructed eyelid, thus aiding vascularization of the graft. The lower eyelid is also splinted upward, thus decreasing the likelihood of lower eyelid retraction. The suture is left in place 3 to 5 days postoperatively.

It has been said that there are no surprises in surgery, only surprised surgeons. Careful planning and thoughtful, precise surgical technique can greatly diminish surgical complications.

REPAIR OF EYELID DEFECTS WITH THE ORBICULARIS OCULI MOBILIZATION TECHNIQUE
NAUGLE-LEVINE PROCEDURE

Constance L. Fry, MD; Thomas C. Naugle, Jr, MD; and Mark R. Levine, MD, FACS

Orbicularis oculi mobilization can be used in conjunction with a variety of eyelid reconstruction techniques to facilitate the vascularization of grafts and overall healing of tissue, especially in potentially compromised situations of tissue loss after excisions of malignancies or in cases of severe trauma. The orbicularis courses in a circumlinear fashion around the eyelid margins with the upper and lower sections of the pretarsal orbicularis intertwining with each other laterally and the preseptal and orbital portions extending from medial to superior and then coursing laterally almost 360° to medial inferior, thus originating and terminating at and near the medial canthal tendon. The eyelids contain a rich blood supply from branches of the ophthalmic, lacrimal, facial, and superficial temporal arteries interconnecting with each other. This facilitates maintenance of the blood supply to the advanced orbicularis muscle flap.

In patients with a full-thickness defect of the upper or lower lid margin involving 50% of the eyelid or more, a tarsal substitute is important to maintain the approximation of the lid to the globe. The orbicularis mobilization technique allows for placement of a free tarsoconjunctival graft and a skin graft to reform the lid, particularly when the defect is shallow vertically. The size of the defect that can be reconstructed is commensurate with the size of the tarsal graft that can be harvested. Tarsal stability is maintained by leaving at least 3 mm of upper tarsus intact at the margin on the side where the tarsoconjunctival graft is harvested. This may result in a tarsal graft as much as 7 mm in vertical height (in the non-Asian eyelid). The limit of the horizontal length of the defect that can be repaired is determined by the horizontal length of the superior tarsus available for harvesting, which may be up to 20 mm or possibly more. The horizontal dimensions of the graft harvested should be 2 mm less than the defect. The defect is measured by gently bringing the 2 edges

together (without pulling on the defect) to prevent pin cushioning or eyelid retraction.

The primary advantage of the orbicularis mobilization technique is that it enables the patient to maintain a functional visual axis immediately after surgery instead of the 4- to 6-week period of occlusion that typically occurs following a lid-sharing procedure. This technique is particularly useful for monocular patients and those whose occupations make unilateral occlusion problematic. Moreover, only one procedure is required with the orbicularis mobilization instead of the 2 separate surgeries for the lid-sharing technique. Additionally, orbicularis mobilization can be used to cover exposed bone in the medial and lateral canthal regions and to allow for skin graft placement or healing of the defect by secondary intention with the aid of directional sutures. Moreover, for larger facial defects, tissue at the same plane as the orbicularis, such as the frontalis, can be mobilized with the orbicularis to close large defects.

Lower Lid Defects

Step 1

A full-thickness lower lid defect of 50% or more of the horizontal extent of the lid is present after tumor resection or tissue loss from trauma (Figure 37-1). Figure 37-2 depicts the defect showing the skin removed and the extent of the underlying orbicularis. The area and surrounding tissue, as well as the donor sites for skin and tarsoconjunctival grafts, are infiltrated with 2% lidocaine with epinephrine (1:100,000), and the region is prepped and draped in the usual sterile fashion. Typically, these procedures are performed with intravenous sedation and local infiltration of anesthetic for pain control. In cases of extensive tissue loss, in which

Levine MR.
Manual of Oculoplastic Surgery, Fourth Edition (pp 237-242).
© 2010 SLACK Incorporated

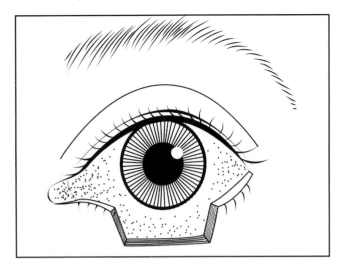

Figure 37-1.

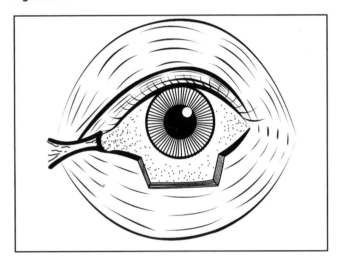

Figure 37-2.

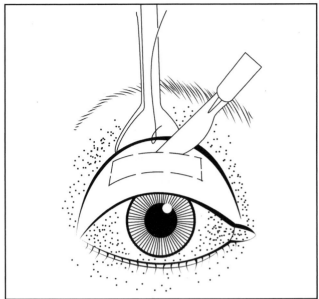

Figure 37-3.

0.5 forceps are used to carefully dissect the tarsal graft from the overlying levator attachments in order to prevent ptosis. Bipolar cautery is used to obtain hemostasis (Figure 37-3).

Step 4
The tarsoconjunctival graft is secured to the medial and lateral edges of the recipient bed and inferiorly to the lower lid retractors with 6-0 polyglactin (Vicryl) on a gently curved spatulated needle, such as S-29; care is taken not to pass the suture full-thickness to avoid corneal irritation.

Step 5
Fine skin hooks are placed in the skin immediately adjacent to the defect and the orbicularis muscle is separated from the overlying skin with blunt dissection utilizing a spreading technique with blunt Stevens scissors. Hemostasis can be achieved with a combination of low-energy bipolar cautery, cold saline irrigation, and Gelfoam soaked in thrombin. It is imperative to be gentle with the overlying skin and minimize cauterization to avoid unnecessary scarring. Thus, bipolar cautery at low energy settings is usually preferable to monopolar cautery. The dissection extends inferiorly to include a section of orbicularis that is approximately 2 to 3 times the height of the defect. The medial and lateral extent of the dissection is at least half of the width of the defect on each side (Figure 37-4).

Step 6
The orbicularis is then grasped with forceps or skin hooks by the assistant. The underlying orbital septum is grasped with 0.5 forceps and is separated from the overlying orbicularis with blunt dissection using Stevens scissors, taking care not to buttonhole the orbicularis. Meticulous hemostasis is again maintained with electrocautery, which may be monopolar or bipolar The dissection is carried

a lengthy surgical time is anticipated, there rarely may be a need for a general anesthetic.

Step 2
The edges of the defect are grasped with 2 pairs of 0.5 forceps and brought gently toward each other, avoiding any traction, and the horizontal and vertical dimensions of the defect are measured with calipers or a ruler.

Step 3
A 4-0 silk suture is passed full-thickness through the lid margin of the ispilateral or contralateral upper lid, which is then everted on a Desmarres retractor. A 15° Supersharp or #15 Bard-Parker blade is used to incise the tarsoconjunctival graft, 1 mm shorter in the horizontal dimension than the primary defect; the slight shortening is done to prevent ectropion. Care is taken when harvesting the graft to begin no closer than 3 to 4 mm from the upper lid margin in order to preserve the normal lid architecture and prevent ectropion, entropion, and trichiasis. Also, the vertical dissection of the graft does not extend above the tarsal plate, to avoid inducing ptosis. Sharp Westcott scissors and

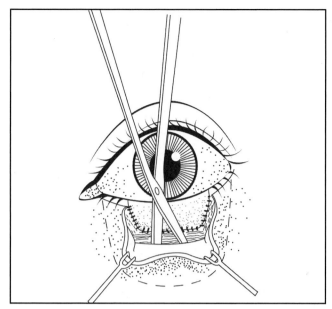

Figure 37-4.

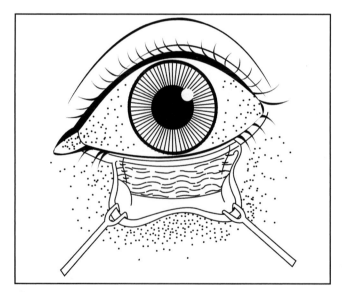

Figure 37-5.

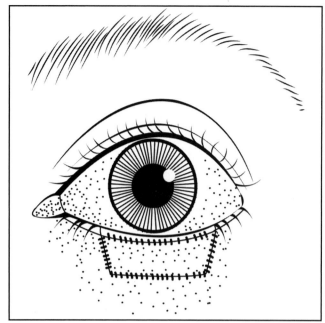

Figure 37-6.

out to the same extent in each direction as the subcutaneous dissection. Care should be taken in the area of the infraorbital nerve not to dissect below the septum and to use bipolar cautery.

Step 7

Once the orbicularis has been mobilized anteriorly from the skin and posteriorly from the orbital septum in both an inferior direction as well as medially and laterally, it may be grasped and gently elevated to cover the tarsoconjunctival graft that has been secured to the eyelid margin and lower lid retractors. The orbicularis should lie without any tension over the tarsoconjunctival graft. If there is any tension, either further mobilization of the orbicularis is required or, in the case of large defects, vertical relaxing incisions should be made on either side of the defect extending inferiorly until the tension is released.

Step 8

Once the orbicularis lies without tension on the tarsoconjunctival graft, it may be secured to the graft. Multiple interrupted sutures of 6-0 polyglactin are used to secure the orbicularis to the graft, while recessing the orbicularis approximately 1 mm from the superior border of the graft. Care is taken to take partial-thickness bites in the graft (Figure 37-5).

Step 9

A skin graft is then harvested to complete the closure of the anterior lamella. The graft should be somewhat larger than the primary defect to allow for shrinkage. Skin may be harvested from the contralateral upper lid (if sufficient skin is present to avoid lagophthalmos), the retroauricular, supraclavicular, or inner arm regions. The skin graft is fenestrated and thinned to the rete pegs and is then secured to the advanced orbicularis. It is not necessary to use a thick skin graft as the mobilized orbicularis fills the volume deficit; a thinned graft will have better color and texture match. Care should be taken to recess the skin graft slightly so that the conjunctiva can epithelialize the newly formed lid margin. The skin graft may be secured with a running 6-0 chromic gut suture at the recessed lid margin and interrupted 6-0 chromic gut or 6-0 silk sutures along the remainder of the graft (Figure 37-6).

Step 10

Once the edges of the skin graft are secured, the graft may be further fixated to the orbicularis with quilting sutures. A 6-0 chromic gut suture on a P-1 needle is passed through the skin graft, into the orbicularis, and out through the skin graft and tied. Several quilting sutures may be placed to facilitate vascularization of the graft.

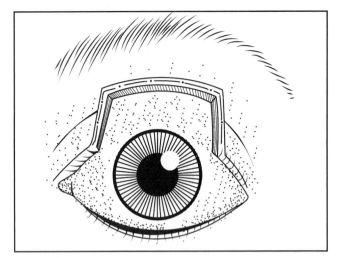

Figure 37-7.

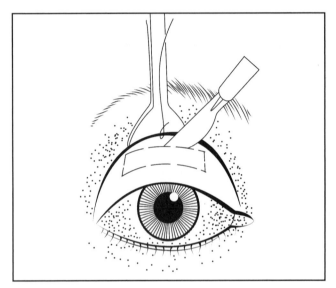

Figure 37-8.

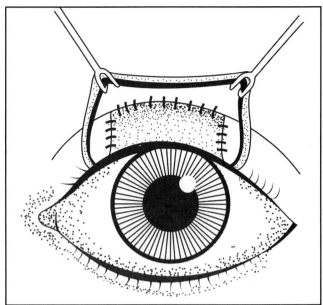

Figure 37-9.

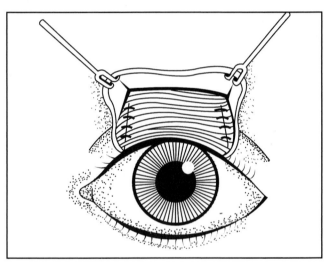

Figure 37-10.

Step 11 (optional)

The graft may be covered by a Telfa pad cut slightly smaller than the graft, and a cotton bolster may be placed over the Telfa and secured to the skin adjacent to the graft with interrupted 6-0 silk or chromic sutures tied over the bolster. If a bolster is used, it is left in place 7 to 10 days, and ointment is placed at its periphery to allow seepage onto the graft. Two reverse Frost sutures or suture tarsorrhaphies may be placed for 7 days to keep the lid on traction and prevent lower lid retraction.

Upper Lid Defects

Steps 1 to 3

See Steps 1, 2, and 3 of repair of lower lid defects with orbicularis mobilization (Figures 37-7 and 37-8).

Step 4

The tarsoconjunctival graft is secured to the medial and lateral edges of the recipient bed and superiorly to the levator aponeurosis with 6-0 polyglactin on a spatula needle; care is taken not to incorporate the septum while securing the levator and not to extend full-thickness through the recipient tarsus and cause corneal irritation.

Steps 5 to 12

See Steps 5 to 12 of repair of lower lid defects with orbicularis mobilization (Figures 37-9 through 37-11, with quilting sutures depicted in the skin graft).

Medial and Lateral Canthal Defects

For defects in the medial and lateral canthus with exposed bone, the following steps should be performed.

Step 1

The defect and surrounding tissue, as well as the areas for skin graft (if used), are infiltrated with 2% lidocaine with epinephrine (1:100,000), and the

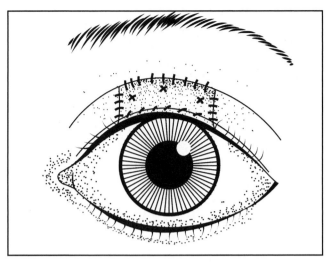

Figure 37-11.

region is prepped and draped in the usual sterile fashion.

Step 2

Fine skin hooks are placed in the skin immediately adjacent to the defect, and the orbicularis muscle is separated from the overlying skin and the underlying fascial attachments with blunt dissection using a spreading technique with blunt Stevens scissors. Hemostasis can be achieved with a combination of low-energy bipolar cautery, cold saline irrigation, and Gelfoam soaked in thrombin. It is imperative to be gentle with the overlying skin and minimize cauterization to avoid unnecessary scarring, thus bipolar cautery at low energy settings is usually preferable to monopolar cautery in areas adjacent to the skin and when near the infraorbital, supraorbital, and supratrochlear neurovascular bundles.

Step 3

The orbicularis is mobilized in one or more directions from the edges of the defect. If only one direction is mobilized, the area mobilized will encompass about 2 to 3 times the area of the defect. Alternatively, if orbicularis is mobilized above and below the defect, the area in each direction should be about twice the size of the defect. Then, the upper and lower mobilized orbicularis can be secured together with multiple, interrupted 5-0 polyglactin suture with buried knots. Particularly in the medial canthal region, quilting sutures should be used to secure the advanced orbicularis posteriorly to prevent tenting forward of the area and a loss of the medial convexity.

Step 4 (option 1) Skin Graft

A skin graft is then harvested to complete the closure of the anterior lamella. The graft should be somewhat larger than the primary defect to allow for shrinkage. Skin may be harvested from the excess tissue in the upper lids, retroauricular, supraclavicular, or inner arm regions. The skin graft is fenestrated and thinned to rete pegs and is then secured to the advanced orbicularis. Quilting

sutures of 6-0 chromic gut are placed from the skin graft to the orbicularis to further prevent webbing or tenting of the graft, particularly medially. It is not necessary to use a thick skin graft as the mobilized orbicularis fills the volume deficit; a thinned graft will have a better color and texture match. The skin graft may be secured with interrupted 6-0 chromic gut or 6-0 silk sutures along the remainder of the graft.

Step 4 (option 2) Healing by Secondary Intention With Directional Sutures

Horizontal mattress sutures of 5-0 or 6-0 chromic gut are placed at the skin edges of the defect in order to lessen the anterior lamellar defect by 25% to 50%. The sutures are placed from the skin edge inferior to superior and superior to inferior. Each inferior limb is tied to shorten the area of the defect that will fill in by secondary intention. Care must be taken not to create adverse directional forces on the lid margins that could cause lagophthalmos, lid retraction, or ectropion; occasionally, the orientation of the mattress sutures must be altered to avoid placing adverse tractional forces on the eyelids.

Postoperative Care

Ophthalmic ointment of choice is placed on the graft 3 times a day and continued several days after suture removal. Sutures are typically removed 7 to 10 days after surgery, depending on healing.

Complications

EYELID RETRACTION

Using 2 reverse Frost sutures on either end of the graft, making the horizontal dimension of the graft 2 mm less than the defect, and ensuring the appropriate tension on the 2 ends of the recipient bed are the best ways to prevent eyelid retraction. Additionally, care should be taken to avoid incorporating any of the septum into the attachment of the lower lid retractor complex to the tarsoconjunctival graft in the lower lid or in the attachment of the levator to the graft in the upper lid. Should significant lid retraction occur, the lateral canthal region should be evaluated and any laxity corrected with a tarsal strip procedure.

A unique group are patients with relative globe proptosis. They are at greater risk of eyelid retraction, and care should be taken to avoid shortening the lid excessively; instead, the graft should be made sufficiently tall and wide to allow coverage of the globe.

GRAFT FAILURE

Skin grafts may fail for multiple reasons. The orbicularis mobilization technique helps to prevent this by supplying a rich blood supply to the graft. Prevention of hematoma formation by good preoperative and intraoperative planning is preferable. This begins with cessation of smoking and cessation of medications and herbal products that promote bleeding. Intraoperative measures include fenestrating the graft, placing quilting sutures, and, if necessary, placing a bolster to aid in preventing graft failure. If a hematoma occurs under the graft, it should be drained. If the graft continues to look dusky for several days, hyperbaric oxygen treatment can be used to attempt to reverse a failing graft.

CORNEAL ABRASIONS

Corneal abrasions may occur from deep sutures securing the tarsoconjunctival graft extending posteriorly and touching the cornea, or from the skin graft riding too high at the lid margin. If the cause is a deep suture eroding posteriorly, the wound may be revised and the suture replaced, or a simpler solution is to place a bandage contact lens in the eye until the suture dissolves. The patient should receive topical antibiotic solution 3 times daily in the eye and have the contact lens replaced every 2 weeks until the suture has resorbed. If the skin graft is riding too high and rubbing on the cornea, it should be trimmed and recessed below the lid margin and resutured with 6-0 chromic gut. If the skin edge is found to rub the cornea weeks to months after the reconstruction, the edge should be recessed, and an amniotic membrane graft or buccal mucosal graft can be sewn to the lid margin to promote an epithelial surface.

INADEQUATE HORIZONTAL LENGTH OF TARSOCONJUNCTIVAL GRAFT

If the tarsoconjunctival graft is not adequately long enough to cover the defect at the time of the primary repair, a periosteal flap can be elevated and rotated from the lateral or medial orbital rim and attached to the edge of the tarsoconjunctival flap.

RECONSTRUCTION OF MEDIAL CANTHAL DEFECTS

Joseph A. Mauriello, Jr, MD

The soft tissues of the medial canthal area are anatomically complex and include the bony attachments of the medial canthal tendon and the lacrimal drainage system. Therefore, the multicontoured medial canthus requires special reconstructive considerations. The soft tissues may be reconstructed with a full-thickness skin graft. Laterally based upper lid and lower lid full-thickness advancement flaps mobilized after canthotomy and cantholysis of the superior and inferior crus of the lateral canthal tendon augmented by a semicircular lateral canthal flap serve to close the eyelid portions of medial canthal defects.

In addition, various flaps, most importantly, V-Y advancement flaps, glabellar, and rhomboid flaps, are described.[1-5]

Certain caveats are necessary for successful repair of medial canthal defects after tumor excision. First, the defect should be covered with as thin a flap as possible to avoid masking a recurrence of the tumor. The author, therefore, does not generally use midline glabellar flaps and prefers full-thickness skin grafts harvested from the retroauricular skin. Second, any modality, whether a full-thickness skin graft or a flap, should ideally not bridge a multicontoured area; the eyelid portion should ideally undergo reconstruction by a technique that is separate from the medial canthus in order to avoid webbing and frank ectropion of the medial aspect of the upper or lower lid. In other words, a full-thickness skin graft should not extend from the eyelid tissues to the medial canthal and nasal tissues. Third, the integrity of the lacrimal drainage system usually requires insertion of a silicone stent in the upper and lower canaliculus. Ideally, at least 6 mm of normal canaliculus are necessary for reconstruction; a Jones bypass may be necessary if there are not significant canalicular remnants to allow reconstruction. Fifth, reconstruction of the medial canthal tendon is necessary and is discussed.

Modalities for medial canthus reconstruction will be considered:

* Full-thickness skin graft from retroauricular donor site
* Local upper and lower lid full-thickness advancement flaps augmented by lateral canthal semicircular flap
* Glabellar flap—A "V" to a "Y" flap.
* Rhomboid flaps
* Glabellar flap combined with nasolabial V-Y advancement flap
* Tarsoconjunctival flaps from the upper and lower lid

Full-Thickness Skin Graft

This technique is extremely useful for medial canthal reconstruction. Specific surgical techniques to optimize full-thickness skin grafting are outlined elsewhere (Figure 38-1).[1]

Step 1

The author prefers to place a pressure patch over the treatment eye to avoid inadvertent trauma to the operated eye.

Step 2

Patients must call the physician if pain or bleeding develops under the patch.

Flaps

Flaps can be either local upper and lower lid full-thickness semicircular advancement flaps combined with a lateral canthal semicircular flap or local upper and lower lid full-thickness semicircular advancement flaps augmented by a lateral canthal semicircular flap. Local advancement flaps of entire upper or lower lid may be used. These flaps are characterized by residual tarsus at the medial extent of the tumor resection.[1] The flaps only serve to reconstruct

Levine MR.
Manual of Oculoplastic Surgery, Fourth Edition (pp 243-246).
© 2010 SLACK Incorporated

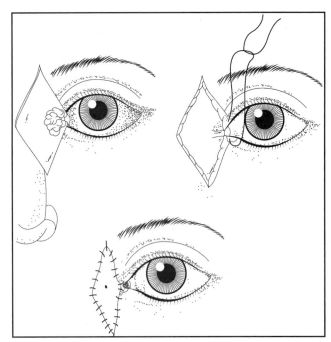

Figure 38-1. (Adapted from McCord CD, Nunnery WR. Reconstruction of the lower eyelid and outer canthus. In: McCord CD, Tanenbaum M, eds. *Oculoplastic Surgery Second Edition*. New York, NY: Raven Press; 1987:93-115.)

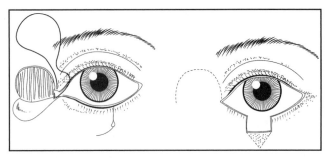

Figure 38-2. (Adapted from McCord CD, Nunnery WR. Reconstruction of the lower eyelid and outer canthus. In: McCord CD, Tanenbaum M, eds. *Oculoplastic Surgery Second Edition*. New York, NY: Raven Press; 1987:93-115.)

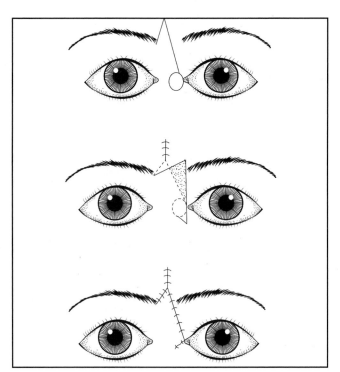

Figure 38-3. (Adapted from Collin JRO. *A Manual of Systematic Eyelid Surgery*. New York, NY: Churchill Livingstone; 1989:73-98.)

the lateral aspect of the medial canthal defect; the author prefers a full-thickness skin graft to reconstruct the main portion of the medial canthal defect.

Step 1

A lateral canthotomy with cantholysis of the inferior crus of the lateral canthal tendon along with recession of the retractors of the lower (or upper) lid is employed for full-thickness lower eyelid defects (Figure 38-2).[1] Additional tissues may be mobilized medially by use of a lateral semicircular flap. This technique may be combined with a full-thickness skin graft to reconstruct the medial portion of the eyelid defect and is discussed elsewhere in this text.

Step 2

It is important to close the eyelid defects by advancement of the tarsus of the upper and lower lid with 4-0 chromic double-armed, horizontal

mattress sutures. Each arm is secured to the deep medial canthal tissues to avoid medial ectropion.

The Mustarde flap[1] is mentioned in an effort to provide completeness, but advancing a Tenzel lateral semicircular flap is generally sufficient to reconstruct the medial aspect of the lower lid. Any further deficiency of anterior lamellar tissue may be treated by use of a full-thickness skin graft. The author has not used a Mustarde flap in his practice in more than 25 years.

Glabellar Flap—"V" to a "Y" Flap

This technique is best for medial canthal defects that involve the most medial portion of the upper lid. The glabellar flap is a significantly thicker flap and, therefore, is often too bulky to reconstruct the natural concave shape normally present at the medial canthus. Secondary debulking procedures may be performed. The V-Y advancement flap from the medial canthus is useful for relatively small defects (3 x 3 cm) (Figure 38-3).[2] As with all flaps, the degree of mobility of a V-Y advancement flap depends on the laxity of the skin and subcutaneous tissue. The technique results in a fairly good color and textural result.

The surgical technique involves undermining and rotating the flap from the glabellar region as described (see Figure 38-3)[2,3]:

Step 1

An inverted "V" incision in the midline of the brow with one limb extending down to the defect.

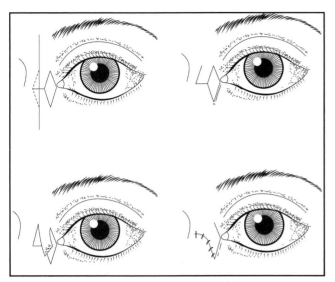

Figure 38-4. (Adapted from Ng SGJ, Inkster CF, Leatherbarrow B. The rhomboid flap in medial canthal reconstruction. *Br J Ophthalmol.* 2001;85:556-559.)

Step 2

Undermine the flap, and leave it attached by a broad pedicle across the bridge of the nose.

Step 3

The brow defect is closed to make the stem of an inverted "Y" using a 4-0 chromic absorbable suture to close the subcutaneous tissues. The advanced flap is rotated on the pedicle across the bridge of the nose.

Step 4

The flap is sutured after it is thinned. Generally, the superior tip of the flap is excised.

Rhomboid Flap

The defect should generally form a rhomboid with its long axis oriented vertically. As with all transpositional flaps, the rhomboid flap is ideal for older patients with thin, lax, less sebaceous skin so that less traction is required to pull the flap into the defect (Figure 38-4).[4]

Step 1

The rhomboid defect should consist of 2 equilateral triangles that are placed base to base (see Figure 38-4). For medial canthal defects, there are 2 possible rhomboid flaps. A line of the same length as the bases of the triangles is drawn horizontally across the nose from the base of the triangles. Two lines are then drawn from the tip of the horizontal line at an angle of 60° to a vertical line that bisects the horizontal line. These lines are of the same length and are parallel to each side of the rhomboid defect. The upper flap is mobilized because of the greater laxity of the upper nasal skin and because the resultant scar is more easily hidden.

Step 2

The skin and subcutaneous tissue at the base of the flap are undermined to enable it to stretch down-ward into the defect. The edges of the defect are also undermined. Buried 4-0 or 5-0 chromic sutures are used to secure the flap in position.

Step 3

The undersurface of the flap is anchored to periosteum to support the medial commissural tissues in an appropriate position in order to recreate its normal concavity. The nasal skin is closed with 6-0 plain sutures.

Step 4

A Telfa dressing with moistened cotton sutured over the medial canthus serves to apply pressure, avoid hematoma formation, and reform the concave contour of the medial canthus. Massage of the flap may be necessary to limit web contracture upon healing 2 months after surgery.

The technique may be modified for inferiorly placed defects in that the flap may be extended inferiorly by lengthening the vertical incision. To close defects that extend laterally into the upper or lower lid, the lateral lid skin can be undermined and pulled medially to join the rhomboid flap.

Tarsoconjunctival Flaps

Tarsoconjunctival flaps from the upper and lower eyelids are used to reconstruct the posterior lamella of the eyelid portion of medial canthal defects (Figure 38-5).[3] Local advancement flaps of skin and muscle from the upper and lower lids may be used to reconstruct the anterior lamella with caution to avoid vertical shortening of the lower lid and cicatricial ectropion. For this reason, a full-thickness skin graft may be necessary. The canaliculi may require reconstruction as well.

Step 1

After excision of the tumor, the remnant of the upper lid is everted on a Desmarres eyelid retractor after a 4-0 silk transmarginal traction suture is applied to the upper lid (see Figures 38-5A to 38-5C).

Step 2

The tarsoconjunctival flap is mobilized from the upper lid after incising the tarsoconjunctiva 3- to 4 mm above the eyelid margin and parallel to the eyelid margin for a horizontal distance necessary to reconstruct the lower eyelid medially with some horizontal tension to avoid postoperative ectropion.

Step 3

The medial aspect of the tarsoconjunctival flap is secured to the posterior aspect of the medial canthal tendon (at the level of the posterior lacrimal crest) and to the inferior periosteum. The medial tarsus of the lower lid is sutured directly to the lateral tarsal conjunctival flap (see Figures 38-5D and 38-5E).

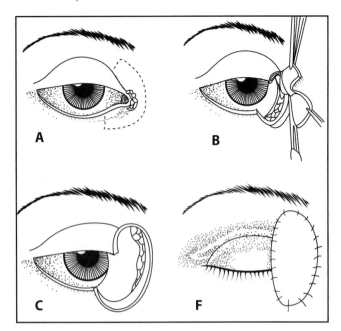

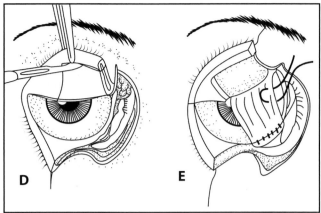

Figure 38-5. (Adapted from McCord CD, Wesley R. Reconstruction of the upper eyelid and medial canthus. In: McCord CD, Tanenbaum M, eds. *Oculoplastic Surgery Second Edition.* New York, NY: Raven Press; 1987:73-91.)

Step 4

A skin graft harvested from the left retroauricular skin is sutured to the skin edges and secured in place with sutures tied over Telfa and moistened cotton, 2 eye patches, and fluff that are secured by 1-inch tape (see Figure 38-5F). The flap is horizontally divided in 6 weeks to where the new medial canthal angle is to be.

CHAPTER 39

COMPOSITE ADVANCEMENT FLAP (CUTLER-BEARD PROCEDURE)

Richard D. Lisman, MD and Christopher I. Zoumalan, MD

The Cutler-Beard procedure is indicated in the reconstruction of large defects of the upper eyelid. Typically, defects of more than 60% of the eyelid require repair with this 2-stage reconstruction using full-thickness tissue from the lower eyelid.[1-4] In the first stage, a full-thickness flap from the lower eyelid is advanced posterior to an intact lower eyelid margin. This includes the conjunctiva of the lower fornix, deep tissue of the lower eyelid, and skin. It attains collateral vascularization and lengthens over a period of 3 to 8 weeks. In the second stage, the flap is divided at the level of the palpebral fissure, and the lower eyelid is reconstructed. The fornices are moderately foreshortened after this procedure.

Preoperative Contraindications

If a monocular patient's visually useful eye is involved in an upper eyelid defect, closure of that eye is performed only if no other alternative exists. In addition, if continuous local medication is needed for an ocular condition such as severe glaucoma, complete eyelid closure as part of a 2-stage reconstruction is performed only under exceptional circumstances. Prior use of the lower eyelid for a 1- or 2-stage reconstruction of an upper eyelid defect may result in a shortage of tissue for further reconstructive procedures. In these cases, alternative procedures such as midline glabellar and temporal transposition flaps may be the only options left to the surgeon.

Preoperative Indications

If a defect of the upper eyelid is large enough to prohibit primary closure, closure with a release of the lateral canthal tendon, or closure with the use of lateral canthal tissue (Tenzel or inverted semicircular flap procedure), a 2-stage procedure is indicated. Additionally, smaller defects in a previously reconstructed eyelid lacking ample adjacent tissue for advancement require a 2-stage procedure.

Anesthesia

The procedure may be performed under local or general anesthesia as indicated by the surgeon's preference and the patient's medical condition.

Surgical Procedure

In 1955, Cutler and Beard initially described the procedure for partial and total upper eyelid reconstruction. This technique is often called the 2-stage advancement flap, the bridge flap technique, the composite advancement flap, or the Cutler-Beard procedure.[1]

If a carcinoma is present in the upper eyelid, it is resected through the eyelid margin such that a margin of at least 2 to 3 mm of normal, uninvolved meibomian gland is excised on either side with the lesion. This may be done with a razor blade, a cataract knife, or scissors. A razor blade knife provides a straight cut edge on the uninvolved tarsal surface to aid in the subsequent upper eyelid reconstruction. Frozen sections can be taken from the host or the specimen. If a Mohs' fresh tissue technique has been used, wound margins are débrided and appropriately trimmed before reconstruction. The tumor-free recipient bed is prepared as illustrated in Figure 39-1.

Levine MR.
Manual of Oculoplastic Surgery, Fourth Edition (pp 247-252).
© 2010 SLACK Incorporated

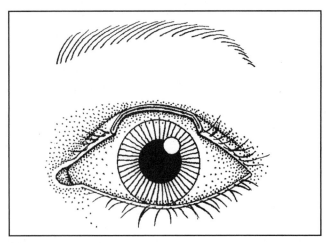

Figure 39-1.

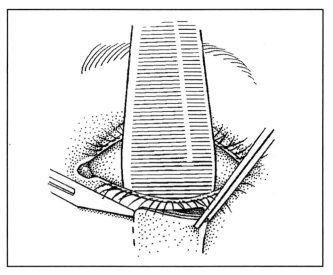

Figure 39-2.

FIRST STAGE

Skin Incision

Step 1

A corneal protective lens is placed on the globe, and 1% lidocaine (Xylocaine) is injected into the surgical site. Epinephrine 1:100,000 is also used for maximum hemostasis if the patient is not hypertensive.

Step 2

Initially, an attempt is made to minimize the size of the upper eyelid defect by bringing the wound edges together with 2 skin hooks. The residual width of the defect is then observed, and a marking pen is used to translate that distance to the advancement flap from the ipsilateral lower eyelid. The markings are made on the lower eyelid approximately 4 to 5 mm below the eyelid margin to preserve its marginal arcade, thus preventing ischemia of the remaining lower eyelid margin. The surgeon must avoid incision closer than 4 mm to the eyelid margin. Two vertical relaxing incisions are drawn from each side of the horizontal incision, extending inferiorly toward the inferior orbital rim (Figure 39-2). The advancement flap does not contain tarsus. The tarsus of the lower eyelid measures only 4 to 5 mm in height, and it remains with the lower eyelid margin to maintain stability. A number of investigators have proposed that additional tissue be inserted between the skin-muscle and conjunctival layers of the advancement flap as a substitute for upper eyelid tarsus and to lend stability to the reconstructed upper eyelid. Some authors believe that this substitution is necessary[5-7] and recommend the use of autogenous cartilage to recreate this skeleton of the upper eyelid. We do not believe this is necessary and have had success using the standard Cutler-Beard procedure.[6] Furthermore, we have observed eyelid necrosis with all types of tissue inserted into the flap, presumably compromising its vascular supply. Donor sclera has been used, with a few cases resulting in eyelid necrosis.

Advancement Flap

Step 3

To obtain a perpendicular incision in the leading edge of the lower eyelid advancement flap, the incision is created in 2 steps. The skin and orbicularis are incised with a #15 Bard-Parker blade, 4 to 5 mm below the lower eyelid lash line (see Figure 39-2). The eyelid is then everted on a Desmarres retractor, and the conjunctiva is similarly incised 4 to 5 mm from the lash line. A straight Stevens scissors can be used to join the incisions on either side of the eyelid, creating a perpendicular, full-thickness blepharotomy. It is important that the initial skin and conjunctival incisions are created the same distance from the eyelid margin so that they will meet in a perpendicular fashion deep within the lower eyelid. A Stevens scissors is used to lengthen the flap inferiorly with vertical incisions at each end of the blepharotomy. They should be directed toward the inferior orbital rim and slightly outward (medial and lateral) so that the flap's base is wider than the apex. This mobilizes more tissue for advancement superiorly. It is important to incise the advancement flap inferiorly, toward the orbital rim, because this flap must be further stretched over a period of 3 to 8 weeks, and a maximum amount of tissue may be needed for the second-stage reconstruction. If the vertical incisions are angled outward, some additional tissue is available to fill some or any defect created by canthal resections. The corneal protective lens is now removed, and the full-thickness advancement flap is placed posterior to the full-thickness lower eyelid margin (the "bridge"). The advancement flap is sutured directly into the upper eyelid defect in layers (Figure 39-3A).

Step 4

The flap's conjunctiva is directly approximated with the conjunctiva remaining in the upper eyelid defect. Interrupted or continuous 6-0 plain or chromic sutures can be used. It is often possible to locate

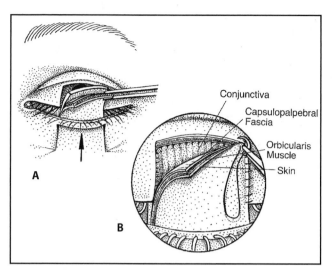

Figure 39-3.

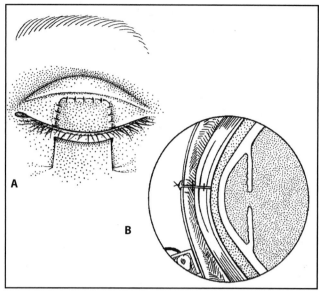

Figure 39-4.

fragments of the levator muscle or aponeurosis that have been left after the upper eyelid resection (Figure 39-3B).

Step 5

The levator or its aponeurosis is sutured to the capsulopalpebral fascia of the advancement flap just anterior to the conjunctiva. Three or 4 5-0 polyglactin (Vicryl) sutures are used for this closure. Skin is now closed with 6-0 nylon continuous sutures, and attention is directed to the eyelid margins (see Figure 39-3B). The nasal and temporal eyelid margins are sutured to the flap in a fashion similar to any eyelid marginal laceration: 6-0 silk sutures are used to approximate posterior and anterior margins of the approximated tissue. In simple eyelid lacerations, normal landmarks are observed; for example, the lash line, gray line, and mucocutaneous junction are easily approximated. In the advancement flap technique, the intact host lash line, gray line, and mucocutaneous junction are sutured with 6-0 silk to the corresponding anatomic locations within the advancement flap (Figure 39-4).

Occasionally, after upper eyelid reconstruction, the fine lanugo hairs at the new upper eyelid margin can result in trichiasis. Instead of advocating insertion of any foreign material to stabilize the eyelid margin, we prefer leaving the conjunctival edge slightly longer than the dermal edge to avoid trichiasis.

A significant amount of lower eyelid laxity must remain at the base of the advancement flap. The flap must pass easily under the lower eyelid margin and into the upper eyelid defect without undue tension to prevent vascular compromise of the bridge or advancement flap. Closure is not performed at the inferior base of the bridge; this site is left to granulate. If additional tissue is needed to restore lateral or medial canthi, the bridge flap can often be stretched in that direction. Surrounding tissue can be mobilized to fill the defect of the eyelid extremi-

ties. The first-stage reconstruction only places tissue into the defect, where the tissue is left to stretch and revascularize. If necessary, canthoplasty or additional surgical revisions are performed during the second stage. Only light dressings are placed on the eye in order to prevent vascular compromise of the newly reconstructed upper eyelid. Skin sutures are removed after 7 days, and the eyelid margin sutures of 6-0 silk are removed at 9 to 10 days.

SECOND STAGE

Step 6

The lower eyelid flap is kept in place for 3 to 8 weeks. Collateral vascular channels infiltrate the periphery of the flap usually in 3 to 4 weeks in a healthy patient. Additional time is needed only if the patient has an extremely tight lower eyelid (because of relative youth) or if there was prior skin damage (sun exposure, surgery). The purpose of the second-stage procedure is not only to open the eye, but also to restore and contour the upper and lower eyelids.

Opening the Flap

Step 7

A grooved director is placed beneath the advancement flap often through the nasal and temporal extremities of the eyelid palpebral fissure.

Step 8

A marking pen is used to locate the position of the flap at which a good upper eyelid height would be attained. It is much more advantageous to leave slightly more tissue on the upper eyelid, which can be trimmed later, because upper eyelid retraction and subsequent corneal exposure is difficult to treat.

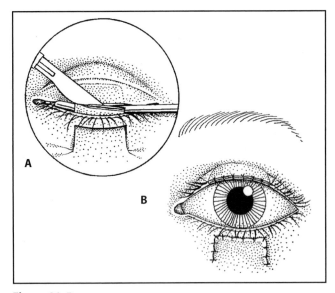

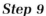

Figure 39-5.

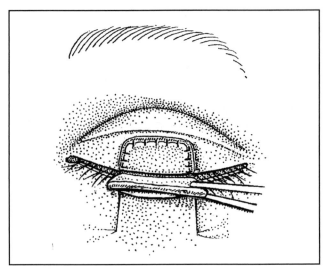

Figure 39-6.

Step 9

The skin of the flap is incised over the grooved director with a #15 Bard-Parker blade. This incision is not curvilinear. A straight cut produces a good eyelid contour with levator contraction. The initial incision is not full-thickness (Figure 39-5A). Sharp iris or blepharoplasty scissors are used to incise deep tissue posterior to the initial incision. A sharp, beveled cut can be created at the appropriate eyelid height. The iris scissors are angled slightly to bevel the incision, leaving the conjunctival edge more inferior than the skin edge. If the skin edge overhangs the conjunctiva, fine lanugo hairs from the advanced lower eyelid skin may produce a trichiasis that is difficult to treat. The conjunctival and skin edges can be loosely approximated with a running 6-0 plain suture or left unsutured to granulate within a few weeks (Figure 39-5B). Contour irregularities or excess length of the upper eyelid can be revised at a later date, often as an office procedure with the use of sharp iris scissors.

Restoration of the Lower Eyelid

Step 10

Attention is next directed to the restoration of the lower eyelid. The inferior border of the lower eyelid "bridge" must be denuded to allow for reapproximation to the incisional site. A razor blade knife can be used to trim this edge, which has by now granulated. The superior edge of the flap is sutured to the inferior border of the lower eyelid margin site if there is no subsequent formation of an ectropion (see Figure 39-5B).

Correction of Any Secondary Ectropion

Step 11

The lower eyelid can often undergo sufficient tissue loss, resulting in a cicatricial ectropion. This should be corrected at this time. Often, securing the lower eyelid with a tarsal strip procedure or other form of tightening procedure at the lateral canthus can restore normal eyelid positioning. Though not performed commonly, skin grafting or a suborbicularis oculi fat pad lift may be necessary if tissue loss is excessive.

Alternative Procedures

The advancement flap we describe involves only soft tissue without tarsus. As previously mentioned, we do not advocate "strengthening" the new upper eyelid with any tarsal substitutes because we have found that upper eyelid stability is acceptable without it. However, some surgeons believe that the traditional composite advancement flap technique of creating a new upper eyelid lacks appropriate stability. To reinforce the new eyelid, a number of alternative techniques can be used. For instance, advancing tarsoconjunctival flaps from the same eyelid, the use of autogenous cartilage, and, most recently, donor Achilles tendon have been reported as effective techniques. In contrast, donor sclera should be avoided because of the risk of antigenic reaction and eyelid necrosis resulting from the induced inflammation.[5-7]

Autogenous cartilage is used from either the posterior auricular area or nasal-septal region, and the tarsal substitute is placed anterior to the conjunctiva and sutured to the surrounding fragments of the eyelid that remain after the initial resection (Figure 39-6). Cartilage is sutured to the surrounding tarsal remnants with 6-0 or 7-0 silk interrupted sutures. The skin-muscle flap is then advanced over the cartilage and sutured into place as described previously. Donor Achilles tendon has recently been reported as an effective substitute to autogenous cartilage. Advancing local tarsoconjunctival flaps from the same eyelid has been reported with success. A free skin graft is then used to repair the skin defect.

Complications: Postoperative Management

As with any surgical procedure, the best treatment of a complication is prevention. Careful preoperative and intraoperative evaluation, coupled with a sound knowledge of anatomy and surgical technique, achieve this goal in most cases.

Necrosis of the lower eyelid bridge can occur if the incision is too close to the eyelid margin. The minimum amount of tissue that must be left at the eyelid margin is 4 mm, but 5 mm is preferred. This avoids damage to the marginal arterial arcade. The bridge should be manipulated as little as possible. If necrosis occurs within this bridge, the medial and lateral stumps can be left to granulate. At the second stage, these 2 ends can be reunited, often with the help of a lateral cantholysis or semicircular flap procedure.

Entropion of the upper eyelid rarely occurs, and it is not usually a result of instability of the eyelid margin. Thus, we do not advocate insertion of any tarsal substitute within the upper eyelid for routine Cutler-Beard procedures. Entropion can be prevented during the second stage of the procedure. The incision is subtly beveled so that the conjunctival edge rests more inferior than the skin edge. Granulation then occurs from posterior to anterior, forming the new mucocutaneous junction anteriorly on the new upper eyelid margin. This keeps the skin surface away from the globe.

However, retraction of the upper eyelid is a common complication. The flap can be reunited once again with the previous lower eyelid advancement flap and left in place for another 3 to 4 weeks to elongate the foreshortened upper eyelid. This complication may be avoidable with foresight and judgment. If uncertain, the surgeon can reconstruct the upper eyelid longer than intended with subsequent revision later if necessary.

Retraction of the upper eyelid can occur even if the advancement flap has been left long at the second-stage procedure. Furthermore, cicatrization with retraction is possible if the second stage was performed before appropriate development of peripheral vascular ingrowth into the flap. A loss of soft tissue can only be rectified by additional placement of soft tissue. This is a difficult situation to improve without resorting to reconstructive procedures such as median forehead, glabellar, or temporal transposition flaps.

Ptosis of the new upper eyelid usually spontaneously corrects with time as the upper eyelid tissue retracts. If this does not correct the ptosis, more tissue can be judiciously excised at a later time.

If the surgeon incorporates a posterior lamellar graft (ie, autogenous cartilage), it is safer to use these at or after the second-stage reconstruction. The advancement flap's vascular supply is compromised at the first stage, and necrosis of the entire new upper eyelid has been reported. This is a devastating complication, and reconstruction is largely limited to the use of multistage forehead flaps.

Lanugo hairs may still cause trichiasis even after a properly performed second stage. In these cases, the offending hairs can be removed. The affected skin can be surgically resected or treated with electrolysis. Either method removes the hairs and their follicles. This area is then allowed to heal by secondary intention.

Dry eye syndrome is commonly encountered after a large full-thickness eyelid resection. Production of all 3 components of the tear film decreases because of a loss of the accessory lacrimal glands, meibomian glands, and conjunctival goblet cells. Although the Cutler-Beard procedure shortens the superior and inferior fornices, dry eye syndrome is a common complication of this operation. However, care should be taken not to exacerbate a shortened fornix. If the second stage of the reconstruction yields a relatively ptotic upper eyelid, a dry eye is certainly less likely. Ptosis may not be aesthetically satisfactory for the patient, but it can provide a favorable environment for dry eye syndrome.

Prolonged postoperative edema is common after Cutler-Beard procedures because of extensive disruption of lymphatic vessels in the upper and lower eyelids. This resolves, but it may take several months to do so.

The lack of cilia along the new upper eyelid margin can result in aesthetic and functional problems. There is no mechanical barrier preventing debris from falling into the eye. Patients may complain of chronic foreign body sensation. Patients are remarkably comforted by wearing false eyelashes, trimmed to match any remaining upper eyelid cilia.

FREE TARSOCONJUNCTIVAL GRAFTS AND COMPOSITE GRAFTS

Gil A. Epstein, MD

Free tarsoconjunctival and full-thickness composite grafts are useful in eyelid reconstruction made necessary by trauma, tumor removal, or congenital coloboma. Free tarsal grafts have also been advocated in the treatment of severe cicatricial ectropion.

Tarsus provides eyelid support, and support is necessary when doing large upper or lower lid reconstruction. Obtaining tarsus by advancement, sliding, and transposition techniques as well as use of alternate tissue (cartilage, sclera) are discussed in Chapters 32, 35, 36, 37, 39, and 41.

The advantages of a free tarsoconjunctival graft in eyelid reconstruction include the following: (1) it is a one-stage procedure; (2) physiologic tissue is used; (3) there is minimal corneal irritation; (4) there is accordance of visual obstruction (especially useful in monocular patients); and (5) it is easily obtained. The main disadvantage is the availability of surrounding skin and orbicularis to provide vascular nourishment to the graft.

Composite grafts are full-thickness grafts, including lid margin. They are particularly useful in upper eyelid reconstruction but may be applied to lower lid repair. Advantages are similar to those for free tarsoconjunctival grafts; in addition, the eyelashes are preserved. Composite grafts may have a tendency to fail because of poor blood supply. The failure rate may be reduced by rotating or sliding a skin-muscle flap as a nutrient source.

Free Tarsal Grafts

Because the lower eyelid is too short vertically to be considered a donor site, the upper lid is the usual donor.

Step 1

Local infiltrative anesthesia or a regional frontal nerve block using lidocaine hydrochloride 2% with epinephrine is administered.

Step 2

A traction suture of 4-0 silk or equivalent is placed through skin, orbicularis, and superficial tarsus approximately 2-mm superior to the lashes. The eyelid is then everted over a Desmarres retractor, exposing the tarsoconjunctival surface.

Step 3

A horizontal tarsoconjunctival incision is made with a #15 Bard-Parker blade 4 mm from the posterior lid border with the aid of calipers. This approach avoids the marginal artery and still leaves the donor lid enough of the tarsus for support (Figures 40-1 and 40-2).

Step 4

Meticulous dissection between the anterior tarsus and levator superiorly is done with iris scissors. The levator aponeurotic attachments to tarsus should be avoided (Figure 40-3).

Step 5

Vertical tarsoconjunctival incisions are made with the scalpel corresponding to the recipient defect to be filled.

Step 6

When the superior tarsal border is reached, the graft is excised with scissors. Hemostasis is achieved with unipolar or bipolar cautery. I prefer wet-field bipolar coagulation because of less charring.

Step 7

The donor area is left to granulate and usually does so within 2 to 4 weeks. Topical antibiotic ointment is used, and the eye is patched for 24 hours. The defect should not be closed; otherwise, lid retraction or entropion may ensue.

Levine MR.
Manual of Oculoplastic Surgery, Fourth Edition (pp 253-258).
© 2010 SLACK Incorporated

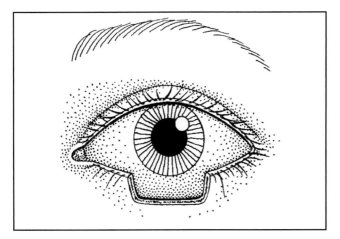

Figure 40-1.

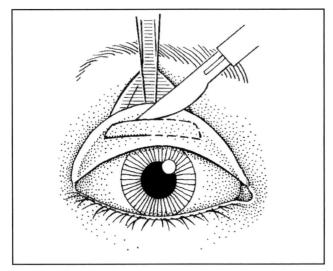

Figure 40-2.

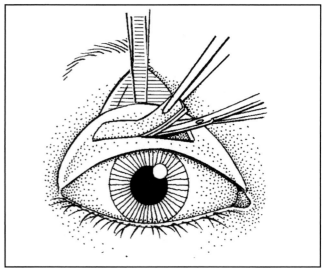

Figure 40-3.

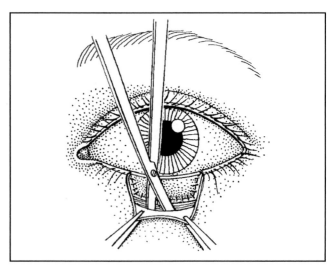

Figure 40-4.

Placement of the Tarsoconjunctival Graft in Eyelid Reconstruction

To survive, it is essential for the tarsoconjunctival flap to receive blood supply. Skin and muscle are rotated to provide nourishment. The defect size should be minimized so as to require as small an area of graft as possible. For lower eyelid repair, a canthotomy and cantholysis may be done. The following procedure is for a lower eyelid reconstruction.

Step 1

The tarsal conjunctival graft is placed with the conjunctival surface touching the globe (Figure 40-4).

Step 2

The vertical arms are sutured to adjacent tarsus with 6-0 polyglactin (Vicryl) or equivalent material. Care is taken to place these sutures intratarsally to prevent corneal irritation. If no adjacent tarsus is present, the tarsoconjunctival graft may be attached to the medial or lateral orbital rim with 4-0 Vicryl sutures. A periosteal hinge flap may be helpful in making the attachment.

Step 3

The inferior graft border is then united to conjunctiva, tarsus (if any remains), Müller's muscle, and capsulopalpebral fascia with running 6-0 Vicryl.

Step 4

The surrounding skin and orbicularis are undermined with spring or iris scissors, and a sliding or rotational flap is performed to cover the graft (Figures 40-5 and 40-6). If there is a skin deficiency, it may be necessary to perform a skin graft in the area where the sliding or rotating flap arose (Figure 40-7). In the lower eyelid, retroauricular skin is preferred for the free skin graft.

Step 5

Skin is united to conjunctiva on the new eyelid margin with running or interrupted 6-0 silk. Mattress sutures may be used to tack the skin flap to the tarsus.

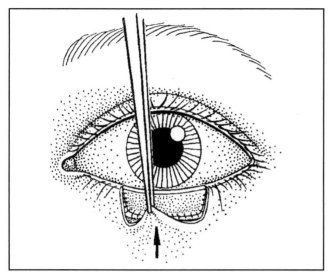

Figure 40-5.

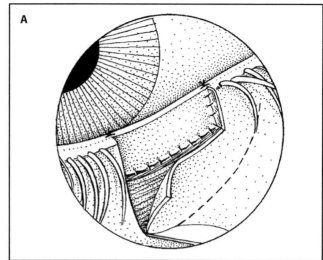

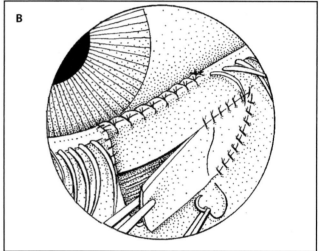

Figure 40-7.

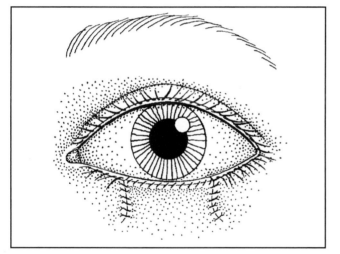

Figure 40-6.

Step 6

Antibiotic ointment is applied, and the eye is patched for 24 to 48 hours. If a skin graft was necessary, a Telfa bolster is used. Skin sutures are removed in 5 to 7 days. Upper lid defects may be handled in a similar manner as that for the lower eyelid. I generally prefer composite grafts from the lower eyelid or a Cutler-Beard procedure for large upper eyelid defects.

Use of Tarsoconjunctival Graft for Severe Cicatricial Entropion

A free tarsoconjunctival graft has been advocated in severe cases of cicatricial upper lid entropion. The graft may be harvested from the ipsilateral or contralateral upper eyelid. In either case, a 3- to 4-mm full-length graft is placed 1.5 to 2.0 mm superior to the mucocutaneous junction. Attempts are made to place sutures intratarsally or to externalize them to prevent corneal rubbing. The donor site is allowed to granulate spontaneously (Figure 40-8).

Composite Graft for Eyelid Reconstruction

Composite (full-thickness, including eyelid margin) grafts are particularly useful in upper eyelid reconstruction and temporal lower lid repair when a canthotomy and cantholysis cannot be performed. The viability of a composite graft is increased when a vascular supply can be provided. This usually takes place by rotating or sliding skin or skin and orbicularis over the tarsoconjunctival aspect of the composite graft.

The donor site usually is from the contralateral eyelid. Care is taken to preserve the tarsal contour and to maintain orientation of the lashes. If the defect is in the temporal portion of the upper lid, a nasal contralateral composite graft is preferred. Composite grafting may be done in conjunction with canthotomy and cantholysis if necessary. The following procedure is for an upper lid defect.

Step 1

The proposed donor site is infiltrated with 2% lidocaine with epinephrine.

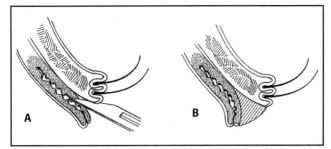

Figure 40-8.

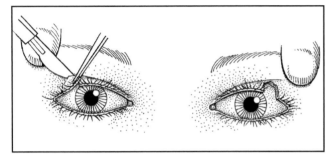

Figure 40-9.

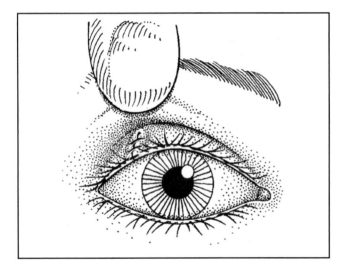

Figure 40-10.

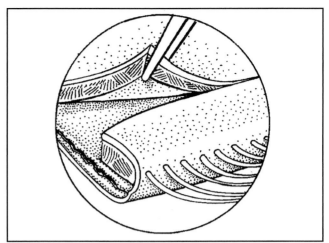

Figure 40-11.

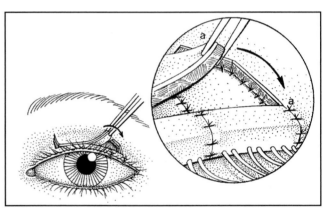

Figure 40-12.

Step 2

A #15 Bard-Parker blade or Stevens scissors is used to make a full-thickness vertical incision from lid margin to the superior tarsal border. A Westcott scissors is then used in an oblique direction to form a pentagon (Figure 40-9).

Step 3

The lid margins are then crossed to test the amount of available tissue. A canthotomy and cantholysis may allow a great horizontal amount of tissue. A scratch may be made so as to mark the point of overlap. Minimal tension is suggested for the upper lid, whereas more tension can be applied when dealing with the lower eyelid.

Step 4

The pentagon is completed with blade and scissors.

Step 5

The donor lid margin is closed with 3 6-0 silk sutures. The first passes through the anterior lash line, the second through the gray line, and the third through the mucocutaneous junction. The tarsus and levator are closed with interrupted 6-0 Vicryl sutures. The skin is closed with interrupted or running 6-0 silk sutures. The lid margin sutures are tacked to the skin surface to prevent corneal rubbing (Figure 40-10).

Step 6

The skin and orbicularis from the donor tissue are dissected and discarded, leaving 2 mm of skin and muscle from the lash margin (Figure 40-11).

Step 7

The graft is sutured with the colobomatous defect using the same procedure as in Step 5 (Figure 40-12).

Step 8

Skin and orbicularis are undermined and rotated or slid over the tarsal component of the composite graft (see Figure 40-12). A skin graft may be necessary if skin is deficient from the area in which the rotating or sliding flap arose (Figure 40-13).

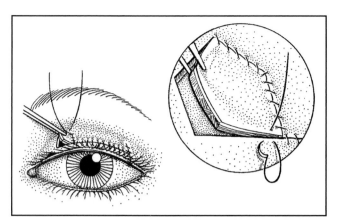

Figure 40-13.

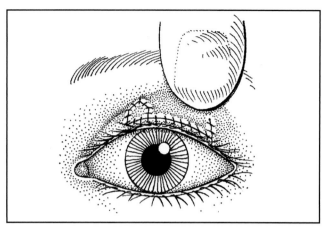

Figure 40-14.

Step 9

Skin is sutured to the flap with 6-0 silk (Figure 40-14).

Step 10

Antibiotic salve is applied to the donor and recipient sites. A light pressure patch over the recipient site is used. Ice may be applied to the donor site if bilateral patching is undesirable. When repairing lower lid defects, especially temporal ones, the composite graft may need to be anchored to the lateral orbital wall directly or with the aid of a periosteal flap using 4-0 Mersilene or 4-0 Vicryl sutures.

Complications

Complications of free conjunctival grafts are rare but can occur in the donor or host eyelid. Retraction of the donor eyelid can be attributed to the tarsal vertical shortening caused by cicatrix. Müller's muscle or levator may be resected, which could also lead to retraction. This can usually be avoided with proper dissection of the donor site. Upper donor eyelid retraction has been reported when the host ipsilateral lower lid has a traction suture placed within it, causing the upper lid to heal in a fixed position. A levator recession may be needed for upper lid retraction. Ectropion of the donor lid occurs when the graft is harvested too close (within 3 mm) to the margin and is substantially long horizontally. Horizontal shortening may be necessary to correct this problem.

Complications of the graft at the host site include separation, which can lead to lid malposition. Necrosis rarely occurs unless there is an inadequate blood supply or infection to the graft. This occurs more commonly with composite grafts. Notching of the lid, as well as trichiasis, is seen when there is necrosis or absorption of the graft. Providing good vascularity to the graft in the host site best avoids these complications.

CHAPTER 41

ADVANCING TARSOCONJUNCTIVAL FLAPS FROM THE SAME LID

Milton Boniuk, MD

In eyelid reconstruction in which primary closure is not possible, a variety of techniques can be used to repair the skin defect. These include free skin grafts, advancing vertical and temporal flaps, and a rotating semicircular flap.

For tarsoconjunctival repair, my preference is my own technique, which uses an advancing tarsoconjunctival flap from the same lid. I have used this technique since 1966 in more than 250 patients, with excellent results. This technique, in combination with a lysis of the lateral canthal tendon, can be used to repair defects of up to 60% of the eyelid. Other techniques include the Hughes tarsoconjunctival flap from the upper eyelid and the transpositional tarsoconjunctival flap from the upper to lower eyelid, free tarsal grafts, and the use of nasal cartilage. In addition, 2 techniques are available for combined skin and tarsoconjunctival repair: the tunnel flaps as described by Cutler-Beard and the use of full-thickness composite grafts from the opposite side.

In dealing with a lesion involving the lower lid, it should be excised and the margins evaluated with frozen sections. Once free margins are obtained, an attempt should be made to approximate and close the defect primarily with the help of a lysis of the lower arm of the lateral canthal tendon. If primary closure cannot be obtained and if there is sufficient tarsus in the adjacent eyelid, the patient would be an excellent candidate for an advancing tarsoconjunctival flap from the same eyelid (Figure 41-1A). The amount of residual defect is measured after an attempt has been made to approximate the margins with toothed forceps. The tarsoconjunctival flap used in repair of the residual defect should be 2 to 3 mm larger than the residual defect measurement.

Surgical Technique

Step 1

The lower lid is everted, and an incision is made through the conjunctiva and tarsus 2 mm from the lid margin and parallel with it (in using this procedure in the upper lid where more tarsus is available, this incision can be made 3 mm from the lid margin). This incision should be several millimeters longer than the defect to avoid tension on the wound.

Step 2

Vertical incisions are made through the conjunctiva and tarsus and are continued through the conjunctiva into the inferior fornix.

Step 3

The tarsoconjunctival flap is undermined from the overlying orbicularis, and the conjunctiva is undermined into the fornix so that the flap can be mobilized into the area of the defect. One must not twist or rotate the conjunctival flap, for it should be continuous with the conjunctival surface on each side of the defect (see Figure 41-1).

Step 4

Each edge of the tarsoconjunctival flap is attached to the adjacent lid margin with 2 or 3 interrupted 6-0 polyglactin (Vicryl) sutures (Figure 41-2). These sutures are placed so that the knots are tied superficially and do not irritate the cornea or ocular tissues. It is important that the sutures be properly placed, with good alignment of the new lid margin and no notching. If they are not placed properly, the sutures must be removed and replaced.

Levine MR.
Manual of Oculoplastic Surgery, Fourth Edition (pp 259-262).
© 2010 SLACK Incorporated

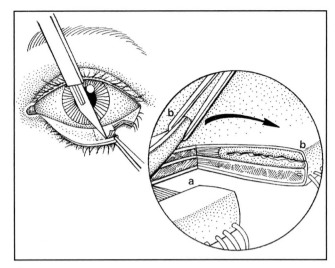

Figure 41-1.

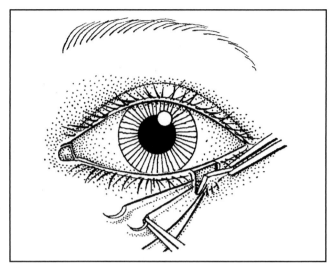

Figure 41-3.

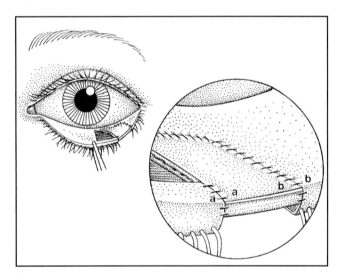

Figure 41-2.

Step 5

To obtain a better blood supply for the advancing flap, the lateral margin of the flap is sutured to the adjacent normal conjunctiva with interrupted 6-0 or 7-0 chromic catgut sutures. The knots are tied superficially so they will be buried and not cause any ocular irritation.

Step 6

In most patients, the skin defect is repaired with a free skin graft from the upper lid or retroauricular region (Figure 41-3). In selected patients, an advancing vertical or temporal skin flap or rotating flap of Mustarde can be used. For smaller skin grafts and flaps, I like to use interrupted 7-0 rather than 6-0 silk sutures because of the lesser reaction incited by these smaller sutures. In suturing the skin to the tarsoconjunctival flap, the skin should be allowed to remain 0.5 to 1.0 mm below the lid margin in an attempt to prevent keratinization and trichiasis at the eyelid margin.

Discussion

I first started using this technique for lesions involving the lateral aspect of the upper and lower lids in combination with some type of skin flap, mainly an advancing temporal skin flap. Vertical skin flaps are not recommended for the lower lid because of the high incidence of ectropion and lower lid retraction. These vertical flaps, however, can be used for defects of the upper lids in selected patients (Figure 41-4).

Initially, it was thought that a free skin graft might not survive over an advancing tarsoconjunctival flap because of poor blood supply. However, this has turned out not to be the case; graft viability has been excellent.

This technique can be used for lesions involving the medial or lateral canthal regions. In these cases in which the upper and lower lids are involved, tarsoconjunctival flaps can be prepared from the adjacent upper and lower eyelid (Figure 41-5). In some patients with large defects in the central portion of the upper and lower eyelid (50% to 60% defects), not enough tarsoconjunctival tissue is present laterally or medially. These defects can be repaired with advancing tarsoconjunctival flaps from the medial and lateral portions of the eyelid (Figure 41-6). The flaps are sutured together and then sutured to the medial and lateral aspects of the remaining eyelid as previously described. In addition to its use for malignant neoplasms, I used the technique in early 2002 with good results for a patient with trichiasis and entropion of the medial third of the upper eyelid associated with atrophy of the underlying tarsus. The atrophic tarsal tissue was excised, and the defect was repaired with an advancing tarsoconjunctival flap from the temporal lid. The eyelashes and lid margin were excised, and a vertically advancing skin flap of the upper eyelid was used to cover the skin defect.

Complications

Complications have been few in number and of minimal significance. Symblepharon can be avoided by keeping 2 raw opposing surfaces from each other. Suturing the

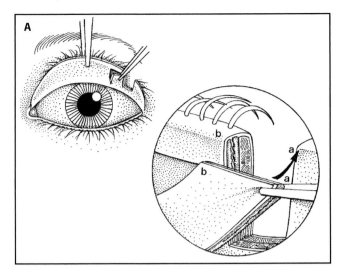

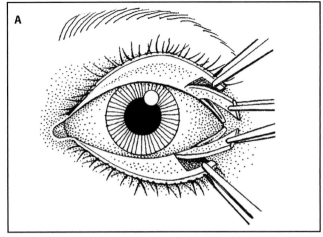

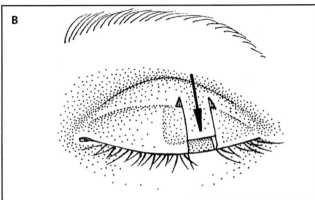

Figure 41-4.

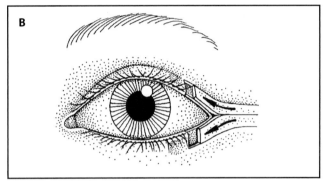

Figure 41-5.

distal margin of the tarsoconjunctival flap to the adjacent conjunctiva or temporarily placing a small silicone rod in the fornix at the time of surgery can help avoid this complication. With lower lid defects, there has been some slight retraction of the lower lid, but this can be avoided by using a flap that is only 2 to 3 mm larger than the forceps. Notching of the lid margin can be avoided in most patients by proper alignment of tissues and attention to suturing details. Trichiasis and keratinization of the lid margin can be avoided in most patients by suturing the skin flap or graft 0.5 mm below the edge of the tarsoconjunctival flap so that the lid margin may become epithelialized with nonkeratinizing epithelium. A few patients have developed pyogenic granulomas at the site from which the tarsoconjunctival flap has been obtained, but these have responded to topical steroid therapy or local excision.

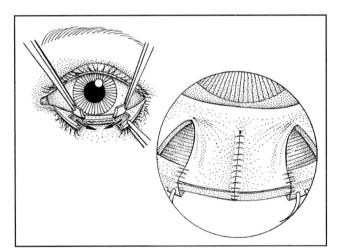

Figure 41-6.

SECTION IX

ORBITAL SURGERY

CHAPTER 42

ENUCLEATION

Jay Justin Older, MD and William P. Mack, MD

Enucleation is performed to remove a blind, painful eye; a traumatized eye; or an eye that is thought to harbor a malignancy. The goal of the surgeon is to remove the eye in the most appropriate manner (eg, remove sufficient optic nerve tissue if a retinoblastoma is present) and to create a socket that will accommodate a properly designed prosthesis. The best possible cosmetic result is achieved in cooperation with an ocularist, but the surgeon must also consider movement of the prosthesis and such potential complications as extrusion of the implant or a contracted socket. The technique presented in this chapter is designed to result in a good cosmetic appearance, as well as minimize such postoperative risks as implant extrusion and contracted socket. The characteristics of the ideal socket and eyelid on the anophthalmic side are (1) a centrally placed, well-covered, buried motility implant of adequate size, fabricated from an inert material; (2) deep fornices; (3) an inferior lid and cul-de-sac that can support the weight and pressure of a prosthesis; (4) a superior lid and supratarsal fold that simulates the fellow eyelid; (5) an anophthalmic socket that is on the same plane as that of the normal side; and (6) normal position of the eyelashes.

Procedure 1

Step 1

The patient is given a general anesthetic and is then prepared and draped in the usual sterile manner for eye surgery. Either one or both eyes can remain in the sterile field. If both eyes remain in the sterile field, the surgeon should re-examine the eyes before beginning the surgical procedure to verify that the proper eye is being removed. The surgeon may evaluate the position of the conformer by comparing both eyes at the end of the operation.

Step 2

The eyelids are retracted with a speculum or with sutures. A 360-degree peritomy is made at the limbus to preserve as much conjunctiva as possible and to permit adequate fornices in the anophthalmic socket (Figure 42-1). If a malignancy is present, for example, a ciliary body melanoma with possible scleral extension, the peritomy should be made in an area posterior to the ciliary body to prevent leaving any malignant cells in the conjunctiva that remain in the socket. In this case, the potential risk of a shortened socket should be outweighed by the potential gain of removing the entire tumor.

Step 3

Tenon's capsule is separated from the globe between the rectus muscles, but it is left attached to the muscles (Figure 42-2).

Step 4

Each rectus muscle is then isolated by passing a muscle hook behind it from either side. Once the entire muscle is isolated, a double-armed 5-0 chromic gut or 5-0 polyglactin 910 (Vicryl) suture is passed through the muscle in a serpentine fashion approximately 2 mm behind the insertion to the globe. The suture is locked on each side of the muscle. The muscle is then severed between the suture and the globe. The ends of the double-armed suture can then be used to retract the muscle away from the globe (Figure 42-3).

Step 5

After the 4 rectus muscles are isolated, tagged with sutures, and cut from the globe, the oblique muscles are located. A muscle hook can be passed in a posteroinferior direction on the medial aspect of the globe to find the inferior oblique muscle, which is

Levine MR.
Manual of Oculoplastic Surgery, Fourth Edition (pp 265-272).
© 2010 SLACK Incorporated

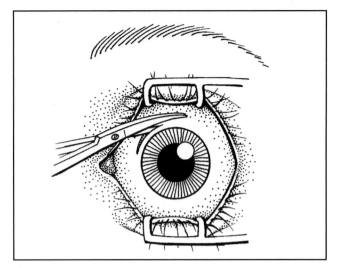

Figure 42-1.

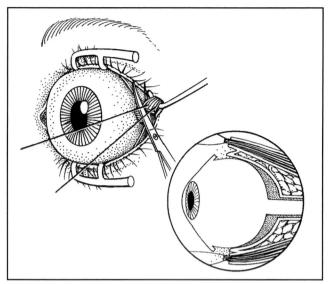

Figure 42-3.

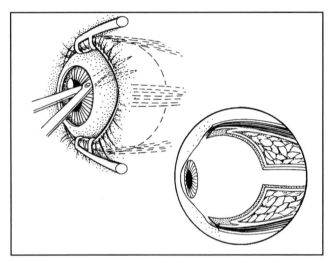

Figure 42-2.

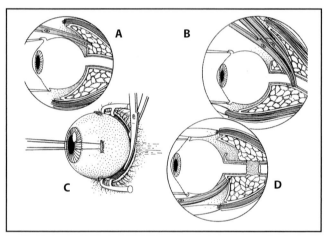

Figure 42-4.

cut and allowed to retract. Similarly, the superior oblique muscle can be approached by passing a muscle hook in the superonasal quadrant next to the globe. Once the tendon is found, the sheath and tendon are cut and allowed to retract. Next, 4-0 silk sutures are passed through the stumps of the medial and lateral rectus muscles. These sutures are used for traction when the globe is removed.

Step 6

Once the 6 muscles have been removed from the globe, another attempt is made to sweep the globe free of Tenon's capsule. A smooth instrument, such as a muscle hook, can be passed along the globe to ensure that Tenon's capsule is completely removed from the globe posteriorly to the optic nerve.

Step 7

Curved clamps can then be passed behind the globe and used to identify the optic nerve and its associated vessels by strumming the nerve. The clamps can be passed along the medial or lateral wall. When using the lateral approach, care must be taken to avoid penetrating the thin medial orbital wall with

the tips of the clamp. The clamps are closed over the nerve and its associated vessels approximately 3 to 10 mm behind the globe and left in place for 5 minutes. The surgeon can be reassured that the proper structure has been clamped by moving the clamps and watching the globe move in the appropriate direction (Figure 42-4A and 42-4B)

Step 8

The clamps are removed; a curved enucleation scissors is then placed such that it will cut the optic nerve and its associated vessels in the previously crushed area (Figure 42-4C and 42-4D). The globe can then be removed. Any other attachments that were not previously removed can be cut at this time. A sterile test tube with iced sterile saline is then placed in the socket to encourage vasoconstriction. This should be held in the socket under moderate pressure for several minutes. If bleeding persists, a clamp with a small piece of gauze can be inserted into the socket to aid in vasoconstriction by pressure. After the eye has been removed, the socket is irrigated with injectable gentamicin (Garamycin) solution and then rinsed with saline.

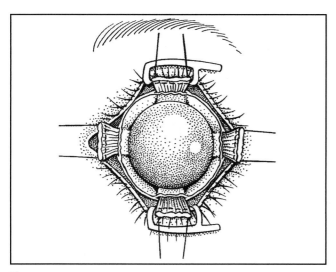

Figure 42-5.

Step 9

When hemostasis is achieved, a methylmethacrylate sphere is placed within the socket. Orbital fat should be seen through the posterior opening in Tenon's capsule. The implant is then placed through this opening into the orbital fat (Figure 42-5).

Step 10

Since the 1940s, various implants have been designed to fill the orbital space after enucleation. The implants with protuberances around which the muscles can be tied tend to have a higher extrusion rate than spheres. Although some surgeons believe that better movement can be obtained with these implants, many ophthalmologists achieve satisfactory movement of the prosthesis using spherical implants. To decrease the extrusion rate, some surgeons use dermis fat grafts to fill the orbit at the time of enucleation. We have not found the additional surgery required to obtain the dermis fat graft necessary because, in our experience, the synthetic spheres have had an extremely low extrusion rate. The implant we prefer to use is a smooth sphere made of methylmethacrylate or other inert substances.

Step 11

The size of the sphere should be such that when it is placed within the orbit, the muscles can be tied over the implant with no evidence of tension. If it looks as if the implant might "pop out of the orbit" and must be held down by tying the muscles firmly, it is either too big or there is significant orbital pressure because of swelling or hemorrhage. In our experience, a 16- to 18-mm methylmethacrylate or a 20-mm hydroxyapatite sphere is the appropriate size for most adults.

Comments

Recent oculoplastic literature has focused on achieving optimal orbital volume replacement after enucleation or evisceration to avoid superior sulcus deformity and enophthalmos. Research by Kaltreider et al[1] suggested the use of A-scan ultra sonography of the fellow healthy eye to provide a tool for correct orbital implant size to replace 80% of the volume removed at enucleation.

Further studies have shown that the ocular prosthesis should not be depended on to increase orbital volume, but instead the focus should be on the placement of the appropriate size orbital implant. Recently, an algorithm has been developed for use with the above-mentioned preoperative method of assessing the optimal orbital implant size through the use of preoperative A-scan ultrasonography of the fellow healthy eye (Table 42-1). This method allows space in the anterior socket for an ocular prosthetic volume of 2 mL when the orbital implant is placed posteriorly in the intraconal space.

Table 42-1

PREOPERATIVE SCAN VALUES

GLOBE SIZE	ENUCLEATION (MM)	EVISCERATION (MM)
A.L. <24 mm (hyperopes)	A.L. -3	A.L. -4
A.L. >24 mm (emmetropes, myopes)	A.L. -2	A.L. -3
Children	A.L. -2	A.L. -3

A.L.= axial length

As seen in Table 42-1, the algorithm divides the preoperative A-scan values into hyperopes and emmetropes/myopes for final orbital implant size calculations. The algorithm can be used for both adults and children for precise preoperative planning for orbital implant calculations for patients undergoing enucleation or evisceration procedures.

Custer et al[2] have focused on the volumetric determination of enucleation implant size. The volume of implant used should be equal to the volume of the enucleated eye (predisease if phthisical) minus the volume of the prosthesis. If the prosthesis size is 2.5 cc and the volume of an eye is 7.2 cc with an axial length of 24 mm, then the implant volume should be 4.7 cc. If spherical, the diameter is 21 mm (Table 42-2).

Globe volume - prosthesis volume = implant volume

7.2 cc (24 mm axial length) - 2.5 cc = 4.7 cc (21 mm diameter)

A scleral wrap adds approximately 1.5 mm to the diameter of the implant.

Table 42-2

CALCULATING IMPLANT SIZE

NATURAL EYE DIAMETER (MM)	NATURAL EYE VOLUME (CC)	PROSTHETIC EYE VOLUME (CC)	IMPLANT VOLUME REQUIRED (CC)	IMPLANT DIAMETER REQUIRED (MM) UNWRAPPED
20.0	4.19	2.5	1.69	15.0
20.5	4.51	2.5	2.01	15.5
21.0	4.85	2.5	2.35	16.5
21.5	5.21	2.5	2.71	17.5
22.0	5.58	2.5	3.08	18.0
22.5	5.97	2.5	3.47	19.0
23.0	6.37	2.5	3.87	19.5
23.5	6.80	2.5	4.30	20.0
24.0	7.24	2.5	4.74	21.0
24.5	7.70	2.5	5.20	21.5
25.0	8.18	2.5	5.68	22.0
25.5	8.69	2.5	6.19	23.0

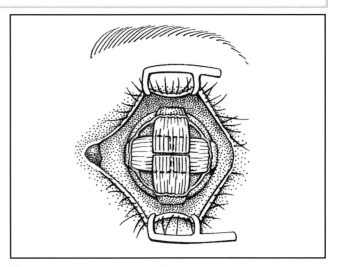

Figure 42-6.

Step 12

The muscles are then attached in the following manner. The medial rectus muscle is tied to the lateral rectus muscle in front of the sphere. The superior rectus muscle is gently advanced and loosely attached to the inferior rectus muscle. Ptosis may occur if the superior rectus is advanced too far inferiorly (Figure 42-6).

Step 13

The anterior aspect of Tenon's capsule is closed with interrupted 5-0 Vicryl sutures (Figure 42-7).

Step 14

The conjunctiva is closed with a running 6-0 plain gut suture (Figure 42-8).

Step 15

After the conjunctiva is closed, an antibiotic ointment is put in the socket; a small to medium conformer is then placed in the socket. The size of the conformer should permit complete eyelid closure with no tension on the fornices. With this method, the conformer does not cause pressure on the conjunctival wound or the closure of Tenon's capsule. The conformer should be transparent and have several holes at least 2 mm in size to allow for the egress of fluid. The surgeon can then examine the socket during the postoperative period without removing the conformer.

Step 16

The eye is then patched firmly with 2 or 3 eye pads. Unless there is some clinical reason to change the dressing sooner, the dressing is changed on the first postoperative day.

Step 17

Antibiotic ointment is continued for 1 to 2 weeks. The patient is examined periodically for 6 weeks, after which time the ocularist can fit the patient for a prosthesis.

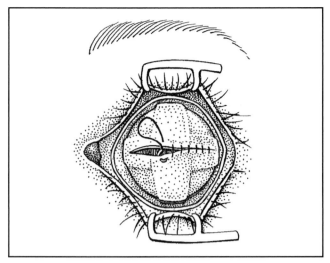

Figure 42-7.

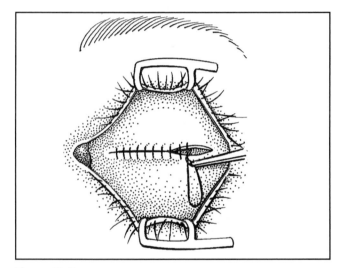

Figure 42-8.

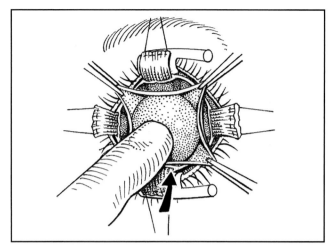

Figure 42-9.

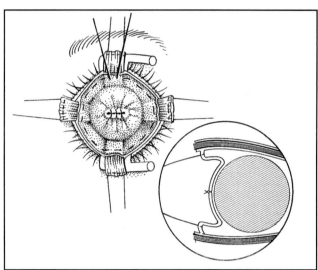

Figure 42-10.

Procedure 2

The ocularist may have difficulty fitting a prosthesis if the ball in the muscle cone migrates. Migration of the implant may occur inferotemporally or superotemporally. Moreover, faulty suturing technique or poor wound healing may result in a thinly covered sphere that has moved anteriorly. An alternative method is to place the sphere posterior to the posterior layer of Tenon's capsule within the orbital fat.

Steps 1 through 8

These steps are the same as in Procedure 1.

Step 9

A 16- or 18-mm sphere is inserted posterior to the posterior layer of Tenon's capsule within the orbital fat (Figure 42-9).

Step 10

The posterior layer of Tenon's capsule from around the optic nerve is then sutured over the sphere with 5-0 Vicryl sutures (Figure 42-10).

Step 11

The layer of Tenon's capsule immediately behind the rectus muscle is closed with 5-0 Vicryl sutures (Figure 42-11).

Steps 12 through 15

These steps are the same as in Procedure 1.

Procedure 3

HYDROXYAPATITE ORBITAL IMPLANT

Since the Food and Drug Administration's approval in 1989, the hydroxyapatite orbital implant has gained popularity as an alternative implant to the conventional methylmethacrylate sphere. Currently, hydroxyapatite is the most widely used orbital implant, with the most common varieties including Bioeye (Kolberg Ocular Prosthetics, San Diego, CA), Molteno MSphere (IOP Inc, Costa Mesa, CA), and the FCI3 synthetic hydroxyapatite (FCI Ophthalmics, Marshfield Hills, MA). The coral

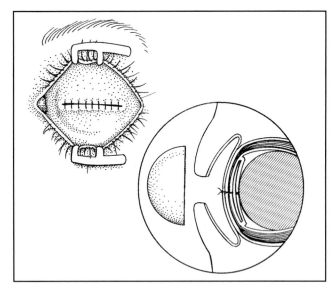

Figure 42-11.

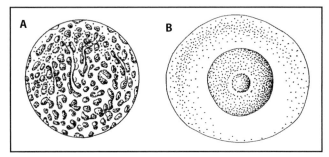

Figure 42-12.

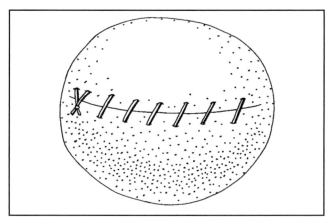

Figure 42-13.

line-derived hydroxyapatite sphere is an integrated implant that is designed to offer improved motility with decreased migration and extrusion rates.

The porous hydroxyapatite implant is derived from the skeletal structure of a specific marine reef-building coral. Hydroxyapatite is composed of interconnecting pores of approximately 500 µm in diameter. After implantation into the orbit, the interconnecting pores provide a framework for fibrovascular ingrowth, which is important for improved motility, decreased migration and extrusion rates, and, possibly, decreased infection rates.

In today's medical economic situation, a major disadvantage of the hydroxyapatite implant is the increased cost of the procedure. Alternative implants to the hydroxyapatite include porous polyethylene (Medpor) and bioceramic orbital implants.

Steps 1 through 8

These are the same as previously described in Procedure 1.

Step 9

Most adult patients can be successfully fit with a 20-mm hydroxyapatite sphere, whereas children may require a 16- or 18-mm sphere (Figure 42-12). The preparation of the hydroxyapatite implant involves wrapping a fresh or banked scleral shell, OcuGuard, or autogenous fascia lata, which has been soaked in antibiotics and povidone iodine,

around the sphere. Like donor corneal tissue, the banked scleral tissue is screened using a national protocol.

Step 10

A "baseball" covering is formed as the scleral shell is sutured around the hydroxyapatite implant with a running 5-0 Vicryl suture (Figure 42-13). Scleral tissue is excised anteriorly, forming 4 rectangular windows (approximately 6 mm x 4 mm) 90 degrees apart for attachment of the rectus muscles (Figure 42-14). A circular opening (approximately 10 to 12 mm in diameter) is also formed in the posterior aspect of the implant. These scleral windows are fashioned with the use of a scalpel to pierce the sclera and Westcott scissors to extend the excisions. Drilling 1-mm diameter holes through the implant windows into the core of the hydroxyapatite implant is advocated by some surgeons to stimulate more rapid vascularization.

Step 11

The hydroxyapatite implant is inserted into the orbit in the same fashion as a silicone or acrylic sphere. With the preplaced double-armed 5-0 Vicryl sutures, the 4 rectus muscles are attached to the anterior lips of the rectangular scleral windows (Figure 42-15). The 2 oblique muscles are attached directly to the sclera in their correct anatomic positions with 5-0 Vicryl sutures.

Step 12

Closure of anterior Tenon's layer is accomplished with 5-0 Vicryl sutures followed by closure of the conjunctiva with a running 6-0 Vicryl suture. A conformer is inserted, antibiotic ointment is applied, and a pressure dressing is worn for 1 to 2 days.

Step 13

Once fibrovascular ingrowth is complete, the patient who desires further motility may undergo a secondary drilling procedure for placement of a connecting peg. Some surgeons advocate that young children wait until at least 6 years of age before having secondary drilling, as cooperation with the

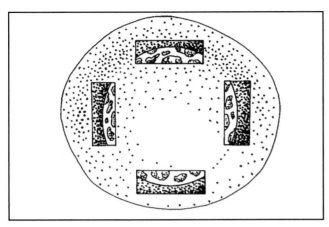

Figure 42-14.

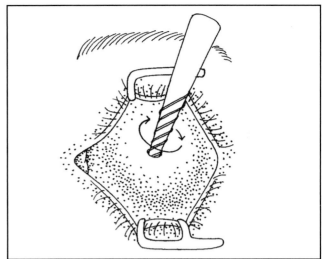

Figure 42-16.

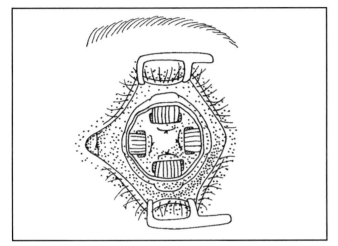

Figure 42-15.

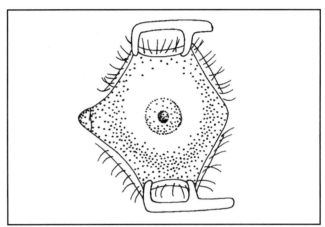

Figure 42-17.

ocularist is necessary for future revisions. Various radiologic studies have been used to assess fibrovascular ingrowth into the hydroxyapatite implant, including bone scans and gadolinium diethylenetriamine penta-acetic acid-enhanced magnetic resonance imaging. The timing of the secondary drilling is usually at least 6 months after insertion.

Step 14

The site for secondary drilling is marked in the center of the hydroxyapatite implant as the patient fixates with the normal eye in primary gaze. Local anesthetic (2% lidocaine with epinephrine 1:100,000) is infiltrated into this area. Conjunctiva and Tenon's layer are cauterized to expose the underlying hydroxyapatite implant.

Step 15

The implant is drilled with a 3-mm cutting burr on an electric drill to a depth of 10 to 11 mm (Figure 42-16). The hole is irrigated with balanced salt solution to remove debris, and a temporary peg with a flat head is inserted (Figure 42-17).

Step 16

After 3 to 6 weeks, the temporary peg is replaced with a permanent peg, which has a round head. The posterior surface of the prosthesis is designed by the ocularist to conform to the contour of the permanent peg, thereby establishing a "ball and socket" joint for improved motility (Figures 42-18 and 42-19).

Complications

Intraoperatively obtained autogenous fascia lata is an alternative to scleral wrapping of the hydroxyapatite implant if there is any concern of human immunodeficiency virus transmission. Although drilling holes through the implant windows may stimulate rapid vascularization, it also may contribute to implant absorption secondary to a foreign body reaction and volume reduction.

Critical care in suturing anterior Tenon's capsule over the implant, combined with vaulting the prosthesis, reduces implant exposure from the coarseness of the hydroxyapatite. Small areas of tissue breakdown may revascularize, whereas large defects may necessitate a fascial or scleral patch with a conjunctival flap. If ocular motility is satisfactory, a peg need not be inserted. If, however, a peg is placed, the drill hole must be centered to enhance movement. Excess motility may result in the

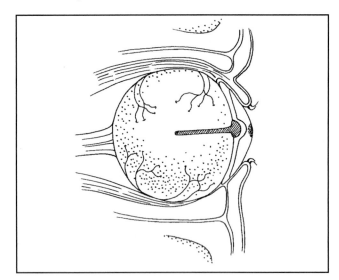

Figure 42-18.

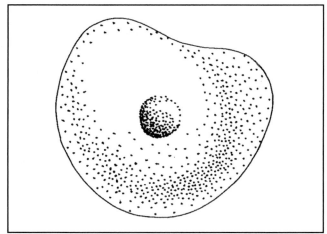

Figure 42-19.

roundheaded peg disarticulating from the depression in the prosthesis and may require a trough to keep the peg in track.

CHAPTER 43

EVISCERATION

Mark R. Levine, MD, FACS and John W. Shore, MD, FACS

Evisceration is a surgical procedure in which the entire contents of the globe are removed through a corneal, limbal, or scleral incision. The extraocular muscles are not detached from the sclera, and the optic nerve and its surrounding meninges are left undisturbed. Depending on the clinical situation, the surgical technique varies; the cornea may be removed (evisceration with keratectomy) or, less commonly, preserved (evisceration without keratectomy). Although most of this chapter is directed toward endophthalmitis, evisceration has become a much more commonly performed procedure today when dealing with the blind painful eye. This may occur following failed retinal detachment surgery, end-stage or rubeotic glaucoma, or trauma. Although sympathetic ophthalmia has always been an underlying concern, the incidence in modern ophthalmic surgery has been extremely rare. In addition, a shortened operating time, minimal orbital disruption, lack of implant migration, and enhanced motility makes evisceration an attractive alternative over enucleation. In any blind eye undergoing evisceration in which the fundus cannot be seen, a B-scan ultrasound is mandatory to rule out intraocular tumor.

Indications

When a diseased eye is to be removed, most ophthalmologists still perform enucleation. With enucleation, the histologic architecture is preserved, the likelihood of cutting through an undiagnosed intraocular tumor is reduced, and all uveal tissue is removed, thereby lowering the risk of post-traumatic or postoperative sympathetic ophthalmia. In the past, evisceration was reserved for cases of suppurative endophthalmitis or panophthalmitis in which there is no chance of preserving an intact functional globe. In this clinical setting, evisceration has several advantages over enucleation: (1) the meninges and optic nerve are not violated, thereby reducing the chance for bacterial seeding of the subarachnoid space and the development of meningitis; (2) drainage of the ocular abscess is performed quickly and easily with excellent operative exposure and superb visualization; (3) excessive bleeding from inflamed orbital soft tissues is avoided; (4) the sclera remains intact and serves as a barrier to progression of the suppurative process (although seeding of the orbit can still occur through emissary and vortex veins); (5) delicate orbital anatomic structures are not disturbed; (6) normal orbital physiology and full ocular motility are anticipated once the infection clears; and (7) the globe remains fixed in position by Tenon's capsule, the extraocular muscles, and the intermuscular septum, so that late migration of the orbital implant is rarely seen. These factors tend to enhance postoperative cosmesis and reduce the incidence of long-term complications of evisceration compared with enucleation.

When suppuration is severe, evisceration provides the surgeon with maximum flexibility. In the most severe cases, the wound is packed open and allowed to heal by secondary intention. Less severely infected wounds are initially packed open, but once the infection and inflammation have subsided and granulation has begun, the wound is closed (delayed primary closure). Wounds in patients with minimal suppuration can be closed primarily, although the risk of implant extrusion remains. Evisceration suffices in most cases of suppurative endophthalmitis, even when significant panophthalmitis is present. If, however, a frank orbital abscess is present, wide drainage of the eye and orbit is indicated. In this situation, evisceration can be combined with orbitotomy. Alternatively, enucleation (which by definition is orbital surgery) can be performed, the orbit widely drained, and the wound packed open.

Levine MR.
Manual of Oculoplastic Surgery, Fourth Edition (pp 273-278).
© 2010 SLACK Incorporated

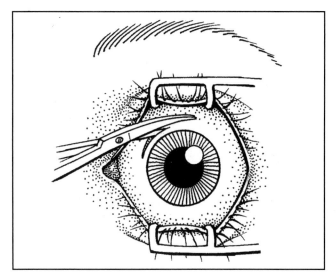

Figure 43-1.

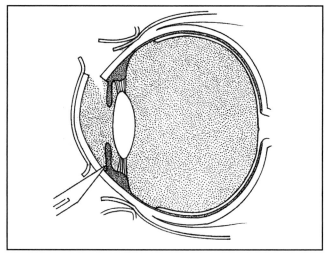

Figure 43-2.

Anesthesia

It is best to perform evisceration with the patient under general anesthesia, but monitored attended local anesthesia works well. A retrobulbar block and frontal block anesthesia must be used for intraoperative and postoperative pain management. This consists of 2% Xylocaine with epinephrine and 0.75% Marcaine. Sedation must be adequate to provide amnesia, because it is difficult to achieve total anesthesia with a regional block or local infiltration in the face of severe suppuration.

Removal of an eye is associated with significant emotional stress. The psychological trauma should not be ignored. Regional facial nerve block is helpful in producing eyelid akinesia and prevents voluntary and involuntary blepharospasm, which complicates technical execution of the surgical procedure. Perioperative antibiotics are indicated when evisceration is performed for endophthalmitis or panophthalmitis. Appropriate microbiologic investigation should precede the initiation of antibiotic therapy.

Surgical Technique

In most cases of evisceration for suppurative endophthalmitis, the corneal stroma is infected and often necrotic. In this situation, it is best to perform keratectomy in conjunction with evisceration. If suppuration is confined to the posterior segment and the cornea is relatively clear, it can be retained. We recommend keratectomy when there is any evidence of corneal infection. If keratectomy is performed, we usually delay closure of the scleral wound for 3 or 4 days to permit inflammation to subside and granulation to begin. Because granulation tissue is resistant to infection, delayed primary wound closure is safe and carries minimal risk of extrusion of the alloplastic scleral implant.

EVISCERATION WITH DELAYED PRIMARY WOUND CLOSURE

Step 1

An eyelid speculum is inserted to provide exposure of the globe. A 360° fornix-based limbal peritomy is performed 2 mm posterior to the limbus, beginning at the 12 o'clock meridian (Figure 43-1). The conjoined Tenon's fascia and conjunctiva are reflected centrally to expose the surgical limbus and can be grasped with forceps to place traction on the cornea during keratectomy. Posteriorly, Tenon's fascia and conjunctiva are separated and dissected off the sclera in 2 layers. The dissection is carried posteriorly to the level of the tendinous insertions of the vertical and horizontal recti muscles. Hemostasis is maintained with bipolar cautery.

Step 2

The sclera is penetrated with a sharp knife at the posterior surgical limbus, and the anterior chamber is entered (Figure 43-2). Care is taken to avoid penetration of the iris, ciliary body, or lens as the sclera is incised. Corneoscleral scissors or a razor blade knife is used to perform the keratectomy. The lens, vitreous, and uveal tract are exposed once the cornea has been removed. It is important to preserve the conjunctiva and Tenon's capsule along the posterior aspect of the wound because this tissue is used to reinforce the wound during delayed wound closure.

Step 3

An evisceration spoon or periosteal elevator, such as a Freer elevator, is introduced into the suprachoroidal space at the scleral spur. The uvea is elevated away from the overlying sclera around the entire inner surface of the globe (Figure 43-3). As the dissection proceeds posteriorly to the optic nerve, bleeding increases because the vortex veins and

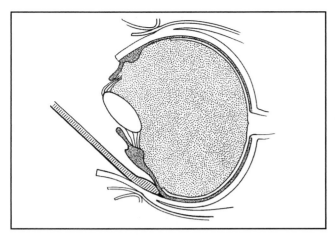

Figure 43-3.

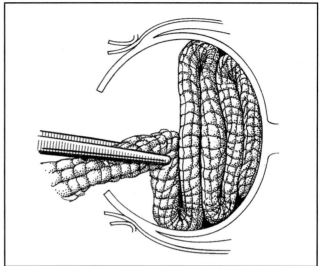

Figure 43-5.

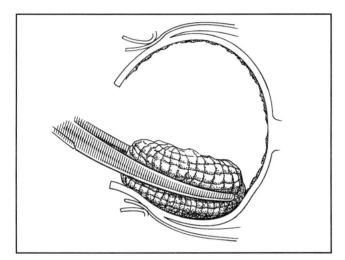

Figure 43-4.

the central retinal artery are severed. Hemostasis cannot be achieved until the entire uveal tract and retina have been removed. The uvea is firmly attached to the sclera at the site of scleral penetration of the vortex veins, at the optic nerve head, and at the scleral spur. These attachments must be severed if the uvea, lens, and vitreous body are to be removed. Once this dissection is complete, the entire contents of the globe are scooped out. All specimens (including the cornea) are submitted for cultures and histopathologic and ultrastructural examination, as indicated. Bleeding is controlled with surgical packing sponges. Surgical thrombin-soaked absorbable gelatin sponge (Gelfoam) and microfibrillar collagen (Avitene) may be used but usually are not required. A light application of bipolar cautery in the region of the vortex veins may be required. Cautery applied near the long posterior ciliary nerves is painful to the patient if the operation is performed under local anesthesia. Unipolar cautery should be avoided because the current can ascend the intact optic nerve, causing proximal axonal damage.

Step 4

Once the bleeding is controlled, residual uveal tissue is removed from the inner surface of the sclera with cotton-tipped applicators or a peanut dissector (Figure 43-4). It is not necessary to evert the sclera to get the uveal pigment off the sclera. The wound is vigorously irrigated with an antibiotic solution such as polymyxin (Neosporin) or povidone-iodine surgical paint mixed 1:1 with normal saline.

Step 5

The scleral shell is packed snugly with a long folded piece of iodoform-impregnated gauze (Figure 43-5). A light turban head wrap is placed to maintain pressure on the orbit. Intravenous antibiotics are continued and tailored to the culture and sensitivity studies previously performed. Dressing changes are initiated on the first postoperative day and continue twice daily under the umbrella of intravenous antibiotics. In most cases, suppuration and inflammation subside rapidly. The wound appears clean and ready for delayed primary closure within 3 to 5 days. A conformer is not used during the period of dressing changes. Oxidative débridement with hydrogen peroxide should be avoided. Frequent dressing changes provide the mechanical débridement necessary to clean the wound without disturbing the development of granulation tissue. The patient may experience some discomfort during dressing changes. During dressing changes, pain and anxiety are easily controlled with appropriate premedication.

Step 6

After keratectomy and at the time of primary or delayed primary wound closure, it is necessary to enlarge the wound slightly so that the proper sized scleral implant can be placed. After the packing has been removed from the wound, a 2-mm x 2-mm triangle of sclera is excised with scissors or scalpel at the 9 and 3 o'clock positions (Figure 43-6).

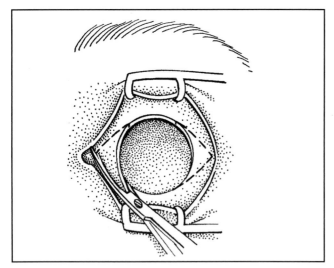

Figure 43-6.

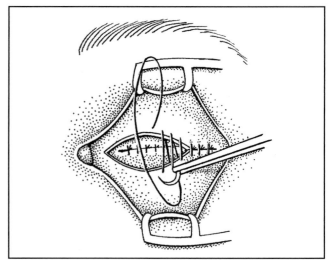

Figure 43-8.

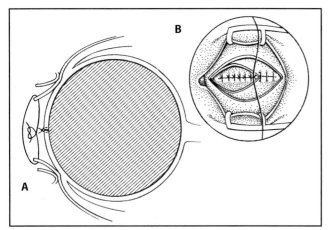

Figure 43-7.

Step 7

A 14- or 16-mm solid silicone sphere is placed within the scleral shell (Figure 43-7A).

Step 8

The sclera is draped over the implant and sutured with interrupted sutures of 5-0 polyglactin (Vicryl) (Figure 43-7B). Alternatively, a horizontal mattress suture technique can be used. If the scleral wound is closed under tension, extrusion is likely. The size of the scleral implant should easily approximate the wound edges and be large enough to fill the scleral shell completely.

Step 9

The conjunctiva and Tenon's capsule should not be incorporated in the scleral closure. Instead, Tenon's fascia is closed with interrupted sutures of 6-0 Vicryl, with the knots buried (see Figure 43-7B), and the conjunctiva is closed with a running suture of 6-0 plain catgut (Figure 43-8). Intravenous antibiotics can be discontinued at this time unless the clinical situation dictates otherwise.

EVISCERATION WITHOUT KERATECTOMY

The surgical technique for evisceration without keratectomy is almost identical to the procedure with keratectomy. Although this procedure was advantageous years ago when sclera volume was needed, the introduction of expansion sclerotomies has made this procedure less practical and eliminates the postoperative problem of potential corneal ulceration and necrosis with prosthetic wear.

Step 1

The peritomy is extended only 180°, centered at the 12 o'clock meridian. The conjunctiva and Tenon's fascia are reflected centrally and posteriorly as previously described; however, it is not necessary to separate Tenon's fascia from the conjunctiva because both are closed in one layer.

Step 2

Once the sclera has been opened, relaxing incisions are made at the 3 and 9 o'clock positions, so that the cornea can be retracted interiorly. A 4-0 silk traction suture is placed through the cornea at the 12 o'clock position, so that the cornea can be retracted to gain exposure during evisceration. The conjoined Tenon's fascia and conjunctiva attached to the cornea must not be damaged or torn because they are used to support the wound during wound closure.

Step 3

The residual uveal tissue is removed after evisceration as previously described. Some surgeons advocate scraping the endothelium off the posterior corneal surface. This is not necessary but can be accomplished with a #15 surgical blade or a clean, dry, cotton-tipped applicator, if desired. Delayed primary closure is not performed if the cornea is preserved; if delayed primary wound closure is indicated, keratectomy should be performed.

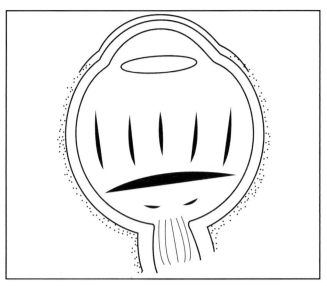

Figure 43-9.

Step 4

The wound is closed primarily after a 16- or 18-mm solid silicone sphere is implanted. Because the cornea is preserved, the globe can accommodate a larger implant. It may be necessary to enlarge the relaxing incisions at the 3 and 9 o'clock positions if an 18-mm sphere is used.

Step 5

The cornea is draped over the implant and sutured to the sclera with interrupted 5-0 Vicryl sutures. The scleral wound must be closed under tension. An implant of proper size must be chosen. The conjunctiva and Tenon's fascia are approximated in one layer with interrupted sutures of 6-0 Vicryl.

EVISCERATION WITH KERATECTOMY AND BORDERLINE TO SMALL SCLERAL POUCH

As mentioned, any kind of wound tension can result in implant extrusion. In these situations, a smaller implant may be placed or, preferably, the scleral pouch may be enlarged with expansion sclerotomies. The sclerotomies may be made vertically or horizontally in the equatorial portion of the sclera. This may be combined with removal of the sclera where the optic nerve enters the eye. These relaxing incisions nicely allow more sclera volume to house a larger implant and also encourage vascularization of porous implants if placed. Porous implants should not be used with any evidence of infection within the scleral pouch (Figure 43-9). In the event that expansions cannot house an adequate implant, the posterior sclera may be totally transected, and an alloplastic sphere placed in the intraconal space. The posterior sclera is closed with 6-0 Vicryl, and the anterior sclera is then closed with Vicryl, taking bites of posterior sclera to collapse it down and provide another barrier for extrusion. The conjunctiva and Tenon's fascia are closed in one layer with 6-0 Vicryl.

Postoperative Management

After primary or delayed primary wound closure, with or without keratectomy, a standard silicone or clear methylmethacrylate conformer is placed within the cul-de-sac to maintain the fornices. The conformer should not be so large as to put undue pressure on the suture line. A light pressure dressing is used to absorb drainage from the wound. The dressing is removed 24 to 36 hours after surgery. Topical antibiotic ointments are used daily to promote wound hygiene and comfort. Swelling is usually minimal and resolves within 5 to 10 days. When the wound is healed and postoperative swelling has subsided, a custom-fit prosthesis is ordered.

In postoperative evisceration cases involving blind, painful eyes, there is a lot of pain and swelling. This is best managed with no conformer, or the smallest one, as fornices have not been surgically disrupted. Medial and lateral suture tarsorrhaphies are performed with 6-0 silk, and a tight patch is applied. The patch is left on for 5 uninterrupted days, which will reduce the swelling considerably. The patch and suture tarsorrhaphy sutures are removed, a small conformer placed if not at the time of surgery, and antibiotic ointment without steroids applied, so as to not retard wound healing.

Occasionally, the conjunctival, Tenon's, and sclera suture line with keratectomy separates with implant exposure. This usually requires taking the patient back to surgery and replacing the spherical implant with a smaller one, or performing expansion sclerotomies if not previously done. The goal is to remove all tension off the sclera suture line with meticulous closure.

EXENTERATION

Charles B. Slonim, MD

Orbital exenteration is an extensive surgical procedure that involves removing the total soft-tissue contents of the orbit. This procedure is performed to prevent the spread of malignant tumors that have the potential to extend beyond their primary ocular or orbital origins.

An exenteration is classified by the amount of soft tissue that is removed. A total exenteration involves the removal of the entire orbital contents, including the periosteum, periorbita, and eyelids. A subtotal exenteration spares some of the periorbita, such as the eyelids, retrobulbar fat, or muscle cone. An extended exenteration involves the removal of the bony orbital walls and sometimes the sinuses in addition to a total exenteration procedure.

Indications for exenteration include malignant tumors of the eye and adnexa, malignant tumors extending into the orbit from its surrounding structures, mucormycosis and related invasive fungal diseases of the orbit, congenital deformities of the eye and orbit (neurofibromas), occasional cases of severe socket contracture, and severe trauma. Any invasive tumor that extends from the juxta-orbital structures into the orbit or that originates within the ocular or adnexal structures and extends outward into the orbit should be considered for this procedure. Other possible modalities of treatment should be considered before proceeding with this disfiguring surgical procedure. A reliable and definitive diagnosis of the pathologic condition must be obtained.

Surgical Procedure

Orbital exenteration is usually done while the patient is under general anesthesia and with the appropriate monitoring systems. Local monitored anesthesia using regional orbital nerve blocks (retrobulbar, frontolacrimal, infratrochlear, and infraorbital) and local infiltrative anesthesia to the anterior thigh for the skin graft along with moderate to heavy intravenous sedation can be successfully used. One gram cefazolin or 600 mg clindamycin (for penicillin-allergic patients) is given intravenously between 30 and 60 minutes before the start of the procedure for antimicrobial prophylaxis.

TOTAL EXENTERATION

Step 1

Two double-armed 4-0 silk bridle sutures are used to secure the globe anteriorly to the back of the eyelids (Figure 44-1). One suture is passed under the medial rectus muscle and the other under the lateral rectus muscle. The superior needle of each pair is passed full-thickness (posterior to anterior) through the upper lid tarsus approximately 1 mm above the lashes. The inferior needle is passed through the lower lid tarsus approximately 1 mm below the lashes and directly across from the upper lid suture. The ends of each bridle suture are tied securely over the lashes and lid margins. The ends of these sutures can be left long to serve as traction sutures later.

Step 2

A marking pen is used to outline the entire orbital rim as defined by palpating its entire circumference (Figure 44-2, solid line).

Step 3

The subcutaneous tissue below the outline can be injected with lidocaine 1% with 1:100,000 epinephrine mixed with 1:10 hyaluronidase to provide vasoconstriction and prophylactic hemostasis. A minimum of 10 minutes should be allowed for the vasoconstrictive effects of the epinephrine to occur.

Levine MR.
Manual of Oculoplastic Surgery, Fourth Edition (pp 279-284).
© 2010 SLACK Incorporated

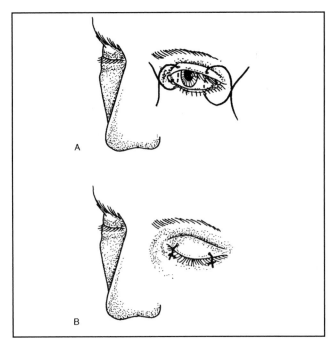

Figure 44-1.

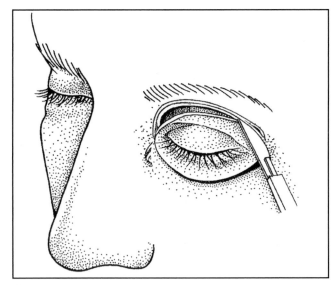

Figure 44-3.

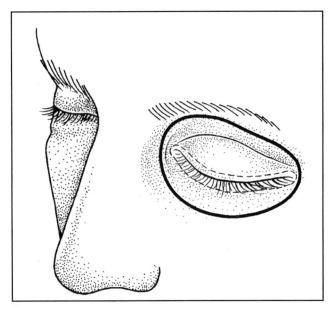

Figure 44-2.

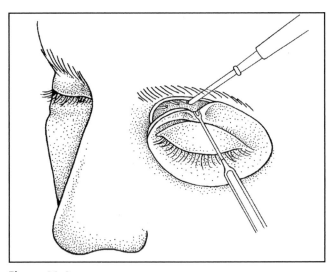

Figure 44-4.

Step 4

An Ellman Surgitron radiofrequency or other solid-state cutting needle or a #15 Bard-Parker blade is used to incise the skin as outlined by the marking pen (Figure 44-3).

Step 5

The subcutaneous tissue is dissected using the fully rectified current of the Ellman radiofrequency cutting needle or the cutting mode of an electrocoagulation unit. The Empire needle (Ellman unit) or the spatula blade attachment (electrocoagulation unit) gives better control of the cutting and a wider area of simultaneous cauterization. The cutting needle or blade should be held perpendicular to the

skin surface with its tip pointed toward the orbital rim below (Figure 44-4). Once the orbital rim is identified, the periosteum of the orbital rim can be incised with the Empire needle, electrocoagulation cutting blade, a #15 Bard-Parker blade, or a solid-state cutting needle (Figure 44-5).

Step 6

A periosteal elevator is used to elevate the periosteum from the orbital walls as far posterior as possible. Further hemostasis is achieved with monopolar or bipolar electrocoagulation or radiofrequency partially rectified current.

Step 7

At the apex of the orbit, a series of right-angled hemostats can be used to clamp the posterior structures before they are excised. This will help reduce the amount of bleeding as the tissues are cut. Identifying and clamping the optic nerve requires special attention. Visualization of the nerve, at this point, is difficult, and the surgeon must rely on the

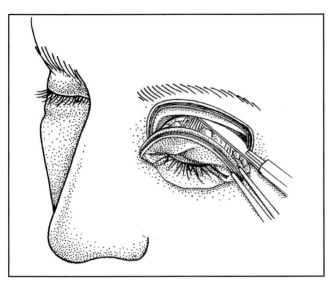

Figure 44-5.

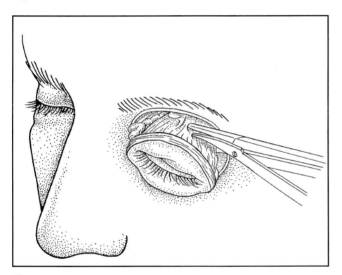

Figure 44-6.

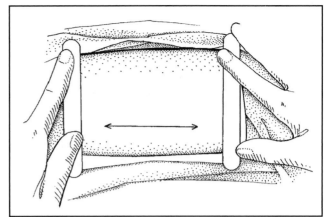

Figure 44-7.

movements of the globe as the nerve is grasped and moved.

Step 8

Enucleation scissors are introduced at this point to sever the optic nerve anterior to the clamp as well as the other soft tissues in the apex of the orbit, which may still have some attachments posteriorly (Figure 44-6). The entire soft-tissue contents of the orbit can now be removed, in total, and sent for further pathologic evaluation. Any remaining apical structure can now be removed by both blunt and sharp dissection. These specimens should be sent to the pathology laboratory separately from the large orbital specimen because these represent the deepest tissue margins to which a possible orbital tumor could have extended. Immediate frozen section evaluation of these deeper margins can be useful. If the results are negative for tumor, the surgeon can avoid removing the apical soft-tissue structures, which can offer the patient a better cosmetic result.

Step 9

The orbit is inspected for bleeding. Microfibrillar collagen, oxidized methylcellulose, topical thrombin, or other hemostatic agents can be used for hemostasis; however, they should be removed before a graft is placed. The orbit is then packed with a saline-soaked gauze pad while the skin graft is harvested.

Step 10a

If a skin graft is not to be used, bacitracin ointment is placed over the orbital walls. Three to 4 feet of petrolatum gauze (0.5-inch) is carefully layered into the entire orbit using bayonet forceps. Two sterile eye patches are taped securely in place after a liquid adhesive solution is placed on the skin around the orbit. This dressing should be left in place for 3 to 4 days after the surgery and changed daily thereafter. Granulation of the orbit will take 2 to 3 months. A delayed skin graft may be applied at a later time.

Step 10b

If a skin graft is to be used, a split-thickness graft will offer the best covering of the recipient site and the best healing of the donor site. A Brown dermatome can be used to harvest the graft from the donor site. This site should be prepared at the beginning of the operation and covered with a sterile drape as the exenteration is performed. With the patient in the supine position, the anterior or inner thigh will yield the best graft.

Step 11

A small amount of mineral oil can be wiped on the surface of the donor site. To ensure a thin layer of oil, the edge of a tongue blade is used to spread the oil along the skin surface (Figure 44-7). The skin graft must be smooth, thin, and uniform. The graft should be approximately 0.04 to 0.05 mm in thickness. This corresponds to a setting of 20 to 25 on the Brown dermatome.

Step 12

The surgeon must hold the dermatome in one hand while applying a flattening "pull" on the donor site

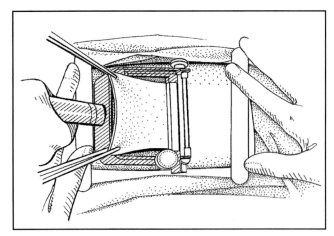

Figure 44-8.

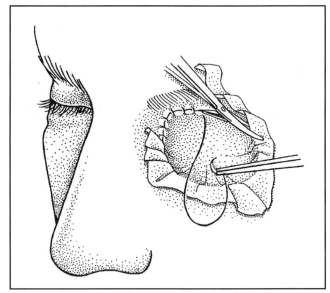

Figure 44-9.

in the opposite direction with the other hand. This can be done by pushing a tongue blade against the upper thigh and pulling superiorly. The palm of the hand with a dry gauze pad is also effective. The dermatome must be pushed slowly and continuously in one motion (Figure 44-8). A total graft length of approximately 10 to 12 cm is sufficient. An assistant can grasp the medial and lateral corners of the graft as it enters the back of the dermatome. This will keep the newly obtained graft from getting caught in the blade mechanism and also will give the surgeon an idea of the size of the graft. Once the appropriate size is obtained, the inferior edge of the graft is cut with a #15 Bard-Parker blade against the bladeguard in the back of the dermatome. The graft is then placed in a shallow saline bath.

Step 13

Attempts to stop the bleeding from the donor site are usually frustrating and do not have to be pursued. The donor site can be coated with a layer of bacitracin ointment and covered with Adaptic gauze. A Telfa pad can be placed over this and taped securely in place with some gauze padding. This dressing should be left in place for 2 to 3 days. When changed, the Adaptic gauze should not be removed until a good epithelium has regrown and the gauze can be removed without causing further bleeding. This dressing should be applied as soon as possible to prevent unnecessary bleeding, which can be difficult to deal with later in the case. If available, topical thrombin (THROMBIN-JMI Spray Kit) can be sprayed on the donor site, which usually produces immediate hemostasis. The donor site can then be covered with a Tegaderm transparent dressing. This dressing can also be left in place until a good epithelium has regrown. A Telfa pad can be placed over this and taped securely in place with some gauze padding. This outer dressing should be left in place for 2 to 3 days.

Step 14

The entire graft is draped into the orbital defect (Figure 44-9). Beginning superiorly, a running 6-0

chromic suture is used to attach the graft to the skin above the orbital rim. As the graft is sutured, the excess skin can be trimmed as needed. It is important to keep the graft deep into the orbital defect and not to allow the suturing to pull the graft away from the apex of the orbit. A saline-soaked cotton ball can be pressed into the orbit on top of the graft to keep it as far posterior as possible. Folds in the graft should be avoided and trimmed away as they occur.

Step 15

Once the graft is sutured in place, 3 or 4 drainage holes are made in the posterior part of the graft. These holes will allow any possible hemorrhage to seep through the graft instead of elevating it away from the recipient site. The holes can be made with sharp scissors. Care must be taken not to cut too deep; otherwise, bleeding might ensue.

Step 16

Bacitracin ointment is then placed on the graft. Three to 4 feet of petrolatum gauze (0.5 inch) is carefully layered on top of the graft to fill the entire orbit. A bayonet forceps is used to layer and press the gauze against the entire graft surface (Figure 44-10). Two sterile eye patches are taped securely in place after a liquid adhesive solution is placed on the skin around the orbit. This dressing is left in place for 5 days.

Step 17

The patient is placed on systemic antibiotics for 5 days postoperatively. Once the dressing and packing have been removed, the patient can be instructed to care for the socket. Cleansing with half-strength 3% hydrogen peroxide daily will help keep the socket clean and free of infection. Patients can normally be fitted with a prosthetic device in 2 to 3 months.

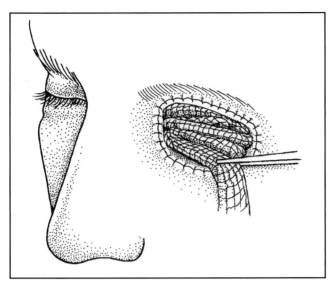

Figure 44-10.

SUBTOTAL EXENTERATION

If some of the eyelid skin can be saved, a subtotal exenteration can be performed. The eyelid margins, tarsal plates, and orbicularis muscles, however, must be sacrificed.

Step 1

Two double-armed 4-0 silk bridle sutures are used to secure the globe anteriorly to the back of the eyelids (see Figure 44-1). One suture is passed under the medial rectus muscle and the other under the lateral rectus muscle. The superior needle of each pair is passed full-thickness (posterior to anterior) through the upper lid tarsus approximately 1 mm above the lashes. The inferior needle is passed through the lower lid tarsus approximately 1 mm below the lashes and directly across from the upper lid suture. The ends of each bridle suture are tied securely over the lashes and lid margins. The ends of these sutures can be left long to serve as traction sutures later.

Step 2

A marking pen is used to outline the eyelid skin approximately 3 to 4 mm superior to the lash line of the upper lid and 3 to 4 mm inferior to the lash line of the lower lid. The lines are connected around the medial and lateral canthal angles (see Figure 44-2, dotted line).

Step 3

The subcutaneous tissue can be injected with lidocaine 1% with 1:100,000 epinephrine mixed with 1:10 hyaluronidase to provide vasoconstriction and prophylactic hemostasis. A minimum of 10 minutes should be allowed to elapse for the vasoconstrictive effects of the epinephrine to occur. This injection will also help create a tissue plane for dissection.

Step 4

An Ellman radiofrequency or other solid-state cutting needle or a #15 Bard-Parker scalpel blade or a solid-state cutting needle is used to incise the skin as outlined. The skin and orbicularis muscle are dissected anterior to the orbital septum until the orbital rim is reached. Vertical relaxing incisions may be necessary in the distal edges of these eyelid skin-muscle flaps to facilitate the dissection. Hemostasis is obtained using monopolar or bipolar cautery.

Step 5

As the skin is retracted, the surgeon can proceed with Step 5 of the total exenteration, as outlined earlier. The required graft will be smaller and its edges sutured directly to the skin of the eyelids as they are draped around the orbital rim into the orbit.

Common Complications

One common complication is harvesting the skin graft too deep. The dermatome must be set so that the dermis layer is not violated. This will result in exposed areas of subcutaneous tissue, which heal poorly. If this should occur, stop immediately and adjust the dermatome. At that point, the thicker harvested skin should be left attached to the unharvested donor skin bed within the dermatome. The harvesting can then continue to the desired length. The thicker portions of the final graft can be thinned out manually.

Another possible complication is graft failure. Areas of graft failure should be treated conservatively, as these "bare" areas of orbital bone will eventually granulate. Problems with wound healing are common in patients who have had previous radiation therapy to their orbits. Large epithelial bullae may occur and should be débrided along with any other dried secretions on the surface of the graft. Care must be taken not to elevate the graft from the recipient bed during this débridement. The graft over the nasolacrimal duct ostium may take many weeks or months to granulate and epithelialize.

A third common complication is folds in the donor graft. Any part of the graft that is not touching the recipient bed will eventually become devitalized and necrose and slough. It can then be removed during routine débridement.

CARUNCULAR APPROACH TO THE MEDIAL ORBIT

Robert A. Goldberg, MD

Several options are available to access the medial orbit in the subperiosteal plane. Traditionally, the cutaneous (Lynch) incision was used to access this space. The coronal incision also provides access to the medial subperiosteal orbit. However, these incisions create visible scars (particularly the Lynch incision) and require dissection through subcutaneous tissues, extending the operative time and prolonging postoperative recovery. The caruncular approach provides rapid access to the medial orbit, floor, and roof and avoids the need for a skin incision. Although the access is slightly more constricted compared to the wide open exposure provided by the coronal or Lynch incision, attention to the details of creation of the surgical wound allows adequate exposure for safe and effective surgery in the medial orbit, including orbital decompression, orbital fracture surgery and bony reconstruction, and medial orbital tumor exposure.

Operative Anatomy

The caruncular incision follows the plane of the posterior surface of the orbital septum, allowing the surgeon to remain posterior to the lacrimal sac (LS) and canaliculi (Figure 45-1). In the medial orbit, the septum is defined by its relationships to Horner's muscle (HM). HM arises from the posterior lacrimal crest and travels forward into the eyelids as it becomes part of the orbicularis sphincter. By following the posterior surface of HM, a plane that is easily entered by gentle blunt dissection, the surgeon is directed to the posterior lacrimal crest, the site of the initial entry into the subperiosteal space, and remains posterior to the lacrimal apparatus. The medial orbital septum is not a well-developed membrane. Therefore, some orbital fat usually spills into the surgical field. By dissecting as carefully and accurately as possible along the posterior

surface of HM, some elements of the fibrous orbital septum remain intact. The less the septum is disrupted, the more the orbital fat maintains some encapsulation, preventing widespread entry of fat into the surgical field.

The anterior ethmoid artery crosses the subperiosteal space 24 mm posterior to the lacrimal crest, usually at or above the level of the medial canthal tendon. In the subperiosteal space, it is identified as a fibrovascular band emanating from a depressed foramen in the orbital wall.

Anesthesia

General anesthesia is required for adults and children. Supplemental local anesthesia is achieved by injecting 1% lidocaine with epinephrine 1:100,000 mixed with an equivalent amount of 0.75% bupivacaine. An injection of 1 to 2 mL is administered to the medial bulbar conjunctiva, caruncle, and superior and inferior fornix.

Surgical Steps

CONJUNCTIVAL INCISION

Step 1

The conjunctival incision is designed to cut across the caruncle at its lateral one-fourth border. The incision should be adequately long: a common beginner's mistake is to make a short incision and then struggle with exposure later on in the case. The incision can be extended into the superior and inferior fornix to the level of the lacrimal puncta, so that the total length is at least 2 cm (Figure 45-2).

Levine MR.
Manual of Oculoplastic Surgery, Fourth Edition (pp 285-288).
© 2010 SLACK Incorporated

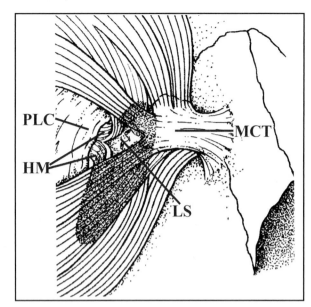

Figure 45-1.

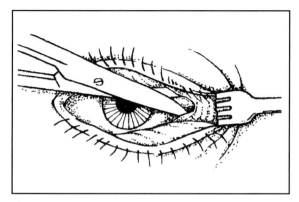

Figure 45-3.

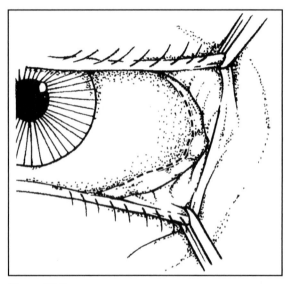

Figure 45-2.

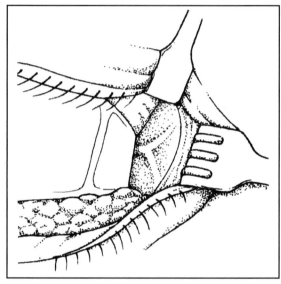

Figure 45-4.

DISSECTION ALONG THE POSTERIOR SURFACE OF HORNER'S MUSCLE

Step 2

After the conjunctival incision is made, dissection proceeds along the posterior surface of HM to the posterior lacrimal crest. The assistant can grasp the skin of the upper and lower eyelid adjacent to the lacrimal puncta to provide exposure. A few snips of sharp dissection through the subconjunctival fibrous tissue allow the surgeon to fall into the plane of the orbital septum. A blunt-tipped Stevens tenotomy scissors can then be gently pushed forward, palpating for the posterior lacrimal crest, which is identified as a "bump" on the medial orbital wall. If too much pressure is placed, the sur-

geon will push through the lamina papyracea into the ethmoid sinus.

Step 3

Once the scissor tips rest on the posterior lacrimal crest, safely posterior to the lacrimal apparatus, gentle spreading of the scissor tips on the bone creates a dissection plane within the orbital septum. The orbital septum is not well defined in this area, and extensive dissection or repeated entry into the wound can cause orbital fat to spill into the field. It is best to create the dissection plane with one single motion, avoiding removing the scissors from the surgical field (Figure 45-3).

Step 4

Without removing the scissors, a malleable retractor is passed along the scissors, so that no new plane is created, and then the scissors are withdrawn while the malleable retractor rests with its tip on the posterior lacrimal crest. The assistant can place a lacrimal rake in the medial cut's conjunctival edge to elevate HM on stretch and expose the wound (Figure 45-4).

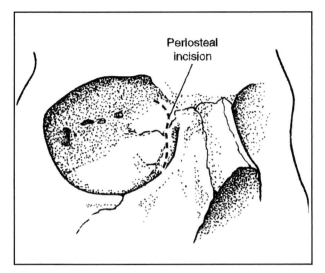

Figure 45-5.

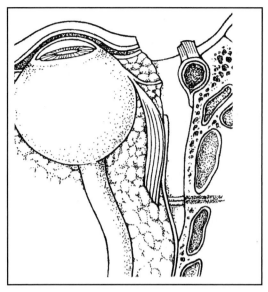

Figure 45-6.

PERIOSTEAL INCISION

Step 5

With some gentle blunt dissection using a cotton-tipped applicator, the surgeon can usually identify the white periosteum overlying the posterior lacrimal crest. This is primarily a blood-free plane, but focused cautery is sometimes needed to control bleeding from bony perforators. The periosteum over the lacrimal crest is incised using sharp dissection or fine-tip cutting cautery. It is extremely important to make an adequately wide periosteal incision. The most common error is failure to create an adequately large periosteal incision before entering the deeper orbit. The periosteum is incised sharply (a sharpened, round-tipped Tenzel periosteal elevator is a good tool for this) to create an opening of at least 2 cm; this typically extends superiorly just deep to the trochlea and inferiorly to the bony orifice of the nasolacrimal duct (Figure 45-5).

SUBPERIOSTEAL DISSECTION

Step 6

After the initial periosteal opening has been made, creating a subperiosteal plane is fairly straightforward (Figure 45-6). The caruncular incision allows wide exposure of the orbital roof and floor, for example, to visualize the stable bone in a large medial fracture. To access the deeper orbit, it is usually necessary to cut across the anterior ethmoid artery. The artery is seen as a fibrovascular structure emanating from a depressed foramen at the frontal ethmoidal suture; I often find approaching the artery from above, coming down from the frontal bone, is the easiest way to identify the structure in preparation for coagulation with bipolar cautery and transection. For the deepest cases, the same technique is used for the posterior ethmoid artery.

INFERIOR OBLIQUE

Step 7

The caruncular incision allows visualization of the medial half of the orbital floor. For wider exposure of the floor, or to create an incision that allows placement of a large implant for an inferomedial fracture, it is necessary to cut through the inferior oblique muscle. This is most easily accomplished if an inferior fornix incision and exposure of the subperiosteal floor is accomplished first. This then leaves a soft tissue bridge between the medial caruncular incision and the inferior fornix incision; this soft-tissue bridge contains the inferior oblique muscle and also the attachments of Lockwood's ligament along the posterior lacrimal crest and posterior edge of the lacrimal duct orifice. The muscle is identified, and an absorbable suture is placed through the muscle 3 mm from its bony origin. Then, the muscle is transected below the suture; at the end of the case, the preplaced suture can be reattached to the muscle stump (arrow). After the inferior oblique is cut, sharp dissection through the remaining fibrous strands of Lockwood's ligament (posterior to the LS and duct) joins the inferior and medial incisions in the subperiosteal plane, providing 270° exposure of the medial, inferior, and superior orbit (Figure 45-7).

CLOSURE

Step 8

Only the conjunctiva should be closed. If the initial incision passes through the caruncle, then a small yellowish portion of the caruncle remains in the lateral wound edge, serving as an alignment point for a single absorbable suture closure to the body of the caruncle. If needed, one additional interrupted absorbing suture can be placed superior and inferior to the caruncular suture.

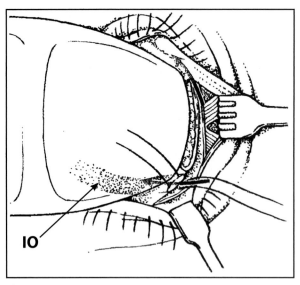

Figure 45-7.

Postoperative Care and Complications

Postoperative antibiotics are not indicated. In potential infectious cases, preoperative antibiotics can be used and continued postoperatively. Poor wound construction, particularly with maceration or damage to the conjunctiva, can lead to scarring, symblepharon, and even limitation of motility. Failure to follow the plane of orbital septum to the posterior lacrimal crest by passing through the orbital septum inappropriately anteriorly results in damage to the lacrimal system; in particular, it is possible to cut across the common canaliculus if the surgeon creates an inappropriate anterior dissection plane.

ANTERIOR ORBITOTOMY

Dale R. Meyer, MD and Thomas C. Spoor, MD

Anterior orbitotomy may be used to access the orbital space for a variety of indications. These include both incisional biopsy and for total excision of a mass, as well as for removal of a foreign body or drainage and culture of an abscess or orbital exploration for trauma or other considerations. The procedure and the placement of the incision are chosen to allow achievement of the surgical goal while minimizing the risk of injury to the patient. Preoperative computed tomographic (CT) or magnetic resonance imaging (MRI) scans, including axial and coronal views of the orbit, are useful to localize the mass (or other pathology) and determine its relationship to important orbital structures: the globe, the extraocular muscles, the optic nerve as well as the adjacent sinuses, and the brain. Proper preoperative localization and identification enable the surgeon to obtain appropriate consultations (eg, neurosurgery or ear, nose, and throat).

With the aid of preoperative CT or MRI scans, the surgeon must decide the goal of the operation and choose the appropriate surgical approach. Major operative complications (eg, blindness, diplopia, and hemorrhage) can be minimized by careful review of the relevant anatomy and attention to fine surgical detail; however, patients should be counseled that the close proximity of the normal structures to orbital pathology within the tight confines of the orbit entails such risks with surgery. Anterior orbitotomy may be used for incisional biopsy or for total excision of orbital masses. Anterior orbitotomy also allows access to the subperiosteal space for drainage of hematomas, abscesses, and sinus mucoceles or to the peripheral and central surgical spaces in the orbit (Figure 46-1). While the term *anterior orbitotomy* refers to anterior surgical approaches to the orbit, access to the middle and deeper portions of the orbit are nevertheless possible. In some cases, anterior orbitotomy may also be combined with a

lateral orbitotomy (with bone flap or removal) to facilitate exposing structures in the deeper orbit. Familiarity with various surgical approaches to the orbit, therefore, is thus essential for successful management of orbital disorders. Because incisions into the anterior orbit may result in visible scarring, the cosmetic effect of incision placement is important. Acceptable access to the orbit may be gained by a transconjunctival incision including a fornix approach (inferiorly) (Figure 46-2), or a partial or complete (360°) limbal conjunctival peritomy; or by transcutaneous (skin) incision including a subciliary incision (inferior orbit), lid crease or sub-brow incision (superior orbit), or Lynch (Z-plasty) incision (medial orbit) (Figure 46-3). A transcaruncular approach can also be used to access the medial orbit. This technique is covered in Chapter 45. Biopsy specimens of lesions may also be obtained with fine-needle aspiration with or without imaging guidance.

Preoperative Management

Blood transfusions are rarely necessary in orbital surgery; however, blood should be available for patients with low hematocrits or with vascular lesions if there is a high risk of significant intraoperative bleeding. For certain highly vascular lesions, preoperative embolization may be considered. Anticoagulants (warfarin [Coumadin]) and platelet inhibitors (clopidogrel, dipyridamole, certain nonsteroidal anti-inflammatory drugs [NSAIDS], and aspirin, or compounds containing hidden aspirin) should be discontinued before surgery if the patient's primary physician considers this acceptable. Certain types of orbital lesions may benefit from consultation with related specialists in the areas of otolaryngology, neurosurgery, and/or neuroradiology.

Levine MR.
Manual of Oculoplastic Surgery, Fourth Edition (pp 289-296).
© 2010 SLACK Incorporated

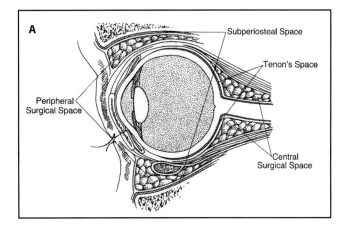

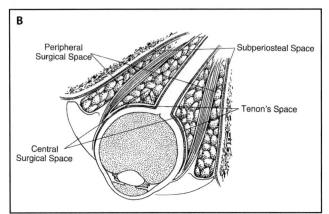

Figure 46-1.

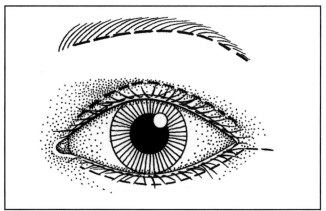

Figure 46-2.

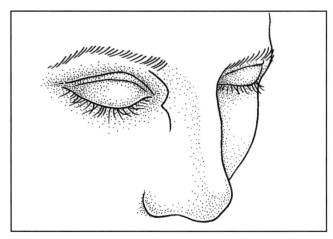

Figure 46-3.

Anesthesia

Most orbital surgery is accomplished under general anesthesia. However, surgery on some anterior lesions including straightforward excisional biopsies may be performed with intravenous sedation ("monitored anesthesia care") or even local anesthesia alone. Infiltrative anesthesia with agents such as lidocaine (Xylocaine) 2% with 1:100,000 epinephrine and bupivacaine (Marcaine) 0.75% allows both immediate and prolonged local anesthesia, enhances hemostasis and separation of tissue planes, and minimizes postoperative incisional pain.

The operative site is prepped in the usual fashion with povidone iodine solution or other suitable agent and is appropriately draped with sterile drapes and towels. If the paranasal sinuses are to be entered or if the procedure is expected to be long, prophylactic intravenous antibiotics such as 1 g cefazolin or 600 mg clindamycin can be given at least 5 minutes before incision.

Magnification and Illumination

Adequate visualization during surgery is important to permit safe access to the orbit, to preserve small vessels and nerves, and to maintain function. Consideration is given to fiberoptic headlight and magnifying loupes for orbital surgery and, in some cases, use of an operating microscope with coaxial illumination. A 200- to 250-mm objective replaces the usual 175-mm objective found on most ophthalmic microscopes. This increases the working distance and minimizes the risk of surgical site contamination. Appropriate microsurgical instrumentation and retractors facilitate orbital dissection.

Transcutaneous Approach

INDICATIONS

A transcutaneous approach allows access to the medial orbit, lacrimal sac, and frontal and ethmoid sinuses. The subperiosteal space may be entered, keeping the periorbita intact without violating the orbital contents. This approach is ideal for medial orbital wall fractures, external ethmoidectomies, transethmoidal optic canal decompression, medial orbital wall decompression for dysthyroid optic neuropathy, and drainage of subperiosteal abscesses and mucoceles of the frontal and ethmoid sinuses.

TECHNIQUE

Step 1

The area of incision is infiltrated with the anesthetic solution with epinephrine to reduce bleeding and minimize postoperative discomfort. Subperiosteal infiltration can facilitate dissection.

Step 2

An incision is outlined (see Figure 46-3) with a marking pen. A "Z" can be placed in the middle of the incision to prevent medial canthal webbing. Superior orbital lesions may be approached subpenosteally through a sub-brow incision made with a #15 Bard-Parker blade through skin and orbicularis to the level of the periosteum. Hemostasis is attained with a large bipolar cautery, and the wound edges are retracted with 4-0 silk traction sutures if necessary. An eyelid crease incision is a cosmetically acceptable way of approaching superior orbit lesions with excellent exposure. After the skin incision, dissection is carried superiorly beneath the orbicularis muscle. The orbital septum is opened, and the fat is pushed aside until the periosteum of the superior orbit is reached.

Step 3

The underlying periosteum is incised with a scalpel and dissected free from the underlying bone with a Freer elevator. The supratrochlear and supraorbital neurovascular bundles are identified and spared if possible.

Step 4

After the subperiosteal space is entered, blunt dissection is carried posteriorly. This is best accomplished with a blunt Freer elevator and a Fraser suction tip.

Step 5

The trochlea and its attached periosteum may be reflected toward the orbit if necessary.

Step 6

A Z-plasty incision through the skin and orbicularis carried down to the periosteum of the anterior lacrimal crest gives access to the medial canthal tendon. The medial canthal tendon can be disinserted by elevating it with its periosteum, or transected. If dissection is behind the posterior lacrimal crest periosteum, the lacrimal sac and insertion of the inferior oblique muscle will not be damaged.

Step 7

As dissection continues posteriorly, the anterior and posterior ethmoidal vessels are identified. They may be cauterized with bipolar cautery and transected or ligated with metal clips as necessary. The posterior ethmoidal arteries serve as a landmark for proximity to the optic canal and sphenoid sinuses. Dissection posterior to this landmark should therefore proceed with extreme caution.

Step 8

Subperiosteal lesions may be biopsied, excised, or drained. If an abscess is drained, a Penrose drain may be left in the subperiosteal space, exteriorized through the skin incision, and removed within 24 to 48 hours postoperatively

Step 9

Lesions in the peripheral surgical space may be palpated through the intact periorbita. After the lesion is localized, the periorbita may be incised with a curved #12 Bard-Parker blade or an anterior-to-posterior incision made with fine orbital scissors. When incising periorbita, one must avoid injuring the underlying medial rectus (medially) or superior rectus levator complex and frontal vessels (superiorly).

Step 10

The exposed lesion can then be dissected from the surrounding tissue using bipolar cautery and moist cottonoids or cotton-tipped applicators.

Step 11

After a biopsy specimen is obtained or the lesion excised, meticulous hemostasis is obtained with judicious use of cautery, and if necessary topical thrombin, absorbable gelatin sponge (Gelfoam), or other hemostatic agents.

Step 12

The periosteal incision is closed with 5-0 polyglactin (Vicryl) sutures. Orbicularis is closed with 5-0 Vicryl sutures with buried knots, and the skin is approximated with a 6-0 suture such as nylon, silk, or fast-absorbing plain gut.

The anterosuperior and superior lateral orbit can be approached in a similar fashion—placing incisions just below the brow (see Figure 46-2). The periosteum may then be incised and dissected as described, exposing intact periorbita and the subperiosteal space. Incision into periorbita exposes the orbital portion of the lacrimal gland. The lacrimal artery and nerves should be avoided. If deeper orbital exposure is necessary, the incision can easily be extended into a Stallard-Wright lateral orbitotomy incision and the lateral orbital wall removed.

Transconjunctival-Medial Orbitotomy

A transconjunctival-medial orbitotomy allows the surgeon access to the intraconal space in the anterior orbit and may be combined if necessary with a lateral orbitotomy to enhance visualization and access to the optic nerve.

INDICATIONS

The transconjunctival-medial orbitotomy approach permits access to the retrobulbar optic nerve for the purpose of optic nerve sheath decompression and to the central surgical space for excision of lesions located medial to the optic nerve. It also allows exposure of medially located lymphangiomas before vaporization with the CO_2 laser or treatment with other measures.

TECHNIQUE

Step 1

A sectoral or complete 360° conjunctival peritomy is performed, which allows the globe to slide freely under the conjunctiva and enhances exposure.

Step 2

The medial rectus is isolated with 2 muscle hooks, and a double-armed 6-0 Vicryl suture is passed through the muscle tendon just behind its insertion. It is tied and double locked on itself superiorly and inferiorly.

Step 3

The muscle is then incised at its insertion site ("disinserted") from the globe.

Step 4

Two 5-0 Vicryl or silk sutures with spatula needles are placed through the small remaining stump of the muscle insertion (globe), looped, and locked several times. Spatula needles minimize the risk of intraocular penetration through the sclera.

Step 5

These sutures are used to retract the globe laterally and may be clamped to the globe with hemostats.

Step 6

The medial rectus is protected with a cottonoid and retracted medially with a malleable or a Sewall retractor (Figure 46-4A). The long ciliary vessels are identified and followed posteriorly, and the optic nerve is located lying between them. The junction of the globe and optic nerve is typically obscured by orbital fat.

Step 7

A key point is that this fat may be packed off with moist cottonoids to provide adequate exposure of a lesion or the optic nerve sheath.

Step 8

Surgical procedure: After adequate exposure, encapsulated lesions may be bluntly dissected and removed (assisted by a cryoprobe if necessary), incisional biopsy may be performed, or the optic nerve sheath may be incised and fenestrated (Figures 46-4B and 46-4C).

Step 8a

In the case of optic nerve surgery, after the orbital fat has been retracted and packed with cottonoids, the optic nerve sheath dura and overlying vessels are exposed.

Step 8b

The short ciliary nerves and vessels must be dissected from the undamaged optic nerve sheath, allowing exposure of dura (see Figure 46-4C). This is accomplished with the operating microscope under high power using blunt orbital dissectors and nerve hooks.

Step 8c

The exposed dura is superficially incised with a fine blade (see Figure 46-4C). Entry into the subdural space is confirmed by the leakage of cerebrospinal fluid.

Step 8d

A blunt nerve hook is inserted into the incision, and the dura is tented away from the underlying optic

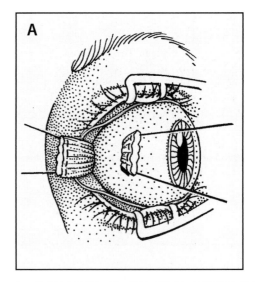

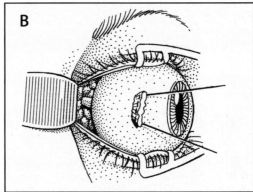

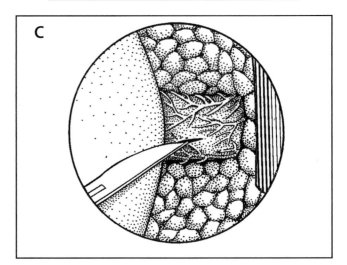

Figure 46-4.

nerve. A portion of the tented dura is excised with long Vannas or Greishaber scissors (Figure 46-4D). The amount of dura excised varies among surgeons.

Step 9

Meticulous hemostasis is obtained with the bipolar cautery and additional hemostatic agents as needed.

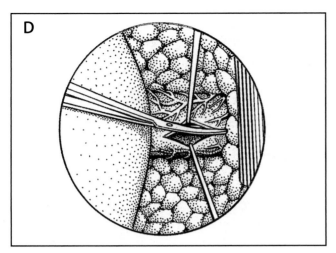

Figure 46-4.

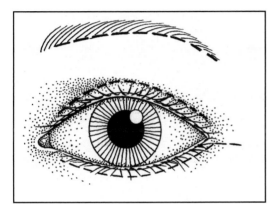

Figure 46-5.

Step 10

The medial rectus is reattached to its insertion site with the 6-0 Vicryl suture, and the conjunctiva is closed with buried 7-0 Vicryl sutures.

Inferior Orbitotomy

The inferior orbit may be approached through a subciliary (blepharoplasty) type of incision or transconjunctivally through the fornix (Figures 46-5 and 46-6). Indications for inferior orbitotomy include repair of an orbital floor fracture, 2-wall orbital decompression for dysthyroid orbitopathy, or lesions in the inferior orbit.

SUBCILIARY SKIN INCISION

Step 1

A subciliary incision is outlined approximately 2 mm below the lid margin and extended into the lateral canthal region hidden in a facial expression line. Excessive lid edema has not been a problem when this incision is kept close to the lid margin.

Step 2

A skin-muscle incision is initiated with a scalpel and completed with scissors and extended along the entire incision line.

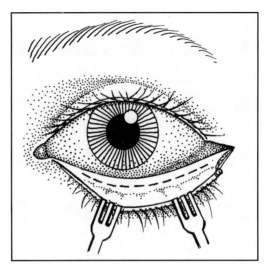

Figure 46-6.

Step 3

A 4-0 black silk suture is passed through the lid margin medially and laterally and is used to place the lid on upward traction.

Step 4

A Westcott or Stevens scissors is used to buttonhole the orbicularis at the lateral portion of the incision.

Step 5

The scissors or a hemostat is passed into the buttonhole and spread, developing a skin-muscle flap anterior to the orbital septum. Scissors are then used to incise the subciliary incision and any areas of adherence between the skin-muscle flap and the underlying orbital septum. Dissection is continued with scissors in the preseptal plane until the inferior orbital rim is exposed.

Step 6

The skin-muscle flap is retracted with Ragnell retractors. Tissue overlying the orbital rim is removed by rubbing with cotton-tipped applicators or a piece of 4 x 4 gauze, which exposes the periosteum.

Step 7

While the globe and orbital contents are protected with a large malleable retractor, the periosteum is incised with a #15 Bard-Parker blade approximately 2 mm from the rim. The surgeon must take care to avoid the infraorbital nerve exiting the infraorbital foramen on the surface of the maxillary bone. This foramen usually lies 5 to 7 mm inferior to the orbital rim but may be variable and is closer to the rim in children.

Step 8

The periosteum is dissected over the orbital rim using a Freer elevator. The periosteum is densely adherent on the anterior surface of the maxilla but loosely adherent along the floor of the orbit.

Step 9

Surgical procedure: The inferior orbital subperiosteal space is now entered. The lacrimal sac and nasolacrimal duct lie well anteromedially. The course of the infraorbital neurovascular bundle is identified. The location of the neurovascular bundle may be variable, but it is usually manifest as a bluish bulge of the mid portion of the orbital floor. The inferior orbital fissure lies posteriorly and laterally approximately 15 to 20 mm from the rim. It is best preserved. Once the floor of the orbit is exposed and the landmarks are identified, a 4-0 Vicryl suture may be placed into the periorbita for retraction, and the surgical procedure—be it tumor removal, orbital decompression, or fracture repair—continues.

Step 10

At the conclusion of the surgical procedure, after perfect hemostasis has been obtained with bipolar cautery and additional measures as needed, the periosteum is closed with interrupted 5-0 Vicryl sutures.

Step 11

The skin-muscle flap may be trimmed of redundant orbicularis along the incision site to prevent bulging and wadding of the incision.

Step 12

The incision is closed with running or interrupted 6-0 nylon, silk, or absorbable suture. A double-armed 4-0 black silk suture can be placed through the lid margin, and the lid placed on upward traction by taping the suture to the forehead if desired to help protect the ocular surface and lessen the potential for postoperative lid retraction.

FORNIX CONJUNCTIVAL INCISION

Access to the floor of the orbit may also be obtained transconjunctivally through the fornix (see Figure 46-6). This incision may be combined with a Berke-type lateral orbitotomy incision to expose the deep, inferior orbit.

Step 1

A lateral canthotomy and inferior cantholysis are performed by clamping the lateral canthus with a hemostat and cutting with scissors.

Step 2

The inferior lateral lid margin is then retracted, exposing the inferior crus of the lateral canthal tendon, which is incised with scissors. The lid can be felt to loosen when cantholysis is accomplished, allowing it to "swing out."

Step 3

A 4-0 silk suture is placed through the lateral portion of the lower lid, which is retracted inferiorly.

Step 4

The fornix is injected with local anesthetic, and the conjunctiva is incised with scissors from lateral canthus to the punctum.

Step 5

The incision is continued deeply through the retractors of the lower lid, and the inferior orbital rim is exposed.

Step 6

The periosteum is then incised and dissected as described previously.

Step 7

At the conclusion of the operation, after closure of the periosteum, the conjunctiva is closed with interrupted or running 6-0 absorbable suture.

Step 8

The lateral canthal tendon is reapproximated with a 5-0 suture. Some surgeons prefer a permanent suture such as polypropylene (Prolene), while others prefer an absorbable such as 5-0 polyglycolic acid (Dexon) or polyglactin (Vicryl) suture. The lateral canthotomy is closed with interrupted 6-0 absorbable sutures. A 4-0 double-armed silk suture can be placed through the lid margin and taped to the forehead, placing upward traction on the eyelid for 24 to 48 hours as previously described; however, the incidence of postoperative lower lid retraction appears to be less with a transconjunctival approach.

TRANS-SEPTAL SKIN INCISIONS

Lesions palpable through the eyelids may be biopsied or removed via a trans-septal approach. This allows direct entry into the peripheral surgical space. Such an approach is useful for excision or biopsy of hemangiomas; lymphomas; and lacrimal gland, dermoid, and epidermoid cysts.

LOWER EYELID

Step 1

In the lower lid, the subciliary blepharoplasty incision is used, and a skin-muscle flap is developed. Gentle pressure on the globe allows prolapse of the orbital fat and septum.

Step 2

The septum is incised and opened along its entire horizontal length.

Step 3

The lesion is then prolapsed forward and dissected free from surrounding structures. The inferior oblique muscle should be avoided. The lesion is dissected using techniques in Transconjunctival-Medial Orbitotomy, Step 8, described on p. 292.

Step 4

At the conclusion of the procedure, the skin-muscle flap is trimmed superiorly and closed with 6-0 absorbable suture. Suturing of the orbital septum is avoided in the inferior orbit because this may result in vertical shortening and lower lid ectropion or retraction.

UPPER EYELID

Step 1

In the upper lid, an incision is outlined in the lid crease and incised with a blade.

Step 2

A double-armed 4-0 silk traction suture is placed through the lid margin and clamped to the drapes, placing the lid on downward stretch.

Step 3

The orbicularis muscle is incised with scissors and may be excised to expose the underlying orbital septum. The orbicularis is tented with forceps and incised with scissors. The preaponeurotic fat is evidence that the orbital septum has been opened.

Step 4

The incision is then extended with scissors, opening the entire orbital septum. The preaponeurotic fat pad and the underlying levator aponeurosis are consistent landmarks. The levator aponeurosis must be positively identified when exploring the superior orbit to prevent inadvertent damage to it during surgery.

Step 5

The lesion in the peripheral surgical space may now be exposed and dissected with appropriate sharp and blunt techniques. Well-encapsulated lesions may be fixated with a cryoprobe if desired and dissected free from surrounding tissue. Use of traction sutures, malleable retractors, and cottonoids facilitates dissection and exposure.

Step 6

At the conclusion of the procedure, meticulous hemostasis is obtained, and the skin is closed with 6-0 absorbable or permanent sutures. The orbital septum need not be closed, and the upper lid orbicularis should not be closed.

Postoperative Management

At the conclusion of surgery, topical antibiotic ointment and a light dressing are applied. In the recovery room, the operative site and eye are examined to assess for any evidence of compromise including check of visual acuity and pupils (afferent defect). Ice packs are applied to the periorbital region, and the head of the bed is elevated 30° to 40°. The patient is examined again several hours later. If prophylactic intravenous antibiotics were administered, they are discontinued within 24 hours after surgery. Intravenous corticosteroids can be considered perioperatively and postoperatively in patients with dysthyroid or idiopathic orbital inflammation, extensive orbital dissections, or significant trauma to the optic nerve. Dosage of intravenous methylprednisolone ranges from 20 to 500 mg every 6 hours during the initial postoperative period, depending on the severity of the inflammation or trauma. Alternative corticosteroids can also be considered. An antibiotic or combination antibiotic-corticosteroid ointment is applied to the incision 4 times a day. Any external nonabsorbable sutures are removed after 4 to 7 days. Patients are seen during the first postoperative week with extended follow-up as determined by the surgeon based on the patient's condition and clinical course.

LATERAL ORBITOTOMY

Jill S. Melicher, MD; Jeffrey A. Nerad, MD; and Jonathan W. Kim, MD

The current definition of lateral orbitotomy encompasses a wide variety of incisions and surgical approaches that involve the creation of a lateral bone flap for enhanced exposure to the lateral orbital wall. As with other types of orbitotomy techniques, adequate surgical exposure is essential to allow safe dissection in this confined region of the orbit. When compared to medial, inferior, and superior orbital approaches, the lateral orbitotomy offers perhaps the most rapid, wide access to the retrobulbar space. The operative risk of the exposure with this procedure is also relatively low, and the cosmesis of the healed incision is typically well accepted. Because of these advantages, the versatile lateral orbitotomy procedure has become the preferred approach for the surgical management of a diverse group of orbital lesions. In this chapter, we stress meticulous technique and individualization of the surgical approach to optimize the surgical outcome for each patient.

Lateral orbitotomy techniques have traditionally been used for lesions in the region of the lacrimal gland fossa and the lateral retrobulbar space, both intraconal and extraconal. Although lesions medial to the optic nerve are usually best approached by a medial orbitotomy, it is also well recognized that a medial approach can be combined with a lateral bone flap to allow intraoperative displacement of the globe, providing significant improvement in the exposure of the medial orbital compartment and vice versa. Posterior lesions confined to the deep orbital apex can be approached by creating a deep, lateral bone flap and contouring the greater wing of the sphenoid bone for additional access. Extensive orbital lesions with intracranial or sinus involvement may require wider exposure than that provided by a typical lateral orbitotomy. Such lesions can be approached by creative configurations of the bone flap to obtain the necessary exposure, such as combining the lateral wall osteotomy with contiguous removal of the zygoma, orbital roof, or both.

Preoperative Evaluation

Adequate preoperative evaluation is essential to allow optimal surgical planning and to minimize intraoperative and postoperative complications. Historic information, such as pain and rate of progression, helps elucidate the nature of the orbital process and provides guidance on the extent of surgical extirpation. Orbital examination for functional deficits may aid in lesion localization and incision placement. Computed tomographic scanning and magnetic resonance imaging are invaluable for defining the extent of the orbital process and planning the surgical approach. The preoperative surgical planning can then be based on the suspected risk of malignancy, presence or expected development of functional compromise, available surgical planes, knowledge of orbital anatomy, and aesthetic considerations.

As with other orbital procedures, aspirin should be discontinued 2 weeks before surgery whenever possible. Nonsteroidal anti-inflammatory medications should be discontinued 7 days prior to surgery. Communication with the patient's primary care physician or cardiologist is essential for patients on warfarin and clopidogrel to safely and effectively discontinue these medications 3 to 5 days before surgery. Herbal medications and supplements can affect bleeding as well and should be reviewed and discontinued prior to surgery. In rare cases, when vascular lesions or significant intraoperative bleeding is anticipated, the patient's blood should be typed and cross-matched preoperatively.

An upper lid crease incision extending into a lateral canthotomy is used in most patients to gain adequate exposure to the lateral orbital wall. This incision has replaced the traditional Stallard-Wright sub-brow incision, which leaves a very visible scar. Other options include the Berke lateral canthotomy incision, a lower eyelid subciliary incision extended into a

Levine MR.
Manual of Oculoplastic Surgery, Fourth Edition (pp 297-302).

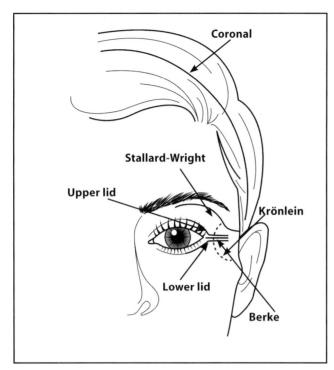

Figure 47-1.

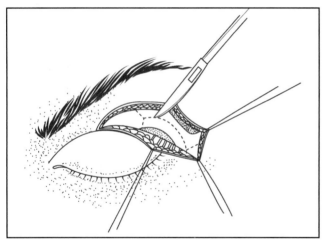

Figure 47-2.

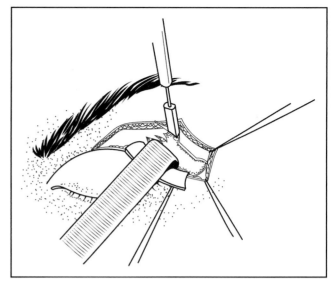

Figure 47-3.

lateral laugh line, and the coronal incision, which allows disinsertion of the temporalis muscle for extensive apical lesions. The Kronlein cutaneous approach results in a prominent scar and is presented for historic significance only (Figure 47-1).

Surgical Procedure

General anesthesia is used routinely. Intravenous steroids (dexamethasone, 4 to 10 mg) are administered preoperatively. Routine antibiotics are not necessary and should be administered on a case-by-case basis. A headlight and surgical loupes are necessary for this procedure.

Step 1

The patient is positioned in the reverse Trendelenburg position, and the head is rotated in the direction away from the operative side. An upper lid skin crease incision is marked with extension into the lateral canthus. Preferably, 10 minutes before the incision is made, a 50:50 mixture of 1% lidocaine with 1:100,000 solution of epinephrine and 0.5% Bupivacaine is injected into the lid crease, lateral canthus, temporalis muscle, and fossa posterior to the lateral orbital rim for hemostasis. Povidone-iodine (Betadine) preparation of the periocular region is accomplished in standard fashion.

Step 2

A traction suture (eg, 4-0 silk) is placed transconjunctivally beneath the insertion of the lateral rectus muscle for later use in identification of this muscle. Other extraocular muscle traction sutures are placed if necessary. A traction suture may be placed in the upper eyelid to maintain closure. We do not use a corneal protective shield routinely.

Step 3

The skin is incised with a scalpel or cutting cautery (Colorado needle). Dissection is carried down to the level of the periosteum of the frontal and zygomatic bones at the lateral orbital rim. Hemostasis is obtained with needle-tipped unipolar or bipolar cautery. After localized undermining, 4 4-0 silk traction sutures are passed through the subcutaneous tissue and muscle and are fixed to the drapes to aid exposure.

Step 4

The periosteum is incised with the Colorado needle or #15 Bard-Parker blade approximately 2 mm posterior and parallel to the lateral orbital rim (Figure 47-2). The incision extends superiorly above the zygomatic-frontal suture and inferiorly onto the superior zygomatic arch. The periosteum and temporalis muscle are elevated and dissected from the lateral orbital rim and then reflected posteriorly away from the orbit (Figure 47-3). The temporalis fascia is incised for 2 cm, and a Dean periosteal elevator is used to elevate the temporalis muscle out of the temporalis fossa. Two 0.5-inch x 3-inch neuro

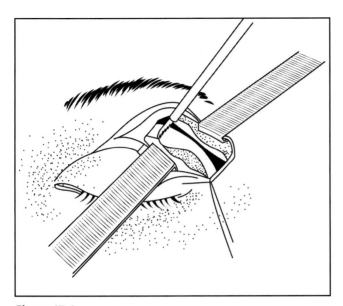

Figure 47-4.

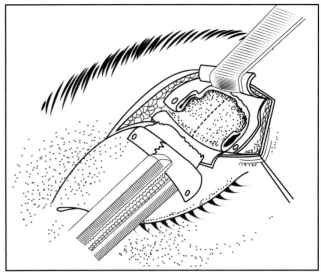

Figure 47-6.

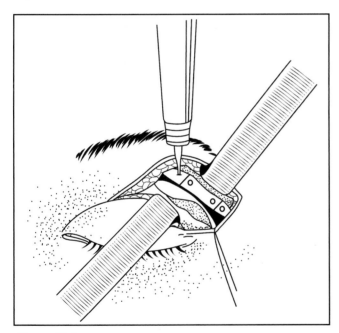

Figure 47-5.

paddies are placed beneath the temporalis muscle in the fossa to assist in hemostasis and exposure. The periorbita is cautiously separated from bone inside the lateral orbital rim for approximately 2 cm using a Freer elevator. Special attention is necessary to avoid inadvertent rupture of the periorbita or injury to the orbital contents. A malleable ribbon retractor and suction are helpful to accomplish this. Bipolar and bone wax may be necessary for hemostasis.

Step 5

Marks are made on the lateral orbital rim at the site of the planned osteotomy. Usually, the superior cut is at or up to 10 mm superior to the frontozygomatic suture. It may be placed further superiorly at the level where the frontal bone of the lateral orbital

rim begins to widen and thicken, if it is anticipated that additional superior exposure will be helpful. A portion of the superior rim can be included with the lateral bone flap. Usually, the inferior osteotomy is just superior to the zygomatic arch but may extend into the zygomatic arch and infraorbital fissure, if it is anticipated that additional inferior exposure will be helpful.

Step 6

A power sagittal or oscillating saw is used to make the bone cuts (Figure 47-4). The osteotomy continues until the thin bone of the posterior lateral orbital wall is encountered. Irrigation fluid and suction improve exposure and prevent heat necrosis of the bone and scattering of bone fragments. Eye protection for the surgical team is essential. A wide malleable ribbon retractor or Sewall retractor can be used to protect the orbital contents and periorbital soft tissue. A power drill is then used to make 1-mm holes from the external to the inner aspect of the rim (Figure 47-5). One hole is placed superior and inferior to each planned osteotomy. During this maneuver, the orbital contents must be protected by a broad malleable retractor. Using this technique, the bone flap can be secured into position at the conclusion of the case with sutures through the drill holes. Alternatively, drill holes for fixation can be placed prior to bone removal using the plate as a template for the drill holes.

Step 7

The lateral orbital wall is grasped at the rim with a Leksell laminectomy rongeur and rocked laterally until it is out fractured (Figure 47-6). The bone is then removed and placed in a saline-soaked sponge.

Step 8

Rongeurs or a cutting burr on the power drill can be used to remove additional bone in the greater wing of the sphenoid bone at the posterior margin of the osteotomy within the temporalis muscle

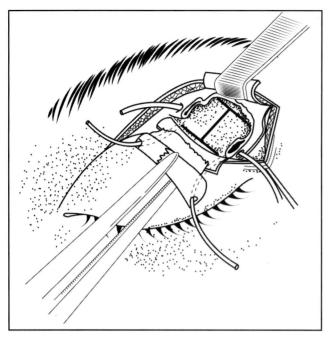

Figure 47-7.

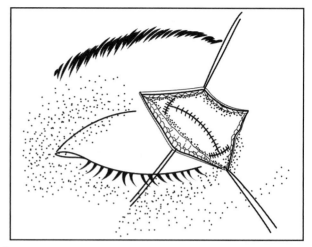

Figure 47-8.

fossa. Medullary bone bleeding arising from the sphenoid bone is controlled with bone wax. The anteroposterior distance from the lateral orbital rim to the middle cranial fossa is usually approximately 3 cm, and bone removal can be safely performed for approximately 2 cm. However, the size and configuration of the diploic space within the greater wing of the sphenoid bone can vary significantly between patients, and this anatomy should be reviewed carefully on the preoperative imaging studies to prevent cerebrospinal fluid leaks.

Step 9

The periorbita is opened as needed to gain adequate exposure. The periorbita in the lateral orbit is usually incised in a T-shaped incision with the anteroposterior limb superior to the level of the lateral rectus muscle. The other arm of the T is placed parallel to the lateral rim. Occasionally, a small tear in the periorbita is observed and may be used as the starting point for the incision. Once the periorbita has been opened, movement of the lateral rectus traction suture allows for identification of the muscle. Typically, gentle manipulation with a malleable retractor will adequately expose the retrobulbar space. Overmanipulation of the lateral rectus may result in postoperative motility problems.

Step 10

Once the proper exposure has been achieved, intraorbital dissection begins. Observation and gentle finger palpation are helpful in locating the orbital lesion. Dissection should be performed with magnification and coaxial illumination, preferably with the operating room microscope. The operating microscope can be advantageous for fine dissection within the orbital apex. Most of the dissection can be accomplished with blunt instrumentation such

as cotton-tipped applicators. Structures should be identified by meticulous dissection and divided under direct visualization. Malleable ribbon or Sewell retractors, in the hands of an attentive assistant, greatly facilitate this portion of the procedure. Frequent blotting with cotton applicators and neurosurgical cottonoids, combined with bipolar cautery and minimal suction, provide displacement of normal structures, provide definition of the tumor or disease, and control bleeding. The placement of neurosurgical cottonoids to prevent orbital fat prolapse into the visual axis once the mass has been identified is helpful to maintain the surgical dissection planes. Dissection of the tumor or capsule can be assisted with tension provided by the placement of a cryoprobe or a traction suture to the mass. Meticulous hemostasis must be maintained at all times. Saline irrigation is helpful to identify bleeding points.

Step 11

Once the tumor is biopsied or removed, the bone fragment is replaced and secured with 3-0 Prolene suture through the preplaced holes (Figure 47-7). Stainless steel wire and other material that may interfere with postoperative computed tomographic scanning and magnetic resonance imaging should be avoided. Microplates and screws are an expensive, sophisticated method of bone fixation and are usually unnecessary.

Step 12

The anterior insertion of the temporalis muscle and periosteum of the lateral orbital rim are closed with 4-0 Vicryl interrupted sutures (Figure 47-8).

Step 13

Traction sutures to the skin-muscle flaps are removed. The muscle and subcutaneous tissue are closed with 5-0 Vicryl interrupted suture. The skin incision is then closed with a running 5-0 fast-absorbing plain gut or Nylon suture (Figure 47-9). The extraocular muscle traction sutures and corneal protector are removed. The eye is

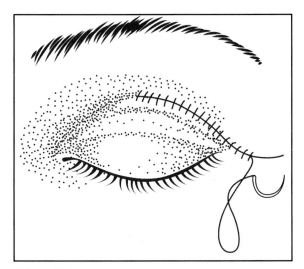

Figure 47-9.

carefully inspected for evidence of injury. Dressings or patches over the eye are typically avoided so that ocular examinations can be performed. Topical ophthalmic antibiotic ointment is applied in the eye and on the incision line at the completion of the case. The visual acuity is checked immediately postoperatively in the recovery room.

Postoperative Management

During the early postoperative period, the vision and pupillary reactions are monitored. The head of the bed is elevated to 30°. The patient is typically admitted to the hospital for 23-hour observation with frequent vision and pupil checks. Intravenous steroids followed by oral steroids are given postoperatively to reduce edema. Antibiotic ointment is placed on the wound 3 times a day for 1 week.

Complications and Management Considerations

Complications after lateral orbitotomy are infrequent and typically resolve spontaneously with supportive measures. Lateral rectus weakness and diplopia may occur but usually resolve without intervention within 6 weeks. A persistent dilated pupil may occur from disruption of the ciliary ganglion and pupillary parasympathetic nerves. This abnormality is usually permanent and untreatable and should not be confused with optic nerve dysfunction. Injury to the levator complex may occur from dissections near the lacrimal gland, resulting in a lateral ptosis. Reduced tear production can also be encountered, owing to disruption of the lacrimal gland ductuli or its innervation. Management of the dry eye condition is usually limited to observation, the use of topical ocular lubricants, and punctal occlusion.

Serious complications, including loss of vision, may occur in rare instances, owing to optic nerve dysfunction. When detected, aggressive and immediate intervention is necessary. Exploration, drainage of blood, and control of hemostasis are required if active bleeding or a large hematoma causes increased orbital pressure or optic nerve compression. Although orbital imaging can be helpful in identifying a hematoma, surgical intervention should not be delayed if there is evidence of acute optic nerve compression. Serious infection may rarely occur and should be treated with appropriate intravenous antibiotics and prompt surgical intervention when indicated.

CHAPTER 48

ORBITAL DECOMPRESSION
GRADED SURGICAL APPROACH

Christine C. Annunziata, MD; Bobby S. Korn, MD, PhD, FACS; and Don O. Kikkawa, MD

Orbital decompression is a surgical technique most often utilized in patients with thyroid-associated orbitopathy (TAO), but may be appropriately applied in such disease states as orbital hemorrhage, hemangioma, lymphangioma, or other space-occupying lesion that causes proptosis or orbital congestion.

TAO is an autoimmune inflammatory disorder that clinically affects 30% to 40% of patients with Graves' disease and poses a threat to vision in 3% to 5% of cases. Orbital volume expansion and proinflammatory disease mediators are responsible for the clinical signs and symptoms of TAO.[1-3] Expansion of the orbital fat is the primary feature of type 1 disease, while extraocular muscle inflammation is characteristic of type 2 disease.[4] In the initial inflammatory phase of the disease, symptoms may be nonspecific and include tearing, foreign body sensation, deep orbital pressure and pain, decreased visual acuity, and diplopia. Typical signs include eyelid retraction, periorbital edema, conjunctival hyperemia, chemosis, punctate epithelial erosions, proptosis, and restrictive strabismus. Severe proptosis or crowding of the orbital apex from enlarged extraocular muscles may result in progressive loss of vision from compressive optic neuropathy requiring urgent surgical intervention.

After a period ranging from 1 to 3 years, the inflammatory phase typically abates, and signs and symptoms gradually improve, albeit not completely to their predisease state. Following regression, patients enter a period of stability, during which time planned surgical rehabilitation can occur.[5]

Goals and Principles

Most orbital surgeons concur that rehabilitative surgery should only be performed in patients who have had inactive TAO for at least 6 months unless vision-threatening complications dictate more immediate intervention.

Planned surgical rehabilitation is staged and typically proceeds in the following sequence: orbital decompression, strabismus surgery, and then lid surgery, because side effects of the preceding step can interfere with the step that follows. Unnecessary steps may be skipped, and, occasionally, multiple steps may be appropriately combined.[6,7]

Orbital decompression has traditionally been indicated for patients with TAO with compressive optic neuropathy and/or corneal exposure.[8,9] However, progressive exophthalmos from TAO may result in marked disfigurement and deep orbital pressure and pain. The social and psychological impact from this disfiguring proptosis can lead to disabling depression, similar to that seen in severe medical conditions such as cancer.[10-12] Consequently, surgical reduction of proptosis for aesthetic reasons is increasing. Advances in surgical technique have improved the efficacy and safety of orbital decompression, and, in experienced hands, the complications of this operation are rare and treatable.[13]

The primary goals of orbital decompression are to expand orbital volume through bony expansion and reduce orbital soft tissue through orbital fat decompression.

Current indications for orbital decompression in TAO are as follows:

- Compressive optic neuropathy
- Exposure keratopathy
- Spontaneous globe prolapse
- Cosmetically disfiguring proptosis
- Orbital pain/pressure
- Orbital congestion
- Reduction of proptosis in preparation for strabismus or eyelid retraction surgery

Levine MR.
Manual of Oculoplastic Surgery, Fourth Edition (pp 303-310).
© 2010 SLACK Incorporated

Preoperative Considerations

All patients being considered for orbital decompression should have high-resolution orbital computed tomography (CT) imaging in both the axial and direct coronal planes. Several factors should be noted on the scan, including presence of sinus disease, extraocular muscle size, orbital fat expansion, thickness of the bony walls, and the position/angle of the cribriform plate in relation to the medial wall.

Standard preoperative medical clearance should be performed, including thyroid function and coagulation studies. A euthyroid state should be achieved for elective surgery given the serious cardiovascular risk of thyroid storm and the hypermetabolic effect on anesthetic drugs. Beta-blockers and antithyroid drugs are useful medications of choice in patients who have not undergone radioactive iodine thyroid ablation.

Accurate exophthalmometry measurements, diplopia documentation, and margin-to-reflex distances should be obtained. Either the Hertel or Naugle exophthalmometer is acceptable, but we find the Naugle device (which measures relative to the superior and inferior orbital rims rather than the lateral rim) to be particularly useful if surgery is performed to remove the lateral orbital rim.

External photographs should be obtained from the patient that provide a chronological depiction of the predisease state and document stability over the previous 6 months. In addition, current external photographs should be taken, including the 9 positions of gaze, full face and profile view, and a view from above and below showing the amount of globe protrusion and lagophthalmos.

A thorough discussion of risks, benefits, and alternatives to the planned surgery should take place. The risks include, but are not limited to, surgically induced diplopia, numbness in the distribution of the infraorbital, zygomaticofacial, and zygomaticotemporal nerves, sinusitis, pain, infection, bleeding, pupil abnormalities, cerebrospinal fluid leak, inadequate proptosis reduction, blindness, and the need for possible further surgery. The risk of surgically induced diplopia varies from 10% to as high as 60% in some studies.[8] One of the most important predictors of postoperative diplopia is the presence of preoperative diplopia or restrictive myopathy in type 2 patients. Serious risks or permanent and untreatable complications such as blindness or intraparenchymal injury are fortunately rare in experienced hands.

Surgical Planning

Orbital decompression comprises removal of bone from one or more walls of the orbit, removal of orbital fat, including intraconal fat, or a combination of bone and fat removal.[14-16] In our experience, the indications for fat-only decompression include patients with very mild proptosis (desired reduction of 2 mm or less). Most other patients will require both orbital fat and bone removal.

The amount of proptosis reduction needed is dependent on both the absolute and relative proptosis measurements. Absolute proptosis refers to the amount in millimeters measured by the Hertel or Naugle device preoperatively.

Relative proptosis refers to cases of unilateral or asymmetric disease as well as the amount relative to the patient's normal state as depicted in predisease photos.

Few guidelines exist in the literature to guide the orbital surgeon with regard to the amount of proptosis reduction relative to severity of preoperative exophthalmos. Traditionally, the amount of proptosis reduction has been related to the number of walls removed, the number and size of cuts made in the periorbita, and the preoperative proptosis.[17] Studies have estimated that orbital decompression reduces proptosis by approximately 2 mm per wall, with an additional 2 to 6 mm provided by fat decompression. Early surgical techniques described removal of the orbital floor and medial wall through a transantral approach.[9] Recently, the use of the deep lateral wall decompression has increased in order to minimize postoperative diplopia. Advances in lateral wall surgical technique have led us to use the lateral wall as our first choice, followed by the medial wall for a "balanced" decompression, and then finally the floor as the last wall to be decompressed.[18-20] The theoretical advantage to a balanced decompression is symmetrical retroplacement of the orbital tissues and symmetric tension on the muscle pulleys with presumably lower incidence of postoperative diplopia. In our opinion, orbital floor removal can be associated with some of the most severe complications (hypoglobus, hypotropia and supraduction deficit, and infraorbital hypesthesia). Therefore, we reserve it as the last wall to be removed. The orbital roof is rarely decompressed.

We advocate a graded orbital decompression approach based on the desired level of proptosis reduction.[21] Presently, our approach is as follows:

❖ For a desired proptosis reduction of up to 4 mm, we perform lateral wall and fat decompression.

❖ To achieve a 4- to 6-mm reduction in proptosis, we perform lateral wall, medial wall, and fat decompression.

❖ To achieve a greater than 6-mm reduction in proptosis, we perform lateral wall, medial wall, posterior orbital floor, and fat decompression with or without lateral orbital rim removal.

Lateral Wall Technique

We perform orbital decompression with bony removal under general anesthesia. Fat-only decompression may be safely and effectively performed under monitored anesthesia care with local anesthesia.

Step 1
The lateral 2 cm of the upper eyelid crease is marked (Figure 48-1) and then infiltrated with 2% lidocaine and 1:100,000 epinephrine mixed 1:1 with 0.75% Marcaine.

Step 2
The eyelid crease is incised with a #15 blade, and the dissection is carried down to the periosteum of the superolateral orbital rim using monopolar cutting cautery (Figure 48-2). The periosteum is incised, and the Senn and malleable retractors are used to reflect the tissues along the rim.

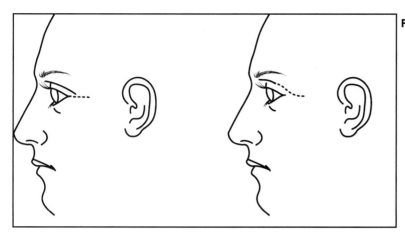

Figure 48-1.

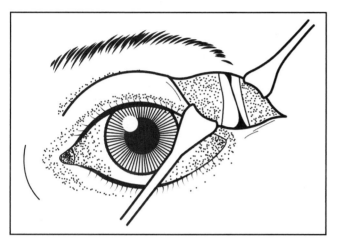

Figure 48-2.

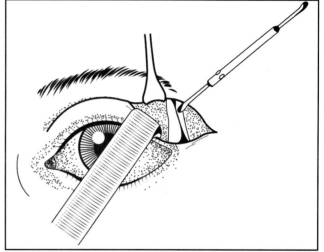

Figure 48-3.

Step 3

A subperiosteal dissection plane is created using a Freer elevator (Figure 48-3), and the periosteum is reflected down to the level of the superior orbital fissure. Particular attention is paid to keeping the periosteum intact, preventing premature prolapse of orbital fat into the surgical field.

Step 4

A 4-mm, high-speed (typically >40,000 RPM), rotating, diamond-tipped burr is used to remove portions of the greater wing of the sphenoid bone, the lacrimal gland fossa, and the area lateral and anterior to the inferior orbital fissure (Figure 48-4). In contrast to the "acorn" style burr, the diamond-tipped burr removes bone at a slower but safer pace. Furthermore, the increased friction and heat generated by the diamond burr provides excellent hemostasis even when decompressing within the highly vascular marrow space. The coagulated blood in the marrow space turns from black in color to white as the inner table is approached, and this color change helps serve as a surgical landmark for the depth limit for bony removal in the lateral wall.

Step 5

Careful hemostasis is then achieved. Hydrogen peroxide is useful for coagulating fine blood vessels. For more persistent marrow bleeding, a gentle polishing motion using the high-speed drill can provide additional hemostasis. Finally, bone wax can be used for recalcitrant bleeding.

Step 6

The periosteum is fenestrated in a posterior to anterior direction, both superiorly and inferiorly using a #12 blade. The intervening segment is slit in a perpendicular fashion, allowing the orbital contents to prolapse into the newly created space. Complete periorbital fenestration is essential to achieve the maximal decompressive effect.

Step 7

In rare cases when the lateral orbital rim is removed, osteotomies are made at a level just above the frontozygomatic suture and just above the zygomatic arch using a long medium oscillating saw (10-mm width). The rim segment is removed using a large rongeur, and the temporalis attachments are released from the bone. The rim is typically not replaced in these cases.

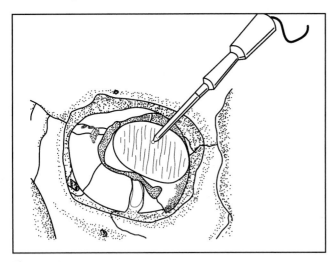

Figure 48-4.

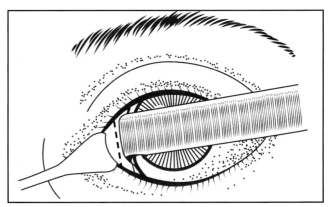

Figure 48-6.

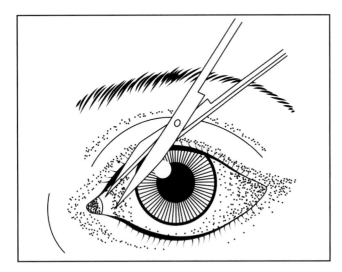

Figure 48-5.

Step 8

Intraconal orbital fat is gently teased from the inferior periosteal incision using monopolar cutting cautery. Care is taken to avoid the lateral rectus muscle as it travels adjacent to this fat. Typically, 2 to 4 cc of intraconal fat can be removed from this lateral access point.[22,23]

Step 9

The orbicularis is closed using 3 interrupted 7-0 polyglactin sutures, and the skin is closed using a running 6-0 fast-absorbing gut suture.

Medial Wall Technique

The medial wall is typically decompressed in conjunction with a lateral wall decompression. An anterior ethmoidal block with local anesthetic is performed, and nasal packing soaked with 4% plain lidocaine and oxymetazoline is placed in the middle meatus. The medial wall is accessed through a transcaruncular incision when lower eyelid retraction repair is not simultaneously performed. However, when lower eyelid retractor recession is to be concomitantly performed, a lateral canthotomy and swinging eyelid approach is performed. In these cases, the inferior oblique muscle is isolated and disinserted with a 6-0 polyglactin suture and reinserted at the conclusion of the case.

Step 1

Traction sutures are placed along the upper and lower eyelid margin using 6-0 silk suture.

Step 2

Westcott scissors are used to make a radial incision in the conjunctiva just lateral to the caruncle. The incision is extended superiorly and inferiorly for several millimeters (Figure 48-5).

Step 3

A curved Stevens scissor is then used to dissect medially until the posterior lacrimal crest is reached. Thin ribbon malleable retractors may help with visualization in this area.

Step 4

The periosteum overlying the posterior lacrimal crest is incised using monopolar cutting cautery, and a subperiosteal dissection plane is created with a Freer elevator (Figure 48-6). The elevator is then used to make a small buttonhole in the lamina papyracea.

Step 5

Using Takahashi forceps and Kerrison rongeurs, the lamina papyracea is removed along with the anterior, middle, and posterior ethmoidal air cells from the posterior lacrimal crest to the sphenoid sinus posteriorly and superiorly to the frontoethmoidal suture. This facilitates the deep apical decompression (Figure 48-7).

Step 6

A wide sinusotomy is performed that communicates the ethmoid, maxillary, and sphenoid sinuses with the nasal cavity to prevent postoperative sinusitis. Communication with the nasal cavity is confirmed with visualization of a Freer elevator through the nares.

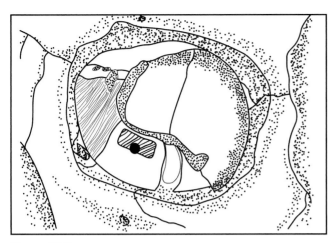

Figure 48-7.

Step 7

The periosteum is slit in a posterior to anterior direction, both superiorly and inferiorly using a #12 blade. The intervening segment is slit in a perpendicular fashion, allowing the orbital contents to prolapse into the newly created space. An additional 2 to 4 cc of intraconal fat may be judiciously removed inferomedially if necessary.

Step 8

Hemostasis is achieved with dilute hydrogen peroxide and cautery. Gelfoam soaked with thrombin may be placed in the ethmoid space if necessary to control bleeding. Alternatively, fibrin glue can be aerosolized into the newly created space.

Step 9

The transcaruncular incision is closed with 6-0 fast-absorbing gut suture.

Inferior Wall Technique

Orbital floor decompression is performed via the inferior fornix/transconjunctival approach. This approach is often made contiguous with the lateral extent of the medial wall decompression. The lower lid retractors are recessed primarily in patients with pre-existing lower lid retraction using the transconjunctival incision.

Step 1

A 2-mm lateral canthotomy and inferior cantholysis is performed using Westcott scissors (as illustrated in Figure 48-1).

Step 2

A transconjunctival incision is created beneath the inferior tarsal border using monopolar cutting cautery (Figure 48-8). The dissection is carried down to the inferior orbital rim, and the periosteum is incised.

Step 3

Subperiosteal dissection continues, using the Freer elevator to expose the posterior half of the orbital floor. Care is taken to avoid disruption of the infraorbital nerve along the orbital floor.

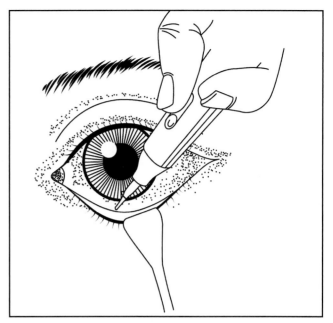

Figure 48-8.

Step 4

A curved hemostat is used to create a buttonhole in the posteromedial orbital floor. Takahashi forceps and Kerrison rongeurs are used to remove the posterior half of the orbital floor, while preserving the anterior portion of the floor and the maxillary-ethmoidal strut (as illustrated in Figure 48-7).

Step 5

The periosteum is fenestrated in a posterior to anterior fashion using a #12 blade in order to allow the orbital fat to prolapse into the maxillary sinus.

Step 6

If the inferior oblique muscle has been disinserted, the imbricating double-armed 6-0 polyglactin sutures may be re-fixated to the muscle stump at the origin along the inferior orbital rim.

Step 7

Lower lid retractor recession can be performed primarily if necessary, or the transconjunctival incision is simply closed using 6-0 fast-absorbing gut suture.

Step 8

The lateral canthus is reconstructed using 6-0 polyglactin sutures to refixate the lateral aspect of the lower tarsal plate to the superior crus of the lateral canthal tendon.

Step 9

The canthotomy skin is closed using multiple interrupted 6-0 fast-absorbing sutures.

At the conclusion of the case, we inject 1 to 3 cc of Kenalog 40 mg/mL mixed 1:1 with Solu-Medrol 125 mg/mL into the retrobulbar space. This may be easily injected using a triport cannula through the lateral orbitotomy incision.

Postoperative Considerations

Most patients undergo unilateral orbital decompression at an outpatient surgical center. Patients are discharged after approximately 1 hour of observation and are checked the following day. However, bilateral orbital decompression can also be performed, and these patients are typically held in the hospital for 23-hour observation. Routine postoperative medications include oral antibiotics, steroids, analgesics, and ophthalmic ointment. Ice pack compresses are used during waking hours for the first 3 days. Patients are informed to call immediately with signs of worsening vision, increased bleeding, or uncontrollable pain.

Outcome Variables

Surgical outcomes vary among surgeons, primarily because surgical techniques are variable. Even with all other things being equal, patient factors also contribute to outcome variability. Examples of these factors include the following:

* Predominate type of disease (type 1 versus type 2). Type 1 patients typically will have greater proptosis reduction than type 2 patients. Theoretically, fat occupies the expanded orbital space easier than enlarged extraocular muscles, leading to a greater decompressive effect in type 1 patients.

* Extraocular muscle fibrosis. The fibrotic and less pliable extraocular muscles in type 2 patients may not fill the newly expanded space well.

* Bony orbit size. Some patients have shallow orbits with less bone to remove. This can be particularly relevant in deep lateral wall decompression that relies upon the amount of bone removed and not on the adjacent air space of the sinus cavity.

Complications

In experienced hands, the rate of complications following orbital decompression is low.[24] Reported complications include the following:

* Postoperative diplopia and globe displacement
* Chronic sinusitis or epistaxis
* Cerebrospinal fluid leak from dural lacerations
* Meningitis
* Tonic pupil from damage to the ciliary ganglion
* Optic neuropathy
* Orbital cellulitis
* Orbital hypoesthesia or pain
* Orbital hemorrhage
* Temporalis wasting with lateral rim removal
* Nasolacrimal duct obstruction
* Inadequate proptosis reduction
* Late enophthalmos due to "imploding antrum" syndrome

Conclusion

Orbital decompression is a highly effective operation to reduce the signs and symptoms associated with proptosis. A graded approach progressing from fat only, to lateral wall, then medial wall, then floor plus fat leads to greater predictability of results and fewer complications in experienced hands. Most of the complications are rare and treatable. Careful patient selection and improved surgical technique have led to a broadening of the indications for this traditionally rare operation.

ORBITAL DECOMPRESSION
ENDOSCOPIC APPROACHES

Steven M. Houser, MD, FACS and Howard Levine, MD

Graves' ophthalmopathy can be effectively managed through techniques to remove the bony walls of the orbit. Orbital fat can then prolapse out of the confined orbit, and the globe will settle back further into the orbit. A retropulsed globe will allow the lids to effectively cover the globe and lessen the risk of corneal exposure and ulceration. Also, removal of the bony walls may relieve pressure from the optic nerve and improve vision.

The previous chapter thoroughly explained the open techniques that an orbital surgeon can employ for orbital decompression. The goals and principles, preoperative evaluation, and operative preparation are identical between open and closed, or endoscopic, techniques.

While the goals are identical, the actual techniques vary a great deal. The open techniques do require significant tissue dissection with greater chance of scarring and a lengthier healing process compared to an endoscopic procedure.

Technique

The ideal arrangement is for the orbital surgeon to work as a team with a skilled sinus surgeon to perform endoscopic orbital decompression. Each surgeon will independently assess the patient and discuss the potential surgery, its risks, and outcomes. The orbital surgeon should perform a complete ophthalmologic examination, especially assessing the visual acuity, degree of proptosis, extent of optic nerve involvement, degree of diplopia, and cornea status. The nasal anatomy can be assessed with headlight and nasal endoscope. Nasal and sinus pathology should be managed either before or as part of the orbital decompression. Among the common pathologies seen are acute or chronic infection, nasal and/or sinus polyps, and deviated nasal septum. A deviated nasal septum may limit adequate access into the sinus endoscopically both at sur-

gery and postoperatively. Infection and polyps may cause postoperative ocular infection and lead to increased complication. An endoscopic orbital decompression requires a transnasal approach, so these tissues are best decongested preoperatively.

In addition to evaluation with nasal endoscopy, a preoperative computed tomographic (CT) scan of the sinuses is of importance. The patient's individual sinus anatomy can be further assessed in conjunction with the physical exam. The surgical route can be planned based on the anatomy.

If bilateral disease is present, surgeons may choose to stage each side by several days or perform bilateral decompression at the same operation. At the time of surgery, if there is any question about injury or status of the optic nerve and vision, surgery should be limited to only one side.

Oxymetazoline 0.05% can be applied per spray several times before surgery to decongest the nasal tissue. In the operating room, either oxymetazoline or 4% cocaine on pledgets placed within the nasal cavity will provide further decongestion and limit bleeding.

Image-guided computer assistance is used to provide the surgeon with information about the landmarks within and about the orbit. This complements the endoscope visualization to ensure complete and adequate decompression.

Surgery is most often performed in an ambulatory surgery center with discharge planned for the same day.

Step 1

The surgeon begins by injecting the middle turbinate and lateral wall with 1% lidocaine with 1:100,000 epinephrine with approximately 4 cc per side. After waiting approximately 7 minutes for the epinephrine to take effect, the surgery can begin.

Levine MR.
Manual of Oculoplastic Surgery, Fourth Edition (pp 309-314).
© 2010 SLACK Incorporated

Step 2

The middle turbinate is typically preserved during endoscopic orbital decompression, although it can be removed if space constraints demand it or the surgeon feels that by leaving it there, scar formation will occur between the lateral middle turbinate wall and the exposed periorbita. The middle turbinate is medialized, or pushed toward the septum, to allow entry into the middle meatus, the space lateral to the middle turbinate. The middle meatus contains the openings to the maxillary, anterior ethmoid, and frontal sinuses and the ethmoid sinus air cells themselves.

Step 3

After medializing the middle turbinate, the uncinate process overlying the bulla ethmoidalis (anterior ethmoid air cells) can be visualized. These structures will be removed to allow the orbital fat to prolapse into this space. The uncinate can be resected through multiple methods: 1) a microshaver can resect the uncinate directly, 2) an uncinotomy with a pediatric-size backbiter forceps may then allow better purchase with a microshaver by creating a raw surface into which tissue is suctioned into the microshaver, or 3) a sharp Freer elevator will allow the uncinate to be separated from the lateral wall, then straight Blakesley-Weil forceps will allow the uncinate to be fully withdrawn from the nasal cavity.

Step 4

The bulla ethmoidalis can be removed with forceps, or per a microshaver instrument. Bony septations within the bulla ethmoidalis are removed up to the lateral ethmoid wall (lamina papyracea). At this point, the bone of the lamina papyracea should be left intact.

Step 5

Below and just anterior to the bulla ethmoidalis is the natural opening to the maxillary sinus, the maxillary ostia. The maxillary sinus has a membranous ostia formed by 2 layers of mucus membrane (one on the nasal and the other on the maxillary sinus side). These fused membranes form the maxillary sinus fontanel. This membranous ostia is within the larger bony maxillary sinus ostia. The membranous ostial opening can usually be visualized during removal of the uncinate process. Using straight through-cutting instruments to remove the fontanel and some of the surrounding bony tissue, the maxillary ostia can be widened posteriorly. A microshaver can further resect the inferior aspect of the maxillary opening to create a very large antrostomy; the tissue is taken down to the superior aspect of the inferior turbinate and anteriorly to the posterior edge of the nasolacrimal duct. This large antrostomy will facilitate removal of bone from the orbit and allow a maximal cavity for the fat to prolapse into.

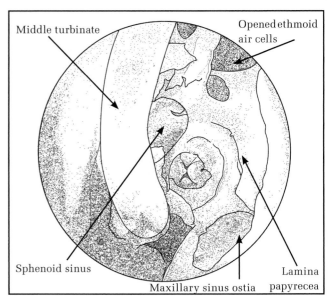

Figure 49-1.

Step 6

Removal of the bulla will expose the basal lamella: the vertical bony wall that separates the anterior from the posterior ethmoid air cells. The basal lamella can be perforated with a suction or microshaver and widely removed from the skull base (fovea ethmoidalis) above to the free edge of the middle turbinate below, and from the lamina papyracea laterally to the middle turbinate medially. Multiple bony septations within the posterior ethmoid cavity should be removed to create a large cavity. Care is taken to open the posterior ostiomeatal complex and sphenoid sinus and the frontal recess and frontal sinus outflow tract to minimize the chances of postoperative rhinosinusitis caused by orbital fat obstructing these areas (Figure 49-1).

Step 7

The sinuses are now maximally opened to first allow bone removal and then incision into the periorbita to permit fatty prolapse for decompression. The lamina papyracea can be carefully removed. The surgeon should take care to avoid transgressing the periorbita as this will prematurely spill fat into the surgical field and limit view. This can be significant because the orbital fat is already under great pressure. Fortunately, the periorbita in patients with Graves' disease is typically tough from inflammation and does not open as easily as the periorbita of a healthy subject. Multiple tools may be needed depending on the angulation and thickness of the bone.

Step 8

The lamina papyracea is palpated with an acorn-shaped perforator (Figure 49-2) looking for a thin or perforated area because this is the easiest place to begin the removal of the lamina papyracea. This permits an assessment of the thickness of the bone

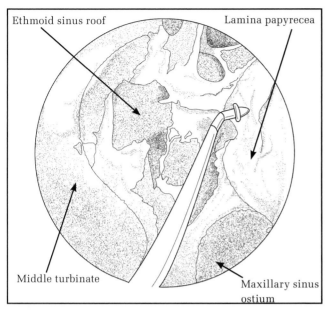

Figure 49-2.

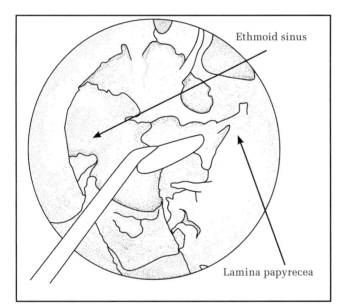

Figure 49-3.

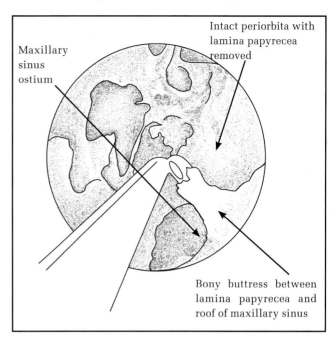

Figure 49-4.

periorbita and display the remaining orbital bone to the surgeon (Figure 49-4). Straight Frazier-tipped suction as well as angled Blakesley-Weil forceps will allow the surgeon to remove bony fragments from within the cavity. Care should be taken to 1) not pull on bone that is still attached and 2) turn any sharp bone fragments in such a fashion during withdrawal as to not injure the periorbita or other nasal structures/mucosa.

Step 10

Thicker bone is encountered at the junction of the ethmoid and roof of the maxillary sinus. This bone is like a buttress protecting the orbit and can be very difficult to remove. An angled ring with suction and a heavy curette usually must be used to fracture this thick bone inferiorly. On occasion, a drill may be needed to thin this buttress before it will fracture. The bone often breaks as far medially as the infraorbital nerve within the roof of the maxillary sinus. Angled forceps can reach into the maxillary sinus to remove fragmented bone (Figure 49-5). It is important to remove such bone; otherwise, the bone may act as a nidus for infection if devitalized, or it may heal in place and limit the fatty prolapse.

Step 11

Posteriorly, within the posterior ethmoid cavity defect, the lamina papyracea approaches the orbital nerve and annulus of Zinn. Great care should be taken to elevate bone in this region. The spatula dissector proves useful in this region as well as a suction curette for thicker bone. Palpation of the orbit will continue to benefit the surgeon by identifying loose or remaining bone.

and any areas of bony dehiscence identified. There are times when the lamina papyracea is thin or even has a perforation in it because of the underlying increased intraorbital pressure secondary to the increased orbital contents. If no natural dehiscence can be identified, the surgeon makes his or her own opening through an area of thin lamina bone. An acorn-shaped perforator will push through the bone with minimal trauma to the underlying periorbita.

Step 9

A spatula dissector and a thinner curette dissector allow careful dissection of thin lamina bone away from the underlying, intact periorbita (Figure 49-3). Pressing on the globe externally will medialize the

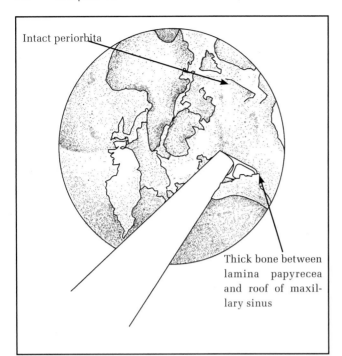

Intact periorbita

Thick bone between lamina papyrecea and roof of maxillary sinus

Figure 49-5.

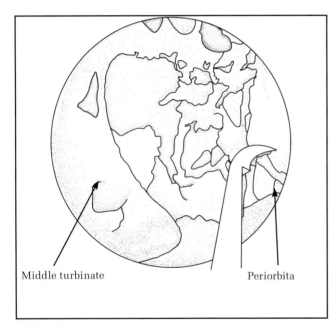

Middle turbinate

Periorbita

Figure 49-6.

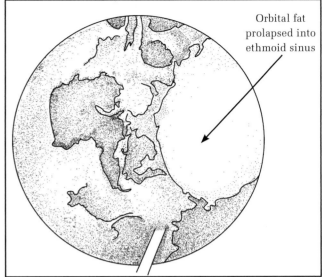

Orbital fat prolapsed into ethmoid sinus

Figure 49-7.

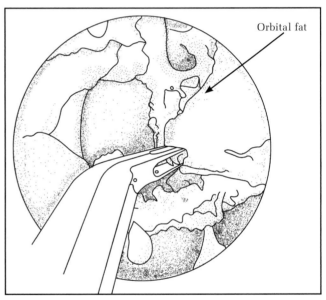

Orbital fat

Figure 49-8.

Step 12

After maximal bone removal, the periorbita medially and inferiorly is fully exposed and ready for opening to allow prolapse of fat into the surgical field. An orbital sickle knife or orbital knife, depending on the angle the patient presents, can be used to incise the periorbita from posterior to anterior (Figure 49-6). The initial cut should be placed as far superior as possible to maximize visualization, with successive cuts moving inferiorly along the periorbita. Beginning inferiorly causes orbital fat to prolapse (Figure 49-7) and blocks visualization superiorly. The knife is not plunged deeply within the tissue to prevent injury to structures embedded within the orbital fat: globe, extraocular muscles, and blood vessels. The fat within the orbit of a patient with Graves' ophthalmopathy is often under pressure; it will spill forth rapidly into the ethmoid cavity as the incisions are made.

Step 13

The fat can be further gently teased into the ethmoid cavity with special alligator forceps (Figure 49-8): the jaws do not fully close so there is less risk of trauma to the vessels or extraocular muscles within the orbit. Great care is taken to inspect the orbital fat, looking for extraocular muscles. Orbital suction picks of various angles (45°, 90°, and 135°)

allow the surgeon to tease fascial bands within the prolapsed fat, allowing further prolapse of fat.

Step 14

No packing is placed at the conclusion of the procedure as this would limit the fatty prolapse. If bleeding needs to be controlled, then various topical gel materials are available to help achieve hemostasis (eg, Floseal). Frequently, a small piece of Telfa is placed into the nasal cavity for about 1 hour after surgery, merely to absorb any blood that may drain from the sinus cavity. This is always removed before discharge.

Step 15

Postoperatively, the patient is asked to refrain from nose blowing for 2 weeks to prevent orbital emphysema. The patient is asked to lavage the nose with saline 6 to 10 times per day to clean crusts and blood clots from the nasal cavity. The surgeon will see the patient in the office on a weekly basis for the next month to carefully clean adherent crusts and blood clots from the surgical site. The nasal mucosa slowly grows to cover over the prolapsed fat.

Complications

An endoscopic orbital decompression presents risks similar to endoscopic sinus surgery. A cerebrospinal fluid leak is possible as the superiorly located lamina papyracea bone is fractured. The firm bone at the junction of the lamina and the fovea ethmoidalis should not be resected to prevent this occurrence. A leak that is recognized should immediately be patched, and consideration should be given to aborting the remainder of the case for a future session.

Orbital injury is possible during sinus surgery, and in particular during orbital decompression. The medial rectus is the closest muscle to the surgical site. Careful use of the instruments as described above should prevent transaction or removal of the muscle. The optic nerve posteriorly should be approached with great care to prevent injury. Transient irritation of nerve or muscle is possible from close dissection.

Nasolacrimal duct injury is rare with an endoscopic approach as the anterior limit of lamina papyracea dissection will naturally stop at the firm bone of the lacrimal region.

Orbital hemorrhage is possible, although decompressed tissue will prevent a localized collection from pressing on the optic nerve and causing ischemic damage.

Diplopia is an expected complication of orbital decompression as the globe position relative to the orbit is altered. Future eye muscle surgery is often necessary to achieve a consensual gaze. It is possible though that some element of diplopic vision will persist long term. Any future surgery for diplopia or eyelid exposure is reserved until all edema from the orbital decompression has resolved.

Recurrent acute or chronic rhinosinusitis is a possibility secondary to obstruction of the sinus outflow from the orbital contents. This, however, is rare because the sinuses are widely opened.

SOCKET RECONSTRUCTION

Meredith Brooke Allen, MD; Perry F. Garber, MD; David A. Della Rocca, MD; and Robert C. Della Rocca, MD

The decision to enucleate or eviscerate a patient's eye is often brought on after a long-standing battle and failure to preserve visual function and eliminate intractable pain. Other indications include tumor resection, penetrating trauma with a threat of sympathetic ophthalmia, and infection. Once the patient has committed to undergo this radical procedure, the next most important issue to consider is the restoration of cosmesis so that the patient can return to a normal social and functional life. Reducing the potential for postoperative complications thus takes on a highly important role. Enucleation alters the dynamics of the orbit into what is classified as the anophthalmic socket. Emphasis during reconstruction should consist of replacement of volume loss, motility considerations, and prosthetic options. In the past, globe removal (volume, approximately 6 to 7 cc) and replacement with an inorganic nonintegrating implant (approximately 2 to 3 cc) plus a prosthesis (approximately 2 cc) did not equal the volume of the orbit preoperatively. Consequently, patients presented with ptosis, sulcus deformities, and often an enophthalmic appearance. Improvements in materials (hydroxyapatite, porous polyethylene [Medpor], and aluminum oxide), a wider array of sizes (14 to 23 mm), and attention to muscle positioning have improved surgical outcomes.

The optimal implant should be lightweight and made of an inert material that sits centrally within the orbit. Inorganic implants larger than 20 mm have been seen by the authors to cause higher rates of extrusion. Wrapping these implants with banked sclera, autogenous fascia lata, or processed pericardium (Tutoplast) may reduce complications. The prosthesis is relatively thin so that it does not weigh too heavily on the lower eyelid and should lie in the plane of the opposite cornea. Decreased motility of the prosthesis, extrusion, a deepened supratarsal sulcus, socket contracture, and eyelid ptosis are problems that still can be seen after enucleation. A coordinated effort by ocularist and surgeon to create the best prosthesis for the patient is important in minimizing these problems.

Evaluating the patient with an anophthalmic socket is done by comparing the enucleated socket to the normal orbit. Exophthalmometry readings may help determine whether the orbital contents are sinking back. The position of the upper and lower eyelids should be examined for evidence of ptosis and laxity. The depth of the supratarsal sulcus should be noted. The surgeon should evaluate the position of the eyelid margin and look for evidence of lashes turning in against the prosthesis. The upper and lower fornices should be of adequate depth to hold the prosthesis. Any socket discharge should be cultured.

Three basic socket problems and their management are discussed in this chapter. The first is that of an extruding implant; the second, contracted fornices; and the third, the anophthalmic enophthalmic syndrome.

Extruding Implant

If extrusion of the implant occurs shortly after enucleation, the patient should be returned to the operating room and the edges of the wound freshened and resutured. Tenon's capsule and conjunctiva are closed in separate layers.

Late extrusion is seen more frequently with oversized (>20 mm), nonintegrated implants, mesh implants, or when socket infection occurs. When implant exposure and thinning of the conjunctiva approaches 3 to 4 mm, Tenon's capsule can be closed and a patch of sclera or fascia placed over it to reinforce and cover the implant. The conjunctiva is then closed over the patch graft.

If the extrusion is profound or the implant is infected, the implant will need to be removed. Reconstruction with a dermis fat graft can be useful in this instance. This

Levine MR.
Manual of Oculoplastic Surgery, Fourth Edition (pp 315-320).
© 2010 SLACK Incorporated

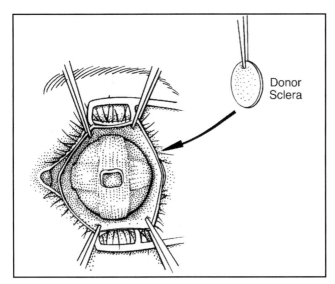

Figure 50-1.

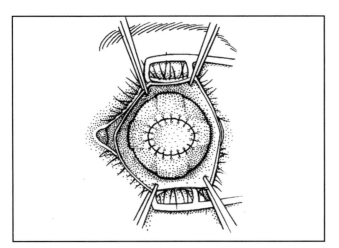

Figure 50-2.

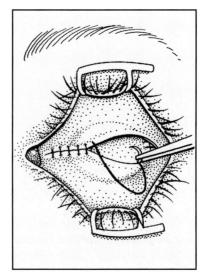

Figure 50-3.

graft can add surface area and a substrate for conjunctiva to grow over the dermis. The posterior fat maintains adequate volume. Dermis fat is an autogenous graft; therefore, it is not rejected and does not migrate. Some absorption of fat may occur over time.

MANAGEMENT OF EXTRUDED IMPLANT

Step 1
The conjunctiva is injected with local anesthetic. The wound dehiscence over the implant is enlarged in a horizontal direction, and the edges are débrided to give fresh surgical margins of conjunctiva and Tenon's capsule.

Step 2
Dissection is performed between conjunctiva and Tenon's capsule toward the depths of the fornices, creating flaps of these layers. Tenon's capsule is then sutured over the implant using 5-0 chromic sutures. If Tenon's capsule cannot be completely closed over the implant, a piece of eyebank sclera or processed pericardium (Tutoplast) is cut to cover the defect and is sutured to the surface of Tenon's

capsule. A margin of sclera 4 mm wider than the defect is recommended (Figures 50-1 and 50-2).

Step 3
Conjunctiva is sutured horizontally over the patch graft using a running 6-0 plain catgut suture (Figure 50-3). A doughnut-shaped conformer may be inserted into the socket to maintain the fornices without putting pressure on the suture line. Antibiotic drops are given 4 times daily for 1 week. A new prosthesis can be fit in 3 to 4 weeks when swelling has subsided.

DERMIS FAT GRAFT PROCEDURE

Step 1
Under general anesthesia, the opening over the extruded implant is enlarged in a horizontal direction, and the implant is removed.

Step 2
The edges of the conjunctiva and Tenon's capsule are freshened. Excision of a capsularized implant is performed with care to avoid damage to the levator complex. An attempt is made to identify the 4 horizontal recti muscles. If they cannot be found, incisions are made in the socket to isolate tissue in the 4 quadrants that may contain them. If they are found, a 5-0 double-armed suture (ie, polyglactin [Vicryl]) is placed through each muscle or quadrant of tissue, and locking bites are taken on each end (Figure 50-4). Saline-soaked gauze is then placed into the socket.

Step 3
The donor site should be prepared and draped at the outset of the operation. It is chosen between the anterior iliac crest and the greater trochanter of the femur, a location that is concealed by a bathing suit. The graft is outlined as a circular area 16 to 20 mm in diameter (Figure 50-5). Then, 1 to 2 mL of saline or lidocaine with epinephrine is injected just beneath the epidermis to facilitate removal of

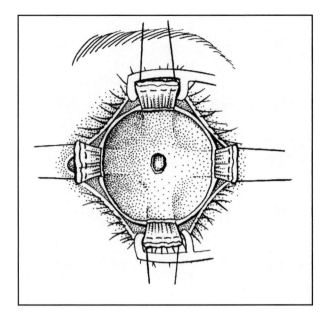

Figure 50-4.

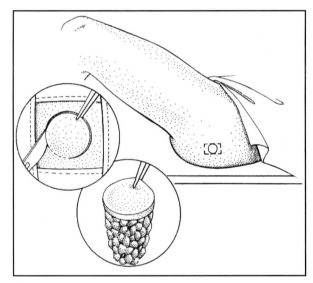

Figure 50-5.

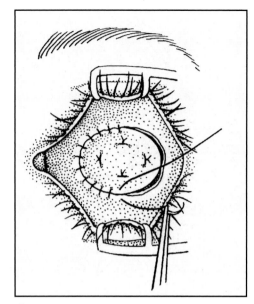

Figure 50-6.

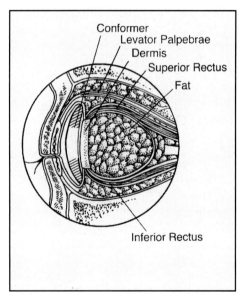

Conformer
Levator Palpebrae
Dermis
Superior Rectus
Fat
Inferior Rectus

Figure 50-7.

the epidermis. The perimeter of the circle is incised with a #15 blade, and the epidermis may be separated with a #11 blade or a diamond burr.

Step 4

The dermis and subcutaneous fat are incised using a #10 blade to a depth of approximately 40 mm. Muscle should be avoided. Alternatively, the button of the dermis can be lifted up and the subcutaneous fat cut with a Stevens scissors under direct visualization to the desired depth (see Figure 50-5). Saline-soaked gauze is inserted into the donor site defect.

Step 5

The dermis-fat graft is then transferred directly to the recipient socket and sutured. Some sizing may be required. The graft is stabilized by attaching each of the recti muscles to the edge of the dermis. Additional absorbable sutures help secure the der-

mis to the adjacent conjunctiva and Tenon's capsule (Figure 50-6).

Step 6

The donor site is closed with multiple layers of 3-0 chromic sutures. The wound is carefully brought together by using the deeper chromic sutures to take tension off of the more superficial tissues and suture passes. Deep, interrupted, buried sutures closing the deep dermis have been particularly helpful in avoidance of wound dehiscence. The superficial skin can be closed with a running 5-0 nylon suture.

Step 7

Antibiotic ointment and a doughnut-shaped conformer are placed into the socket and a sterile dressing applied. The sagittal view shows the dermis-fat graft within the orbit and the conformer in the fornices (Figure 50-7).

Step 8

A pressure dressing consisting of a Telfa pad, gauze fluffs, and Elastoplast is placed on the donor site. Oral antibiotics are administered for 7 to 10 days. Conjunctival epithelium will extend over the dermis in approximately 1 month, and a new prosthesis can be fit in 4 to 6 weeks.

Fornix and Socket Contraction

The fornices can become shallow without loss of conjunctiva, with or without implant migration. Fornix contraction and scarring can also develop from conjunctival insufficiency associated with trauma or chemical injury. In either case, it will be difficult to maintain a prosthesis in the socket. If the fornix is lost but conjunctiva is sufficient, a stent such as a retinal sponge can be sutured in the fornix to deepen it.

We will discuss the techniques to add surface area to the socket with grafted material. A second approach would be to perform a dermis fat graft. The dermis is a useful and healthy substrate for healthy conjunctiva to grow over the center of the graft. We have found that this has added useful surface area to a contracted socket that allows for success in fornix reconstruction. This has been done in combination with the following procedures either combined or in a staged series of procedures.

SURGICAL TECHNIQUE 1

Step 1

The area is injected with local anesthetic. A 3-mm wide retinal sponge is prepared to fit into the horizontal length of the lower fornix.

Step 2

Both arms of a double-armed 4-0 nylon suture on large curved cutting needles are placed through the sponge approximately 5 mm apart. The needles are passed through the fornix to the orbital rim with a bite of periosteum taken before the needles emerge through the skin. The sutures are tied firmly over a silicone band bolster (retinal #240 band).

Step 3

Two or 3 double-armed sutures are inserted in this manner. The patient's prosthesis is then placed into the socket.

Step 4

The silicone bolster is removed in approximately 2 to 3 weeks, at which time a new prosthesis can be fit. If the shallow fornix is caused by a loss or contraction of tissue, other procedures are necessary. With the mildest form of tissue contraction, the tarsoconjunctiva is shortened with the lashes turned inward against the prosthesis. A marginal rotation of the involved eyelid can frequently correct this condition.

More severe contraction of the fornices makes it difficult for the patient to maintain a prosthesis. Additional tissue, such as mucous membrane, must be added to deepen the fornix. If there is associated lower eyelid lax-

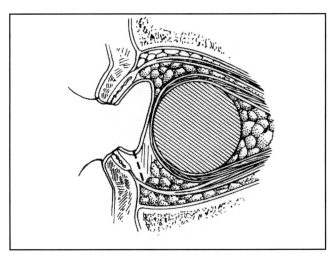

Figure 50-8.

ity, a lateral tarsal strip procedure must also be performed to tighten the eyelid horizontally.

SURGICAL TECHNIQUE 2

Step 1

The procedure can be performed under general or local anesthesia. In addition, a 1:1 mixture of 0.75% bupivacaine (Marcaine) with 2% lidocaine and 1:100,000 epinephrine is injected into the fornix to enhance vasoconstriction and decrease postoperative pain. An incision is made through the conjunctiva of the existing fornix from the caruncle to the lateral canthus. Subconjunctival scar tissue is then excised (Figure 50-8).

Step 2

The size of the graft needed is estimated by cutting a piece of Telfa to the size of the defect. The usual graft measurements are 25 to 30 mm long and 14 to 16 mm wide.

Step 3

The Telfa template is placed on the mucosal surface of the lip and outlined with a marking pen or scalpel. The lip can be inflated with the use of either saline or lidocaine 1% with 1:100,000 epinephrine. The latter agent provides greater hemostasis and reduces postoperative discomfort. If using a mucotome, inject the lip fully until it feels hard to the touch. Care is taken to avoid the buccal sulcus, frenulum, and vermilion border of the lip.

Step 4

The lip is retracted with 2 towel clamps, and the graft is removed using a Castroviejo mucotome with the blade set at 0.5-mm thickness. If a mucotome is unavailable, a #15 scalpel and iris scissors may be used to prepare a full-thickness graft. The graft should be defatted, making it as thin as possible.

Step 5

The graft should be placed onto a block and kept moist in antibiotic solution. It is sutured into the socket using an interrupted 6-0 Vicryl

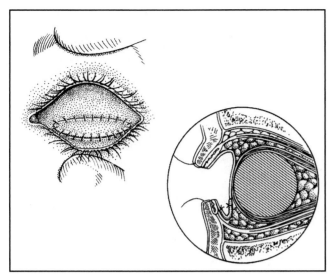

Figure 50-9.

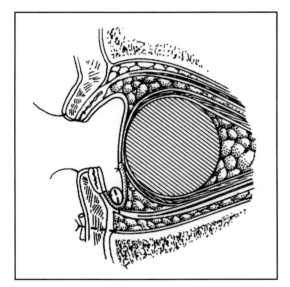

Figure 50-10.

suture at each end. Running 6-0 absorbable sutures are used to suture the graft to the bulbar and palpebral conjunctiva (Figure 50-9).

Step 6

A 3-mm retinal sponge is inserted into the newly created fornix. It is sutured in place with 3 double-armed 4-0 nylon sutures on long, thin cutting needles. The needles are placed through the retinal sponge 5 mm apart. Both arms of the suture are placed through the sponge, through the center of the graft, with a bite of the periosteum being taken before the needles emerge through the skin over the orbital rim. The sutures are tied tightly over silicone bolsters. This holds the graft against its recipient bed and creates a deep fornix (Figure 50-10).

Step 7

The patient's prosthesis, which has been soaking in antibiotic solution, may be inserted into the socket. A traction suture through the lower eyelid

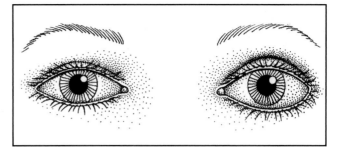

Figure 50-11.

to the eyebrow can be inserted to hold the eyelid in upward traction for several days. Topical antibiotic and a light dressing are applied.

The patient is instructed to eat a soft and bland diet until the mouth re-epithelializes, which takes approximately 10 days. Lidocaine hydrochloride 2% (viscous lidocaine) may be applied to the lip to decrease postoperative pain. Oral antibiotics are administered for 1 week. The stent is removed from the cul-de-sac in approximately 4 weeks. A new prosthesis can then be fit. With severe socket contracture, such as occurs with lye burns, there may be marked loss of both the superior and inferior fornices with a total inability to wear a prosthesis.

Anophthalmic Enophthalmic Syndrome

The anophthalmic enophthalmic syndrome is characterized by (1) enophthalmos, (2) deep superior eyelid sulcus, (3) lower eyelid ptosis, and (4) upper eyelid ptosis. It is caused by loss of orbital volume and redistribution of the orbital contents inferiorly and posteriorly after enucleation, mostly due to gravity and subsequent lid laxity. Both upper and lower lid ptosis may also become evident with time.

When tissue volume insufficiency causes enophthalmos and a deep superior sulcus and there is an adequate but vertically displaced orbital implant, the tissue volume insufficiency can be treated by volume augmentation inferiorly and posteriorly. Clinically, these patients have a deep superior tarsal sulcus with the implant riding low within the orbit and ptosis of both the upper and lower eyelids (Figure 50-11). Medpor plates or wedges can be placed into the inferior subperiosteal space to alleviate some of these problems.

SURGICAL TECHNIQUE

Step 1

This procedure is usually performed under general anesthesia. Lidocaine 2% with 1:100,000 epinephrine is injected into the lower eyelid for vasoconstriction and hemostasis. Traction sutures along the lower lid and upper lid margin are placed, and the lower lid is everted with a Desmarres retractor. A fornix-based conjunctival incision is marked 3 mm inferior to the inferior border of the lower tarsus medially and laterally and 6 mm inferior to the tarsus centrally. A

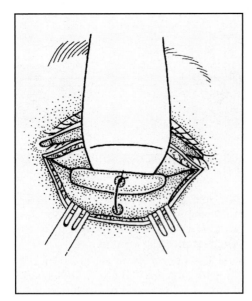

Figure 50-12.

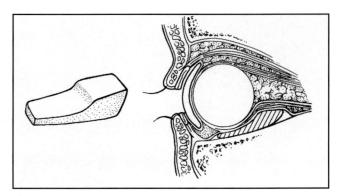

Figure 50-13.

Stevens or Westcott scissors is then used to obtain a plane of dissection anterior to the orbital septum in an inferior direction. Blunt dissection is performed down to the orbital rim. A 4-0 silk traction suture is then placed through the posterior aspect of the conjunctiva and lower lid retractors to facilitate exposure.

Step 2

An incision with monopolar cautery is made in the periosteum 2 mm inferior to the orbital rim. Small, relaxing incisions (H cuts) are used to facilitate mobilization of the periosteum. Periosteal elevators are then used to lift the periosteum in a superior and inferior direction to expose the orbital floor.

Step 3

Medpor, which is well tolerated by surrounding tissue, is prepared in different-sized blocks. The size and shape of Medpor are tailored as required to improve the volume deficit. A #15 Bard-Parker scalpel or Mayo scissors is used to shave or cut the Medpor to an appropriate size and shape. The prosthesis or conformer is inserted into the socket to determine the effect of orbital volume enhancement with Medpor. The superior sulcus depth of the side undergoing the surgery is compared with that of the contralateral side when determining the adequacy of the size and shape of the volume augmentation material.

Step 4

To fix the Medpor in position, a drill hole is made at the orbital rim. A 4-0 polypropylene (Prolene) suture is passed through the rim and the Medpor for fixation (Figure 50-12). The implant should sit just behind the orbital rim, without pushing forward. This limits the possibility of anterior migration of the implant. The suture is then tied.

Step 5

The periosteum is closed over the implant with 5-0 absorbable sutures (Figure 50-13). The conjunctiva is closed with a running 6-0 plain suture.

The patient's prosthesis is reinserted. A mild pressure dressing is applied. Oral antibiotics are administered for 1 week postoperatively.

After volume deficiency is addressed, residual eyelid problems can then be repaired. Lower eyelid ptosis can be corrected by performing a medial canthal tendonplication and/or a lateral tarsal strip procedure. Upper eyelid ptosis can then be addressed by standard procedures. In addition, lateral canthoplasty may also be necessary after socket revision is completed to ensure adequate stability of the eyelid and prosthesis.

Conclusion

The clinical approach to socket problems requires careful evaluation of the orbit, socket, and eyelids. Mild problems may be handled with cooperation between the ocularist and the surgeon. More significant problems including extrusion, socket contracture, and the anophthalmic-enophthalmic syndrome require surgical correction as outlined in this chapter. Eyelid surgery, including ptosis repair, horizontal lid shortening, and lateral canthoplasty, can be done after completion of socket reconstruction.

SECTION X

MISCELLANEOUS

TEMPORAL ARTERY BIOPSY

Robert L. Tomsak, MD, PhD

Giant cell (temporal) arteritis is a vasculitis that usually affects arteries of the head and neck in the geriatric age group. In one autopsy series of patients who died during the active phase of temporal arteritis, the incidence of arterial involvement was superficial temporal, 100%; vertebral, 100%; ophthalmic, 76%; posterior ciliary, 75%; and proximal central retinal, 60%. Because sudden vision loss and even blindness from anterior ischemic optic neuropathy are the most common ophthalmic presentations of the disease, early accurate diagnosis is essential. The superficial temporal artery (STA) biopsy is the "gold standard" for the diagnosis of giant cell arteritis, and, often, the ophthalmologist is called on to do the biopsy.

Presentation and Demographics

The mean age for the clinical presentation of giant cell arteritis is approximately 70 years, and the prevalence increases with increasing age. The disease is more common in women than in men, and whites are most commonly affected; temporal arteritis is less common in blacks, Asians, and Hispanics. Classic symptoms include musculoskeletal pains (polymyalgia rheumatica), headache, scalp tenderness, jaw claudication, fatigue, and vision loss. Headache, fever, and jaw claudication appear to be symptoms with predictive value for positive STA biopsy findings. Pathogenesis is likely immune mediated, but the inciting insults are unknown. Temporal arteritis is a chronic disease that may recur even if treated. It may affect other organ systems and may be fatal.

Preoperative Management

No special precautions are taken. The biopsy can easily be performed in a minor operating room if available. The STA has a main trunk that is quite constant in its location approximately 1 cm anterior to the tragus of the ear. Two to 5 cm superior to this, most STAs divide into a frontal branch and a parietal branch (Figure 51-1). However, the frontal branch is absent or atrophic in approximately 16% of patients. Thus, marking over the main trunk and carrying the line superior and slightly forward for a distance of at least 3 cm ensures locating the artery. A vascular Doppler probe is useful in determining the course of the artery if it cannot be palpated.

Anesthesia

Lidocaine (Xylocaine) 1% or 2% with 1:200,000 epinephrine is the preferred anesthetic. Some state that epinephrine causes vasospasm and difficulty in locating the artery, but the technique described here provides direct visualization of the artery. The added hemostasis from the epinephrine is appreciated. Two to 4 mL of the anesthetic is slowly infiltrated adjacent and parallel to the skin mark—slow injection minimizes discomfort.

Procedure

Step 1

A superficial scratch-down incision is made through epidermis and dermis just until subcutaneous fat is encountered (Figure 51-2).

Step 2

Next, a small curved hemostat is used for blunt dissection perpendicular to the incision (Figure 51-3). Blunt dissection is carried down only to the level of the superficial temporalis muscle fascia. Contrary to popular belief, the STA is actually enveloped by the fascia.

Levine MR.
Manual of Oculoplastic Surgery, Fourth Edition (pp 323-326).
© 2010 SLACK Incorporated

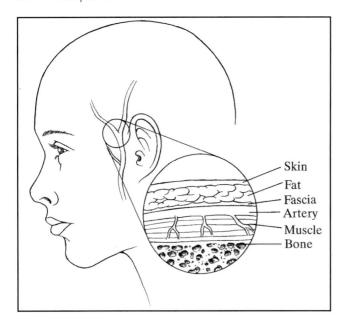

Figure 51-1.

Skin
Fat
Fascia
Artery
Muscle
Bone

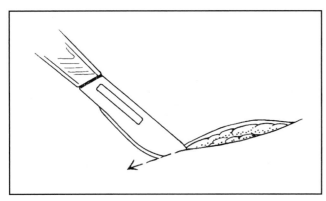

Figure 51-2.

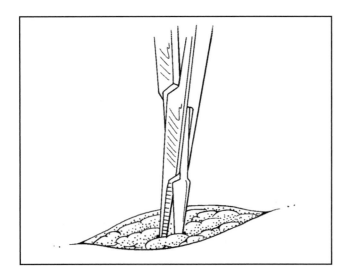

Figure 51-3.

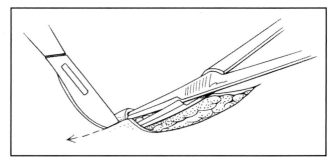

Figure 51-4.

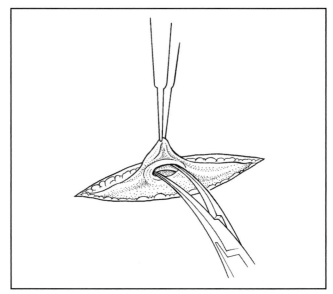

Figure 51-5.

Step 3

The hemostat is turned parallel to the incision, and the instrument is held so that the curved tips are up. It is tunneled underneath the subcutaneous fat but above the superficial temporalis fascia. The hemostat is lifted, and the tips are spread (Figure 51-4). Using the point of a scalpel blade, the incision is extended along its full planned length.

Step 4

After retraction with self-retaining or hand-held instruments, the STA is usually visible through its thin fascial covering. If the STA is not visualized, 0.3-mm Castroviejo forceps are used to tent the fascia, which is carefully buttonholed with blunt Westcott scissors (Figure 51-5). The incision in the fascia is extended to fully visualize the artery. In the region of the main trunk of the STA, the superficial temporal vein often is adjacent to the artery. The wall of the vein is very friable, and care should be taken to dissect it free from the artery. Healthy arteries appear pink and measure approximately 3 mm in diameter. Diseased arteries are often thicker, pale, and rubbery.

Step 5

The exposed length of the artery is clamped on either side with small hemostats, and the specimen is excised between them (Figure 51-6). Thereafter, one 4-0 silk tie is placed around the cut ends of the artery, and the crushed ends are cauterized (Figure 51-7).

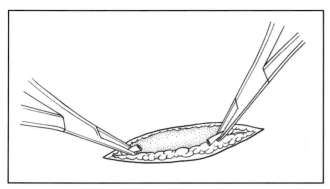

Figure 51-6.

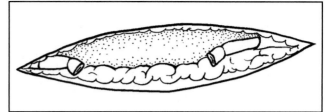

Figure 51-7.

Step 6

A 2-layer skin closure is used with interrupted absorbable sutures (5-0 polyglactin [Vicryl] and 6-0 mild chromic). A pressure dressing is not used.

Complications

Late bleeding has been reported but is obviated by clamping, ligation, and cauterization of the arterial ends.

Comment

The main advantage of the technique of STA biopsy described here is the ease of identification and isolation of the artery even if it is not visible or palpable through intact skin. The extra care taken with the skin incision and subcutaneous dissection minimizes the chances of accidentally transecting the STA or superficial temporal vein or bypassing the artery by going deep into the temporalis muscle.

Length of Biopsy

The need for obtaining long segments of the STA for histopathologic evaluation has been refuted by Chambers and Bernardino. Using statistical analysis, they found that an STA segment as small as 4 mm, if serially sectioned properly, results in a false-negative result rate of less than 1%. The incidence of false-negative biopsy results has ranged from 5% to 61% in various reports. Thus, it appears that careful histologic processing is much more important than the size of the temporal artery biopsy specimen, and close communication between surgeon and pathologist is encouraged.

Interpreting the Biopsy Results

In a recent study of 125 cases of biopsy-proven temporal arteritis, 99% of specimens had fragmentation of the internal elastic lamina, giant cells were present in 66%, and fibrinoid necrosis was observed in 12%. Healed arteritis is characterized by fragmentation and loss of internal elastic lamina, medial fibrosis, and adventitial scarring.

Prior Corticosteroid Treatment and Biopsy Results

A common teaching about temporal arteritis is that the STA biopsy specimen must be obtained before the patient is started on systemic steroids. This is untrue. Achkar, in a series of 535 patients, found that the positive result rate of temporal artery biopsy specimens was unrelated to previous corticosteroid treatment, and To, Enzer, and Tsiaras found positive biopsy results in a woman who had been taking 60 mg of prednisone a day for 4.5 weeks. Therefore, steroid therapy must be begun immediately in any case of suspected temporal arteritis, but the biopsy can be scheduled in a timely, nonemergent fashion.

References and Bibliography

Chapter 11

1. Hester TR Jr, Codner MA, McCord CD Jr. Subperiosteal maler cheek lift with lower lid blepharoplasty. In: McCord CD Jr, ed. *Eyelid Surgery: Principles and Techniques.* Philadelphia, PA: Lippincott-Raven; 1995:210-215.
2. McCord CD Jr. Lower lid blepharoplasty. In: McCord CD Jr, ed. *Eyelid Surgery: Principles and Techniques.* Philadelphia, PA: Lippincott-Raven; 1995:196-209.
3. Putterman AM. Avoidance of needle stick injuries during reuse of surgical needles. *Plastic Reconstr Surg.* 2003;112:333-334.
4. Putterman AM. The mysterious second temporal fat pad. *Ophthal Plast Reconst Surg.* 1985;1:83-86.
5. Putterman AM. Temporary blindness after cosmetic blepharoplasty. *Am J Ophthalmol.* 1975;80:1081-1083.

Chapter 12

1. Chen WPD. Asian blepharoplasty. *Ophthal Plast Reconstr Surg.* 1987;3(3):135-140.
2. Chen WPD. *Asian Blepharoplasty and the Eyelid Crease With DVD.* (A color atlas). Philadelphia, PA: Butterworth-Heinemann/Elsevier Science, Ltd; 2006.
3. Chen WPD. *Asian Blepharoplasty (A Surgical Text).* Oxford, UK: Butterworth-Heinemann; 1995.
4. Chen WPD, Khan JA. Primary Asian blepharoplasty. In: Chen WPD, ed. *Color Atlas of Cosmetic Oculofacial Surgery.* Philadelphia, PA: Elsevier Science, Ltd/Saunders; 2010:73-107.
5. Chen WPD, Khan JA. Revisional Asian blepharoplasty. In: Chen WPD, ed. *Color Atlas of Cosmetic Oculofacial Surgery.* Philadelphia, PA: Elsevier Science, Ltd/Saunders; 2010:251-301.
6. Collin JR, Beard C, Wood I. Experimental and clinical data on the insertion of the levator palpebrae superioris muscle. *Am J Ophthalmol.* 1978;85:792-801.
7. Chen WPD. Concept of triangular, trapezoidal and rectangular debulking of eyelid tissues: application in Asian blepharoplasty. *Plast Reconstr Surg.* 1996;97(1):212-218.
8. Chen WPD. The concept of a glide zone as it relates to upper lid crease, lid fold, and application in upper blepharoplasty. *Plast Reconstr Surg.* 2007;119(1):379-386.
9. Chen WPD. Beveled approach for revisional surgery in Asian blepharoplasty. *Plast Reconstr Surg.* 2007;120(2):545-552.

Chapter 24

Anderson RL, Gordy DD. The tarsal strip procedure. *Arch Ophthalmol* 1979;97:2192.
Frueh BR, Schoengarth LD. Evaluation and treatment of the patient with ectropion. *Ophthalmology.* 1982;89:1049.
Tse DT. Surgical correction of punctal malposition. *Am J Ophthalmol.* 1985;100:339.
Tse DT, Kronish W, Buus D. The surgical correction of lower eyelid tarsal ectropion by retractors reinsertion. *Arch Ophthalmol.* 1991;109:427-31.

Chapter 32

1. Borges AF. The rhombic flap. *Plast Reconstr Surg.* 1981;67(4):458-466.
2. Becker H. The rhomboid to W technique for excision of some skin lesions and closure. *Plast Reconstr Surg.* 1979;64(4):444-447.

Chapter 35

1. Hughes WL. A new method for rebuilding a lower eyelid. *Arch Ophthalmol.* 1937;17:1008.
2. Leibsohn JH, Dryden RM, Ross J. Intentional buttonholing of the Hughes flap. *Ophthal Plast Reconstr Surg.* 1993;9:135-138.

Chapter 36

1. Hewes EH, Sullivan JH, Beard C. Lower eyelid reconstruction by tarsal transposition. *Am J Ophthalmol.* 1976;81:512-514.

Levine MR.
Manual of Oculoplastic Surgery, Fourth Edition (pp 327-328).
© 2010 SLACK Incorporated

Chapter 38

1. McCord CD, Nunnery WR. Reconstruction of the lower eyelid and outer canthus. In: McCord CD, Tanenbaum M, eds. Oculoplastic Surgery. 2nd ed. *New York, NY*: Raven Press; 1987:93-115.
2. Collin JR, ed. *A Manual of Systematic Eyelid Surgery*. New York, NY: Churchill Livingston; 1989:115-145.
3. McCord CD, Wesley R. Reconstruction of the upper eyelid and medial canthus. In: McCord CD, Tanenbaum M, eds. *Oculoplastic Surgery*. 2nd ed. New York, NY: Raven Press; 1987:73-91.
4. Ng SGJ, Inkster CF, Leatherbarrow B. The rhomboid flap in medial canthal reconstruction. *Br J Ophthalmol*. 2001;85:556-559.

Chapter 39

1. Cutler NL, Beard C. A method for partial and total upper lid reconstruction. *Am J Ophthalmol*. 1955;39:1-7.
2. Smith B, Obear M. Bridge flap technique for large upper lid defects. *Plast Reconstr Surg*. 1966;38:45-48.
3. Petersen NC. Reconstruction of the upper eyelid ad modum Cutler and Beard. *Acta Ophthalmol (Copenh)*. 1969;47:228-233.
4. Nesi F, Levine M, Lisman R. *Smith's Ophthalmic Plastic and Reconstructive Surgery*. 2nd ed. St. Louis, MO: Mosby; 1998.
5. Wesley RE, McCord CD. Transplantation of eyebank sclera in the Cutler-Beard method of upper eyelid reconstruction. *Ophthalmology*. 1980;87:1022-1028.
6. Carroll RP. Entropion following the Cutler-Beard procedure. *Ophthalmology*. 1983;90(9):1052-1055.
7. Holloman EL, Carter KD. Modification of the Cutler-Beard procedure using donor Achilles tendon for upper eyelid reconstruction. *Ophthal Plast Reconstr Surg*. 2005;21(4):267-270.

Chapter 42

1. Kaltreider SA, Peake LR, Carter BT. Pediatric enucleation: analysis of volume replacement. *Arch Ophthalmol*. 2001;119(3):379-384.
2. Custer PL, et al. Volumetric determination of enucleation implant size. *Am J Ophthalmol*. 1999;128:489-494.

Chapter 48

1. Kim N, Hatton MP. The role of genetics in Graves' disease and thyroid orbitopathy. *Semin Ophthalmol*. 2008;23:67-72.
2. Kazim M, Goldberg RA, Smith TJ. Insights into the pathogenesis of thyroid associated orbitopathy. *Arch Ophthal*. 2002;120:380-386.
3. Farling PA. Thyroid disease. *British Journal of Anesthesiology*. 2000;85:15-28.
4. Boulos PR, Hardy I. Thyroid-associated orbitopathy: a clinicopathologic and therapeutic review. *Curr Opin Ophthalmol*. 2004;15:389-400.
5. Bartalena L, Baldeschi L, Dickinson AJ, et al. Consensus statement of the European group on Graves' orbitopathy (EUGOGO) on management of Graves' orbitopathy. *Thyroid*. 2008;18(3):333-346.
6. McCracken MS, del Prado JD, Granet DB, Levi L, Kikkawa DO. Combined eyelid and strabismus surgery: Examining conventional surgical wisdom. *J Pediatr Ophthalmol Strabismus*. 2008;45(4):220-224.
7. Shorr N, Seiff SR. The four stages of surgical rehabilitation of the patient with dysthyroid ophthalmopathy. *Ophthalmology*. 1986;93:476-483.
8. Garrity JA, Fatourechi V, Bergstralh EJ, et al. Results of transantral orbital decompression in 428 patients with severe Graves' ophthalmopathy. *Am J Ophthalmol*. 1993;116:533-547.
9. McCord CD Jr. Current trends in orbital decompression. *Ophthalmology*. 1985;92:21-33.
10. Kahaly GJ, Petrak F, Hardt J, Pitz S, Egle UT. Psychosocial morbidity of Graves' orbitopathy. *Clin Endocrinol*. 2005;63:395-402.
11. Lyons CJ, Rootman J. Orbital decompression for disfiguring exophthalmos in thyroid orbitopathy. *Ophthalmology*. 1994;101:223-230.
12. Fatourechi V, Garrity JA, Bartley GB, et al. Graves' ophthalmopathy: results of transantral orbital decompression performed primarily for cosmetic indications. *Ophthalmology*. 1994;101:938-942.
13. Goh MSY, McNab AA. Orbital decompression in Graves' orbitopathy: efficacy and safety. *Intern Med J*. 2005;35:586-591.
14. Kalmann R, Mourits MP, van der Pol JP, Koornneef L. Coronal approach for rehabilitative orbital decompression in Graves' ophthalmopathy. *Br J Ophthalmol*. 1997;81:41-45.
15. Kulwin DR, Cotton RT, Kersten RC. Combined approach to orbital decompression. *Otolaryngol Clin North Am*. 1990;23:381-390.
16. Seiff SR, Tovilla JL, Carter SR, Choo PH. Modified orbital decompression for dysthyroid orbitopathy. *Ophth Plast Reconstr Surg*. 2000;16:62-66.
17. Bailey KL, Tower RN, Dailey RA. Customized, single-incision, three-wall orbital decompression. *Ophthal Plast Reconstr Surg*. 2005;21(1):1-10.
18. Leone CR Jr, Piest KL, Newman RJ. Medial and lateral wall decompression for thyroid ophthalmopathy. *Am J Ophthalmol*. 1989;108:160-166.
19. Goldberg RA, Kim AJ, Kerivan KM. The lacrimal keyhole, orbital door jamb, and basin of the inferior orbital fissure: three areas of deep bone in the lateral orbit. *Arch Ophthalmol*. 1998;116:1618-1624.
20. Shepard KG, Levin PS, Terris DJ. Balanced orbital decompression for Graves' ophthalmopathy. *Laryngoscope*. 1998;108:1648-1653.
21. Kikkawa DO, Pornpanich K, Cruz RC Jr, Levi L, Granet DB. Graded orbital decompression based on severity of proptosis. *Ophthalmology*. 2002;109(7):1219-1224.
22. Olivari N. Transpalpebral decompression of endocrine ophthalmopathy (Graves' disease) by removal of intraorbital fat: experience with 147 operations over 5 years [see comments]. *Plast Reconstr Surg*. 1991;87:627-641;discussion 42-43.
23. Trokel S, Kazim M, Moore S. Orbital fat removal. decompression for Graves' orbitopathy. *Ophthalmology*. 1993;100:674-682.
24. Carrasco JR, Castillo I, Bolyk R, Probitkin EA, Savino PJ. Incidence of infraorbital hypesthesia and sinusitis after orbital decompression for thyroid-related orbitopathy: a comparison of surgical techniques. *Ophthal Plast Reconstr Surg*. 2005;21:188-191.

FINANCIAL DISCLOSURES

Dr. Meredith Brooke Allen has no financial or proprietary interest in the materials presented herein.

Dr. Richard L. Anderson has not disclosed any relevant financial relationships.

Dr. Christine C. Annunziata has no financial or proprietary interest in the materials presented herein.

Dr. Milton Boniuk has no financial or proprietary interest in the materials presented herein.

Dr. James R. Boynton has no financial or proprietary interest in the materials presented herein.

Dr. Daniel E. Buerger has no financial or proprietary interest in the materials presented herein.

Dr. David G. Buerger has no financial or proprietary interest in the materials presented herein.

Dr. George F. Buerger, Jr has no financial or proprietary interest in the materials presented herein.

Dr. John A. Burns has no financial or proprietary interest in the materials presented herein.

Dr. Kenneth V. Cahill has not disclosed any relevant financial relationships.

Dr. Mauricio R. Chavez has no financial or proprietary interest in the materials presented herein.

Dr. William P. Chen has not disclosed any relevant financial relationships.

Dr. Roger A. Dailey receives nonrestricted educational grant support from Allergan, Inc.

Dr. Rodger P. Davies has not disclosed any relevant financial relationships.

Dr. David A. Della Rocca has no financial or proprietary interest in the materials presented herein.

Dr. Robert C. Della Rocca has not disclosed any relevant financial relationships.

Dr. Richard K. Dortzbach has not disclosed any relevant financial relationships.

Dr. Gil A. Epstein has no financial or proprietary interest in the materials presented herein.

Dr. Essam A. El-Toukhy has no financial or proprietary interest in the materials presented herein.

Dr. Steven Fagien has not disclosed any relevant financial relationships.

Dr. Jill A. Foster has not disclosed any relevant financial relationships.

Dr. Tamara R. Fountain has no financial or proprietary interest in the materials presented herein.

Dr. Constance L. Fry has no financial or proprietary interest in the materials presented herein.

Dr. Perry F. Garber has no financial or proprietary interest in the materials presented herein.

Dr. Geoffrey J. Gladstone has not disclosed any relevant financial relationships.

Dr. Robert A. Goldberg has not disclosed any relevant financial relationships.

Dr. Michael J. Hawes has not disclosed any relevant financial relationships.

Dr. Jonathan Hoenig has no financial or proprietary interest in the materials presented herein.

Dr. David E. E. Holck has not disclosed any relevant financial relationships.)

Dr. John B. Holds has not disclosed any relevant financial relationships.

Dr. Steven M. Houser has not disclosed any relevant financial relationships.

Dr. Catherine Hwang has no financial or proprietary interest in the materials presented herein.

Levine MR..
Manual of Oculoplastic Surgery, Fourth Edition (pp 329-332)
© 2010 SLACK Incorporated

Dr. Thomas J. Joly has not disclosed any relevant financial relationships.

Dr. David R. Jordan has not disclosed any relevant financial relationships.

Dr. James Karesh has no financial or proprietary interest in the materials presented herein.

Dr. Don O. Kikkawa has not disclosed any relevant financial relationships.

Dr. Jonathan W. Kim has not disclosed any relevant financial relationships.

Dr. Yoon-Duck Kim has no financial or proprietary interest in the materials presented herein.

Dr. Kimberly A. Klippenstein's work was supported in part by a grant from Research to Prevent Blindness, Inc.

Dr. Bobby S. Korn has not disclosed any relevant financial relationships.

Dr. Jacques G. H. Lasudry has not disclosed any relevant financial relationships.

Dr. H. B. Harold Lee has no financial or proprietary interest in the materials presented herein.

Dr. Bradley N. Lemke has not disclosed any relevant financial relationships.

Dr. Alan M. Lessner has not disclosed any relevant financial relationships.

Dr. Howard Levine is on the scientific advisory boards of Acclarent Inc, Arthrocare Inc, Carbylan Inc, and Ethicon Inc; is a consultant for Acclarent Inc and Medtronic Xomed; is medical director of Rhinosystems Inc; and has equity ownership of Acclarent Inc, Rhinosystems Inc, Rockside Road Surgery Center, and University Hospitals Zeeba Surgery Center.

Dr. Mark R. Levine has no financial or proprietary interest in the materials presented herein.

Dr. Richard D. Lisman has no financial or proprietary interest in the materials presented herein.

Dr. William P. Mack has no financial or proprietary interest in the materials presented herein

Dr. Joseph A. Mauriello, Jr has no financial or proprietary interest in the materials presented herein.

Dr. Jill S. Melicher has not disclosed any relevant financial relationships.

Dr. Dale R. Meyer has no financial or proprietary interest in the materials presented herein.

Dr. Kevin S. Michels has not disclosed any relevant financial relationships.

Dr. Thomas C. Naugle, Jr has not disclosed any relevant financial relationships.

Dr. Jeffrey A. Nerad has not disclosed any relevant financial relationships.

Dr. Frank A. Nesi has not disclosed any relevant financial relationships.

Dr. William R. Nunery has no financial or proprietary interest in the materials presented herein.

Dr. J. Justin Older has no financial or proprietary interest in the materials presented herein.

Dr. Julian D. Perry has no financial or proprietary interest in the materials presented herein.

Dr. Randal Pham has no financial or proprietary interest in the materials presented herein.

Dr. Thu Pham has no financial or proprietary interest in the materials presented herein.

Dr. Allen M. Putterman has no financial or proprietary interest in the materials presented herein.

Dr. J. Earl Rathbun has no financial or proprietary interest in the materials presented herein.

Dr. John G. Rose, Jr has not disclosed any relevant financial relationships.

Dr. John W. Shore has not disclosed any relevant financial relationships.

Dr. Norman Shorr has not disclosed any relevant financial relationships.

Dr. César A. Sierra has not disclosed any relevant financial relationships.

Dr. Charles B. Slonim has no financial or proprietary interest in the materials presented herein.

Dr. Robert G. Small has no financial or proprietary interest in the materials presented herein.

Dr. Thomas C. Spoor has not disclosed any relevant financial relationships.

Dr. Robert L. Tomsak has no financial or proprietary interest in the materials presented herein.

Dr. David T. Tse has not disclosed any relevant financial relationships.

Dr. Ralph E. Wesley's work was supported in part by a grant from Research to Prevent Blindness, Inc.

Dr. Eugene O. Wiggs has no financial or proprietary interest in the materials presented herein.

Dr. Allan E. Wulc is on the speaker's bureau for Medicis and Allergan.

Dr. Christopher I. Zoumalan has no financial or proprietary interest in the materials presented herein.

INDEX

Levine MR..
Manual of Oculoplastic Surgery, Fourth Edition (pp 333-348).
© 2010 SLACK Incorporated

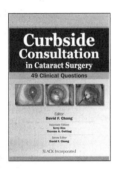
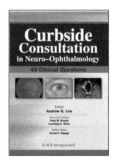
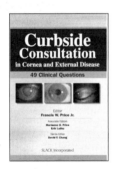
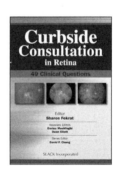
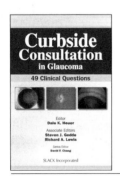

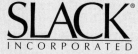